Key Concepts of Pharmacology

Key Concepts of Pharmacology

Edited by **Sean Boyd**

FOSTER
ACADEMICS

New Jersey

Published by Foster Academics,
61 Van Reypen Street,
Jersey City, NJ 07306, USA
www.fosteracademics.com

Key Concepts of Pharmacology
Edited by Sean Boyd

© 2015 Foster Academics

International Standard Book Number: 978-1-63242-253-8 (Hardback)

Printed in the United States of America.

Contents

Preface

The history of pharmacology travels along with that of scientific methodologies and the novel frontiers of pharmacology give way to a novel world in search of drugs and advanced technologies. Constant growth in this field has also altered significantly the way of designing a fresh drug. Modern drug discovery is actually based on profound knowledge regarding the disease and both molecular as well as cellular mechanisms involved in its development. The aim of this book is to provide valuable information on ethnopharmacology and toxicology, and gives an overview of its future applications.

This book is the end result of constructive efforts and intensive research done by experts in this field. The aim of this book is to enlighten the readers with recent information in this area of research. The information provided in this profound book would serve as a valuable reference to students and researchers in this field.

At the end, I would like to thank all the authors for devoting their precious time and providing their valuable contribution to this book. I would also like to express my gratitude to my fellow colleagues who encouraged me throughout the process.

Editor

Part 1

Ethnopharmacology and Toxicology

The Influence of Displacement by Human Groups Among Regions in the Medicinal Use of Natural Resource: A Case Study in Diadema, São Paulo - Brazil

Daniel Garcia and Lin Chau Ming
Universidade Estadual Paulista – Faculdade de Ciências Agronômicas
Brazil

1. Introduction

The migration of human groups around the world and the cultural mix of these people has instigated more researches in the field of ethnobotany/ethnopharmacology in recent years (Pieroni & Vandebroek, 2007). Brazil is an example of blending traditional knowledge combined with the use of natural resources to the cure of various diseases and, therefore, have been the subject of several surveys including ethnobotanical and ethnopharmacological. Given the enormous biological diversity and biochemistry in the several biomes around the world and also in Brazil, it is very difficult to find randomly a molecule on which it is possible to develop a competitive drug, acting on a mechanism known and has significant pharmacological properties (FAPESP, 2011). Therefore, the ethnobotany/ethnopharmacology are among the main strategies used for selecting plants to be investigated in laboratorial studies, those with great chances of success (Spjut & Perdue, 1976; Balick, 1990 as cited in Rodrigues, 2005), and is one of the fastest ways to obtain a safe product and pharmacologically active (Giorgetti et al., 2007).

The ethnobotany looks at how people incorporate the plants in their cultural traditions and folk practices (Balick & Cox, 1997) or, according to Alcorn (1995), is the study of the interrelationships between humans and plants in dynamical systems (as cited in Rodrigues et al., 2005).

The ethnopharmacology was originally defined as a science that sought to understand the universe of natural resources (plants, animals and minerals) as drugs used in the view of human groups (Schultes, 1988). However, over time this discipline has evolved and is defined by the INTERNATIONAL SOCIETY FOR ETHNOPHARMACOLOGY as:

"Interdisciplinary study of the physiological actions of plants, animals and others substances used in indigenous medicines of past and present cultures".

This concept is also currently applied in the case of medicinal substances from non-indigenous people, thus expanding the diversity of information generated in studies ethnopharmacological. The relationship of the biological wealth of the world's diverse ecosystems, sometimes aided by the traditional knowledge of people who directly depend on these places to survive, is ancient for an extensive possibilities of discovering medicinal formulas for curing various diseases. The multiple possibilities resulting from this combination, natural biodiversity and cultural diversity, give richness and complexity in terms of knowledge about the flora and their therapeutic potential, some studies as: Pieroni & Vandebroek (2007) and Garcia et al., (2010) show that this relationship is even more intrinsic when there is displacement of human groups to a new environment.

Brazil offers a favourable environment for studies focused on migration and medicinal plants/animals because it possesses a large area of 8,514,876.599 km^2 (IBGE, 2011) and boasts high indices of cultural and biological diversity. In Brazil, the use of herbs for medicinal purposes is a common practice and very diverse, result of intense mixing that occurred during colonization (Europeans and Africans – sixteen to the eighteen century), added with the ancient knowledge of indigenous people, who ever inhabited these lands (Giorgeti et al., 2007).

Brazil is inhabited by mestizo groups derived from the miscegenation of Indian, Black, European and Asiatic people, 232 indigenous ethnic groups (Instituto Socioambiental, 2011) and 1,342 Quilombola groups (descendants of Afro-Brazilian people) (Fundação Cultural Palmares, 2011). Brazil has the richest flora in the world, with nearly 56.000 species of plants (Ribeiro, 1996; Schultes, 1990). For these and other reasons Brazil may be considered a laboratory *in situ* for a variety of processes that are studied by researchers from diverse fields, including the development of pharmaceutical drugs (Rodrigues, 2007).

However, at present moment, marked by the destruction of natural ecosystems, not only the biodiversity of plants and animals are affected, but also human groups that depend of environments to survive (Davis, 1995).

According to Simões and Lino (2004), the original Atlantic Forest covered approximately 1.3 million km^2, spanning 17 Brazilian states from south to northeast; however, it currently covers only 14 states, and its area has been reduced to 65,000 km^2. Despite alarming fragmentation, the Atlantic Forest still contains more than 20,000 plant species (8,000 endemic) and 1,361 animal species (567 endemic). It is the richest forest in the world in wood plants per unit area; the southern Bahia, for example, holds a record of 454 different species/ha (IBAMA, 2011).

Because of this reality, ethnobotanical and ethnopharmacological surveys make an important role in collecting and valuing traditional knowledge of people about the medicinal use of biodiversity in which they live. This assumption, undoubtedly, is the key to preserve the biodiversity of these sites, as well as cultural traditions, once the ignorance on the potential pharmacological importance for the society becomes absent. While migration has become an integral part of modern globalization is as old as human society (Thomas et al., 2009; Waldstein, 2008). There are many reasons why people decide to leave home and live somewhere else, some having reasons within the place of origin, others with perceived opportunities available from the new environment (Findley & De Jong, 1985; Suzuki, 1996). Whatever the reason for the displacement, the migrants experience some difficulties and opportunities due to its displacement to a new location that those who stay behind may not experience (Lacuna-Richman, 2006). Numerous studies have related information on medicinal plants from human groups who migrated from Haiti to Cuba (Volpato et al., 2009); from Mexico to the U.S.A. (Waldstain, 2006, 2008); from Africa to South America

The Influence of Displacement by Human Groups Among Regionsin the Medicinal Use of Natural Resource:
A Case Study in Diadema, São Paulo - Brazil

5

(Voeks, 2009); from Africa to Brazil (Carney & Voeks, 2003); from Suriname to the Netherlands (van Andel & Westers, 2010); from Colombia to London (Ceuterick et al., 2008); from Germany to eastern Italy (Pieroni et al., 2004); from Albania to southern Italy (Pieroni et al., 2002a, 2002b); and from Europe and Africa to eastern Cuba (Cano & Volpato, 2004; Pieroni & Vandebroek, 2007). However, few studies have focused on migration within a country, such as that described by Rodrigues et al. (2005) and Garcia et al. (2010) regarding migrants from northeastern Brazil who currently occupy the southeast.

Migration between regions encourages contact with the rich biological and cultural diversity and allows interpersonal interactions that contribute to the transformation of local medicinal therapies. As described by Garcia et al. (2010), where the influence of displacement of people from the Northeast and Southeast Brazil to Diadema (São Paulo) resulted in: maintenance, incorporation, replacement and/or discontinued use of natural resources in their medicinal pharmacopoeia. Migrants bring along their traditions, lifestyles, world and health views, such your supporting systems, including knowledge about the use of natural resources to health care and nutrition. These attitudes and practices are held to different ways in the host society (e.g., Nguyen, 2003) and may fall into partial or total disuse, depending of the availability of raw material (Garcia et al., 2010).

This chapter is an attempt to demonstrate the importance that the field ethnobotanist/ethnopharmacological meets in search of new bioactive molecules and how the knowledge about the medicinal use of natural resources can be more diverse and enriched after the displacement of human groups between regions. More broadly and generally, this chapter will also address details of the work done by Garcia et al. (2010) where the authors tried to understand, and comprehend more clearly the extent to which the displacement of people within a country can influence the traditional knowledge about medicinal use of natural resources. We hope this work can contribute significantly to future multidisciplinary research to develop new drugs.

2. Brazilian biodiversity and cultural richness

The Brazilian Atlantic Forest region (Figure 1) was the first to be occupied by European settlers in post-Columbian times (Rodrigues et al., 2008). "Ipe-roxo" (Tabebuia heptaphylla), "cidrão" (*Hedyosmum brasiliensis*), "marcela" (*Achyrocline satureioides*), "estévia" (*Stevia rebaudiana*), "hortelã-do-mato" (*Peltodon radicans*), "espinheira-santa" (*Maytenus* spp), "pata-de-vaca" (*Bauhinia forficata*), "carqueja" (*Baccharis trimera*), "guaco" (*Mikania* spp) and "erva-baleeira" (*Cordia verbenacea*) are some plant species with high chemical and pharmacological potential of the Atlantic Forest biome.

Brazil is very rich in biodiversity, endemism and traditional communities. Is inhabited by diverse ethnic groups, including: Indigenous Ethnic Groups, Quilombo communities, Mestizos, Caiçaras, Fishermen, Rafters, Rubber Tappers, Raizeiros, among other, and the mostly the result of interbreeding between native Indians, Europeans and African elements (Giorgetti et al., 2007).

Native inhabitants of the Atlantic Forest, including non-indigenous, are still in this region, for example, the Caiçaras: people of mixed origin, descendants of European and Native Americans (Rodrigues and Carlini, 2006; Hanazaki et al., 2009). Descendants of Europeans, Africans and Asians settled in Brazil during the colonization and this culminated with cultural miscegenation of many Brazilian communities and ethnic groups, enriching them culturally. All of these groups have traditionally relied on human resources to treat their illnesses and have at their disposal a rich flora.

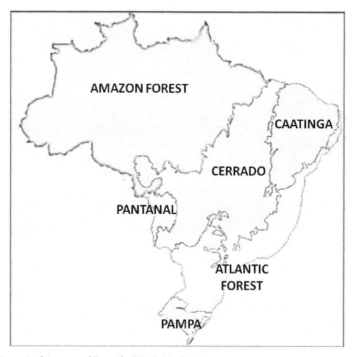

Fig. 1. The six main biomes of Brazil, (IBAMA, 2011)

According to Rodrigues (2005), human groups that live in the forests are still substitutes for laboratory animals, especially in regions where medical treatment is lacking.

The cultural diversity that exists in Brazil is the result of the migration process and miscegenation that begun in the sixteenth century. In this period, were made the first records of the Brazilian medicinal flora (Camargo, 2000; Giulietti et al., 2005; Rodrigues et al., 2008). Little was known about Brazil at the time of the discoveries. The first Jesuits, explorers, scientists, and settlers who arrived in Brazil, reported a lot of characteristics observed on the new environment (Kury, 2001 as cited in Giorgetti et al., 2007).

The first European explorers that arrived in Brazil found a large number of medicinal plants used by indigenous tribes who lived here. Knowledge of local flora was merged those brought from Europe. Those that migrated from Africa (1530-1888) play an important role in traditional popular knowledge in Brazil until today (Rodrigues, 2007). The Africans who came to Brazil adapted your traditions to the new environment (Rodrigues, 2007).

Due the fusion among human groups from different sites of the world and because of the colonization of the Americas, some plants of temperate climate were brought and introduced in tropical locations (Rodrigues et al., 2008), which made these regions,

The Influence of Displacement by Human Groups Among Regionsin the Medicinal Use of Natural Resource:
A Case Study in Diadema, São Paulo - Brazil

7

especially South America, a biologically rich and diverse field, with emphasis on the Brazilian forests. This mixture of traditions associated with the weight of diversity vegetal has led to a traditional medicine and herbal treatment methods and of different researchers (e.g., such as Garcia et al., 2010; Ming, 1995; Pio Correa, 1926).

Sometimes, researchers focus on ethnobotanical knowledge and practices at one moment in time, where little attention has been given to the "drivers" of change over time, and thus the migration becomes widely accepted as one of the principle means by which vegetal genetic material, associated knowledge and practices are diffused on the globe (Carney, 2001; Carrier, 2007; Niñez, 1987 as cited in Volpato et al., 2008).

In this context, the main forces that guide the changes in the traditional medicinal knowledge, as cited by Volpato (2009) are: (a) the adaptation of the original knowledge to the new (host) environment; and (b) the development of strategies to obtain the original remedies (Pieroni et al., 2005b; Volpato et al., 2007).

3. Displacement of human groups

Ethnomedicine/ethnopharmacology normally does not cease to carry with the changes in a new social context, and it can continue to influence the choices of care and health practices. The life experiences of migrants in new land, in general, and their professional life in particular, significantly influence in their attitudes and care about the range of health care seeking (Han & Ballis, 2007).

People, who move from their region of origin to live in somewhere else, are subject to various factors that may influence their health and pharmacopoeias. For example, a group of people moving from the Northeast to the Southeast of Brazil were faced with a new routine of life, different customs, new diseases and most importantly, a distinct vegetation. This last factor induces the need to seek pharmacological learning about local natural biodiversity, which can enrich the knowledge of the information ethnopharmacological.

Bharat et al. (2008) mentions that before Lepcha tribe get in Sikim southwest of Tibet, they migrated to Thailand, Burma, Bhutan and Assam during the course of migration, they could collect important information along the way, which was about the use of wild plants available in these sites and important pharmacological characteristics of plants associated with the welfare of humanity local as well as the efficiency that these drugs had to save his life. In turn, in Sikkim, they encountered many new plant species and developed their pharmacological knowledge about them.

As cited by Ososki et al. (2007), ethnobotanical knowledge is dynamic and may evolves with the exchange, transfer and ownership of information among people adapted to new environments (Lee et al., 2001; Voeks and Leony, 2004). There is often an exchange of knowledge, medicinal plants and cultural traditions when human groups migrate between urban and rural settings (Ososki et al., 2007). Knowledge about the use of medicinal plants is sometimes the only option for many human groups in the treatment of diseases.

Some substances become even promising when they are constantly used by human groups, considering the distances travelled and the consequent exposure to different cultures and vegetal resources(Lee et al. 2001; Ososki et al. 2007).

4. Ethnopharmacological survey among migrants living in the Southeast Atlantic Forest of Diadema, São Paulo, Brazil – A case of study (Adapted of Garcia et al., 2010)

4.1 Methodology

4.1.1 Fieldwork

One of the authors (D. Garcia) spent 14 months (September 2007 to November 2008) in the municipality of Diadema, São Paulo, SP, Brazil (23°41'10"S, 46°37'22"W), selecting, observing and interviewing migrants living in the Atlantic Forest remnants. Diadema is occupied by 394.266 inhabitants (IBGE, 2011), most of whom are migrants from other regions of Brazil. The Atlantic Forest remnants found in this city are rich in plants that are either native or introduced by the influence of those migrants present both in urban and rural areas. Migrants who had relevant knowledge regarding the use of plants and animals for medicinal purposes were selected for interviews following the purposive sampling method (Bernard, 1988). After identifying potential interviewees, the researcher visited them to determine whether they did indeed possess knowledge on medicinal plants and whether they wanted to take part in this study. This ethnopharmacological study was approved by the Ethics Committee of Universidade Federal de São Paulo (UNIFESP's Ethics Committee on Research 1969/07) and Conselho de Gestão do Patrimônio Genético (No. 02000.001 049/2008-71). The interviewees also signed consent forms granting permission to access their knowledge and collect botanical and zoological material. Personal and ethnopharmacological data from the interviewees were obtained through informal and semistructured interviews (Bernard, 1988) that addressed the following topics: personal details and migration history (name, sex, age, religion, marital status, place of birth, migration, main occupation, grade of schooling) as well as ethnopharmacology (name of natural resource, use, part used, formula, route of administration, contraindications, dosages, restrictions of use). Each medicinal plant was collected in the presence of the person who described it during the interviews, in accordance with the methods suggested by Lipp (1989). The plants' scientific names were determined by specialists from the Instituto de Botânica do Estado de São Paulo (IB), and vouchers were deposited at the Herbário Municipal de São Paulo (PMSP). The animals collected were placed in glass vials containing 70% ethyl alcohol, and their subsequent identification and deposit were performed by zoologists from the Museum of Zoology, Universidade de São Paulo (MZUSP) and the Bioscience Institute from Universidade de São Paulo (IB-USP). When interviewees cited plants and animals that were used only in their cities of origin, i.e., not available in Diadema, photos from the literature and other information (e.g., popular name, habits and habitat) were used to identify them to at least the genus level. These organisms are marked with asterisks throughout the text and in Table 1. The Herpetofauna of the Northeast Atlantic Forest (Freitas & Silva, 2005) and The Herpetofauna of Caatingas and Altitudes Areas of the Brazilian Northeast (Freitas & Silva, 2007) were used as identification guides. For plants, the authors also consulted Medicinal Plants in Brazil - Native and Exotic (Lorenzi & Matos, 2008).

4.1.2 Database survey

For the plants and animals identified to the species level, the authors searched the bibliographic databases PUBMED (2011) and SCIFINDER (2011) to determine whether they

The Influence of Displacement by Human Groups Among Regionsin the Medicinal Use of Natural Resource:
A Case Study in Diadema, São Paulo - Brazil

9

had been targets of previous pharmacological studies. To determine the origin of each plant species, was consulted the Dictionary of Useful Plants: exotic and native (Pio Corrêa, 1926).

4.1.3 Dynamics of use

During the field work, the authors made an effort to understand the dynamics of use for each resource and classified them into the following four categories: maintenance of use (resource used for the same purpose in the migrant's city of origin and in Diadema), replacement (resources that were replaced when migrants arrived in Diadema because the original product was not available in Diadema or was less effective than the new resource), incorporation (resources used for the first time in Diadema to treat diseases common to larger cities, such as hypertension, diabetes and anxiety, which were not common in their homeland), and finally discontinued use (resources that are no longer used in Diadema, usually because they are not available).

4.1.4 Data analysis

The level of homogeneity between plant information provided by different migrants was calculated using the Informants' Consensus Factor, Fic (Trotter & Logan, 1986). This term is calculated as $Fic = Nur - Nt / (Nur - 1)$, where Nur is the number of use reports from informants for a particular plant-usage category and Nt is the number of taxa or species used for that plant usage category across all informants. Values range between 0 and 1, with 1 indicating the highest level of informant consent. For instance, if certain taxa are consistently used by informants, then a high degree of consensus is reached and medicinal traditions are viewed as well-defined (Heinrich, 2000).

4.2 Results and discussion

4.2.1 Migrant interviews

Despite the fact that Diadema is composed by thousands of migrants, the authors could observed that only a few had retained traditional knowledge pertaining to medicinal plants and animals. During this time the authors observed that in many cases, this knowledge has fallen into disuse because of: a) a cultural adaptation to the new city, b) the ease of conventional medical care, c) forest degradation, which restricts use of local plants and animals, furthermore d) many migrants have shown concern to participate in the study, since in the past they suffered persecution from government agencies and physicians, who eventually restrained their medical practice. The five selected interviewees migrated from northeast and southeast Brazil and established themselves in Diadema in the 1940s. Three were born in the northeast: two in Pernambuco state (coded as PE1 and PE2) and one in Sergipe state (SE1). The two remaining migrants were born in the southeast: one in Minas Gerais state (MG1) and one in inland São Paulo state (SP1) (Figure 2). All interviewees were Catholic, married and retired, with the exception of PE1 and PE2 who sell medicinal plants. Their average age was approximately 68 years old (ranging from 53 to 80 years old), and their level of education was semi-illiterate to illiterate. They learned about the medicinal uses of plants and animals from their parents and grandparents (Brazilian natives, European and African descendants) in their homelands. All interviewees arrived in the city of

Diadema as adults, and some had migrated through different regions of Brazil, accumulating knowledge on natural resources from human and biological sources. In Diadema, they acquired knowledge from neighbours, books, media (radio, television, magazines), and personal experiences.

4.2.2 Plants: Dynamics of use

The migrants described their knowledge of 85 plant specimens. As can be seen in Table 1, 78 of them were available in Diadema and were collected, resulting in 65 plant species, the remaining 13 could only be identified to the generic level. The plants belong to 37 taxonomic families, with Asteraceae (16 species), Lamiaceae (8) and Euphorbiaceae (7) as the most common. Previous studies have shown that Asteraceae species are the group most commonly reported to have potential pharmacological properties, not only in the Atlantic Forest (Almeida & Albuquerque, 2002; Begossi et al., 1993; Di Stasi et al., 2002) but also in other Brazilian biomes such as the Amazon Forest (Rodrigues, 2006) the pantanal wetlands (Rodrigues & Carlini, 2004) and the cerrado savannahs (Rodrigues & Carlini, 2005). In a review focusing on plants with possible action/ effects on the central nervous system that were indicated by 26 Brazilian indigenous peoples occupying different Brazilian biomes (Rodrigues et al., 2005), Asteraceae was the second most commonly cited family. The same

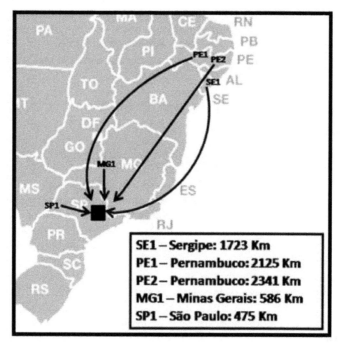

Fig. 2. Location of the Municipality of Diadema, in São Paulo state, southeastern Brazil (black square). Interviewees' migration from their cities of origin to Diadema, being PE (Pernambuco state), SE (Sergipe), MG (Minas Gerais) and SP (São Paulo), and the distance of the displacement (in Km) in each case (adapted of Garcia et al., 2010).

pattern has been detected in other countries, such as Mexico (Díaz, 1977). One factor that may explain the common use of this taxonomic family is the large number of species belonging to it - about 20,000 (Woodland, 1997). Asteraceae also has a wide geographical distribution, both in Brazil and throughout the world (Schultes & Raffaulf, 1990), which facilitates its use by various cultures. From the 65 species identified, it was observed that 33 are native to Brazil while the other 32 are exotic, demonstrating the great floral diversity of the region, which was influenced by European and African people during the civilizing process in Brazil. Furthermore, of the 78 specimens recorded, 54% (42) are spontaneous or were already available in Diadema when interviewees arrived there, while 46% (36) were grown by the migrants, acquired in free markets, or brought from other regions of the country during migration. Below, the authors describe the four 'dynamics of use' categories observed during this study.

4.2.3 Maintenance of use

According to the interviewees, 68 of the 78 specimens cited in the present study, were used in their homelands (highlighted with □ in Table 1). The maintenance of their uses was possible since most of them were available in Diadema, though some were brought from their homelands. SE1 brought four plants from Aquidabã - Sergipe state, for pain relief because they are not available or are more potent than the ones found in Diadema: "bálsamo" (*Sedum* sp.), "anador" (*Alternanthera* sp.), "eucalipto/vick" (*Eucalyptus globulus* Labill.) and "novalgina" (*Achillea millefolium* L.).

4.2.4 Incorporation of use

Fourteen of the 78 specimens listed in Table 1 came to be used by migrants when they arrived in Diadema (highlighted with Δ in Table 1). These incorporations occurred in several ways: through information given by neighbours; through local media, e.g., television, radio, magazines; or through personal efforts, guided by plant organoleptic properties or even by the theory of signatures. This theory, formulated by Paracelsus (XVI century), assumes that characteristics and virtues of herbs can be recognised by their external appearance or "signature" (picture, shape, colour). Finally, observing the relationship between animals and plants can be a valuable guide. PE1 noted that dogs consume "sete-sangria" (*Cuphea carthagenensis* (Jacq.) J. F. Macbr.) when they have diarrhoea; and because it seemed to alleviate their symptoms, he started to use this plant for the same purpose. The migrants incorporated several plants after their arrival in Diadema to treat typical diseases of larger cities: "cipó-cruz" (*Serjania* sp.) to combat high cholesterol; and "guanxuma" (*Sida rhombifolia* L.) and "guiné" (*Petiveria alliaceae* L.) for anxiety. Also included in this category was knowledge concerning local toxic plants, e. g., alamanda-amarela (*Allamanda cathartica* L.) and azaléia (*Rhododendron simsii* Planch.), detailing the risks associated with their consumption.

Similar results were recorded by Volpato et al. (2009), where the use of some plants have been incorporated in Cuban pharmacopoeia by the Haitians. This occurred, according to the authors, as a result of factors such as cultural contact and exchange of information between migrants and host, and personal experimentation or imitation of local practices by migrants. The same authors conclude that Haitians contributed to what is today considered as traditional Cuban medicine by introducing into the dominant Cuban community practices and uses of plants.

Specimen (family) Voucher code	Popular(s) name(s) (migrant) dynamic of use	Origin –geographical distribution - cultivated (C) or spontaneous (S)	Use (part)	Formula and route of administration	Pharmacological studies
Acanthospermum australe (Loefl.) Kuntze (Asteraceae) Garcia 052	Carrapicho (SEI#, MGI□)	Native – Brazilian territory (S)	Wounds in the body (roots)	Medicinal wine - ingestion	Antimalarial activity (Carvalho & Krettli, 1991) and antifungal activity (Portillo et al., 2001)
Achillea millefolium L. (Asteraceae) Garcia 015	Novalgina (MGI, SEI)□	Exotic - south and southeast Brazil (C)	Sedative (leaves)	In natura - ingestion	Antioxidant and antimicrobial activity (Candan et al., 2003)
Ageratum conyzoides L. (Asteraceae) Garcia 010	Mentrasto (PEI)□	Native - southeast to northeast Brazil (S)	Bronchitis* (leaves) Rheumatism* (whole plant)	Infusion – Ingestion Infusion - bath	Anti-inflammatory (Moura et al., 2005), toxic (Singh et al., 2006), antibacterial (Chah et al., 2006) and insecticidal activity (Moreira et al., 2007)
Allamanda cathartica L. (Apocynaceae) Garcia 076	Alamanda-amarela (SEI□, PEI▲)	Native – Brazilian territory (C)	Toxic (whole plant)	Any oral dose is dangerous	Healing activity (Nayak et al., 2006)
Alpinia zerumbet (Pers.) B.L. Burtt & R.M. Sm. (Zingiberaceae) Garcia 018	Brinco-deprincesa (SEI)▲	Exotic – Brazilian territory (C)	Sedative (flowers)	Infusion – ingestion	Antihypertensive effects (De Moura et al., 2005), antinociceptive (De Araújo et al., 2005), anti-amoebic activity (Sawangjaroen, 2006) and hepatoprotector (Lin et al., 2008)
Alternanthera sp. (Amaranthaceae) Garcia 039	Anador (SEI)□	No data (C)	Soothing, headache, pain in the body (leaves)	Infusion - ingestion	Not consulted
Artemisia absinthium L. (Asteraceae) Garcia 049	Losna (SPI, SEI, PEI2)□	Exotic - Brazilian territory (S)	Laxative (aerial parts)	Infusion – ingestion	Acaricidal properties (Chiasson et al., 2001), antifungal and antibacterial (Kordali et al., 2005) and antioxidant activities (Lopes-Lutz et al., 2008)
Artemisia camphorata Vill. (Asteraceae) Garcia 045	Cânfora (MGI, PEI, SEI)□	Exotic - Brazilian territory (C)	Muscle pain (whole plant)	Decoction - massage	No data found
Asclepias curassavica L. (Apocynaceae) Garcia 037	Algodão-domato (MGI, PEI2)□	Exotic - Brazilian territory (S)	Toxic** (whole plant)	Any oral dose is dangerous	Cancer and warts treatment (Kupchan et al., 1964) and poisoning (Radford et al., 1986)
Baccharis dracunculifolia DC (Asteraceae) Garcia 021	Alecrim-docampo (SEI)□	Native - central Brazil (S)	Soothing (aerial parts)	Smoking - inhalation	Bactericidal activity (Orsi et al., 2005), cytotoxic (Fukuda et al., 2006), antiulcerogenic (Klopell et al., 2007), antimicrobial and antifungal (Da Silva et al., 2008) and anti-inflammatory (Paulino et al., 2008)
Baccharis trimera (Less) DC (Asteraceae) Garcia 027	Carqueja (MGI)□	Native - south and southeast Brazil (C)	Diabetes* (whole plant)	Macerate - ingestion	Antihepatotoxic properties (Soicke et al., 1987), anti-inflammatory and analgesic activity (Gené et al., 1996), relaxant effect (Torres et al., 2000), antiproteolytic and anti-hemorrhagic properties (Januário et al., 2004), antioxidant compounds (Simões-Pires et al., 2005), antidiabetic activity (Oliveira et al., 2005) and for losing weight (Dickel et al., 2007)
Bidens pilosa L. (Asteraceae) Garcia 020	Picão-preto (MGI, PEI), Picão-branco (SPI)□	Native - tropical America (S)	Blood purifier (whole plant), Healing wounds* (whole plant), Wounds in the body* (roots)	Infusion – Ingestion In natura – Plaster Medicinal wine - ingestion	Hypotensive effects (Dimo et al., 1999), anti-inflammatory activity (Chang et al., 2005), anticancer and antipyretic activity (Sundararajan et al., 2006), antimicrobial (Rojas et al., 2006) and antitumor potential (Kviecinski et al., 2008)

The Influence of Displacement by Human Groups Among Regionsin the Medicinal Use of Natural Resource:
A Case Study in Diadema, São Paulo - Brazil

13

Specimen (family) Voucher code	Popular(s) name(s) (migrant) dynamic of use	Origin –geographical distribution - cultivated (C) or spontaneous (S)	Use (part)	Formula and route of administration	Pharmacological studies
Bryophyllum pinnatum (Lam.) Oken (Crassulaceae) Garcia 040	Folha-santa, folha-da-fortuna (MG1, SP1, PE1)▫	Exotic - Brazilian territory (C)	Lumbar pain* (leaves) Sedative* (leaves)	In natura - Plaster In natura - plaster	Antibacterial activity (Obaseiki-Ebor, 1985), anti-ulcer (Pal et al., 1991), antimicrobial (Akinpelu, 2000), antinociceptive, anti-inflammatory and antidiabetic (Ojewole, 2005) and neurosedative and muscle relaxant activities (Yemitan et al., 2005)
Cajanus cajan (L.) Millsp. (Fabaceae s.l.) Garcia 003	Feijão-guandu (SP1)▫	Exotic - Brazilian territory (C)	Bronchitis (leaves)	Infusion - ingestion or inhalation	Treatment of postmenopausal osteoporosis (Zheng et al., 2007), antileishmanial and antifungal activity (Braga et al., 2007) and hypocholesterolemic effect (Luo et al., 2008)
Calea sp. (Asteraceae) Garcia 036	Picão (MG1)▫	No data (S)	Diuretic (leaves)	Infusion - ingestion	Not consulted
Carica papaya L. (Caricaceae) Garcia 062	Mamão-papaia (PE1)▫	Exotic - Brazilian territory (C)	Bronchitis* (powder fruit)	Syrup - ingestion	Abortive (Gopalakrishnan & Rajasekharasetty, 1978), antibacterial activity (Emeruwa, 1982), diuretic (Sripanidkulchai et al., 2001) and healing and abortive effects (Anuar et al., 2008)
Cecropia pachystachya Tréc. (Cecropiaceae) Garcia 068	Embaúba (MG1, SEI)▫	Native - south to northeast Brazil (S)	Bronchitis* (powder fruit) Toxic (sap)	Syrup – ingestion Any oral dose is angerous	Antioxidative activity (Velásquez et al., 2003), cardiotonic and sedative effects (Consolini et al., 2006) and anti-inflammatory (Schinella et al., 2008)
Chenopodium ambrosioides L. (Chenopodiaceae) Garcia 006	Mentruz, erva-de- santa-maria (PE1#, SE1▫)	Native - south and southeast Brazil (S)	Muscle pain (aerial parts) Lesions in bone (aerial parts) Worm* (aerial parts) Bronchitis (aerial parts)	Decoction - Massage In natura - Plaster Infusion - Ingestion Syrup - ingestion	Insecticidal properties (Chiasson et al., 2004), antifungal, antiaflatoxigenic and antioxidant activity (Kumar et al., 2007) and mosquito repellent activity (Gillij et al., 2008)
Cissus sp. (Vitaceae) Garcia 053	Sofre-do-rimquem-qué (MG1)*	No data (S)	Kidney stone (leaves)	Infusion - ingestion	Not consulted
Citrus aurantifolia (Christm.) Swingle (Rutaceae) Garcia 063	Limão (MG1)▫	Exotic - Brazilian territory (C)	Fever (leaves)	Infusion - ingestion	Mosquito repellent activity (Das et al., 2003)
Coffea arabica L. (Rubiaceae) Garcia 030	Café (MG1)▫	Exotic - Brazilian territory (C)	Diabetes (ripe fruits) Sinusitis (powder fruit)	Infusion Infusion	Antioxidant (Berson, 2008)
Costus spiralis (Jacq.) Roscoe (Costaceae) Garcia 019	Cana-do-brejo (SP1, PE2)▫	Native - northeast and southeast Brazil (S)	Laxative and Rheumatism (leaves)	Infusion or decoction - ingestion	Antiurolithiatic (Araújo et al., 1999)
Croton fuscescens Spreng (Euphorbiaceae) Garcia 013	Velando (SEI)▫	Native - Brazilian territory (S)	Inhibits the growth of skin stains/ wounds in the body (resin)	In natura - topic	No data found

Specimen (family) Voucher code	Popular(s) name(s) (migrant) dynamic of use	Origin –geographical distribution - cultivated (C) or spontaneous (S)	Use (part)	Formula and route of administration	Pharmacological studies
Cuphea carthagenensis (Jacq.) J. F. Macbr. (Lythraceae) Garcia 007	Sete-sangria (MG1□, SP1□, SE1△)	Native - Brazilian territory (S)	Intestinal infections and heart problems* (aerial parts)	Infusion - ingestion	Antiinflammatory and antinociceptive activities (Schapoval et al., 1998), vasorelaxant properties (Schuldt et al., 2000), treat high levels of cholesterol and triglycerides (Biavatti et al., 2004)
Cymbopogon citratus DC. - Stapf. (Poaceae) Garcia 026	Capim-limão (MG1, SE1, PE2)□	Exotic - tropical countries (C)	Bronchitis* (leaves) / Sedative* (leaves)	Syrup – ingestion / Infusion - ingestion	Anxiolytic (Palmieri, 2000), larvicidal activity (Cavalcanti et al., 2004), antibacterial (Warnissorn et al., 2005), antimalarial activity (Tchoumbougnang et al., 2005), insect repellent (Moore et al., 2007), hypoglycemic and hypolipidemic effects (Adeneye et al., 2007) and antimicrobial activity (Nogueira et al., 2008)
Dieffenbachia sp. (Araceae) Garcia 071	Comigo-ninguém- pode (PE1)□	No data (C)	Toxic (whole plant)	Any oral dose is dangerous	Not consulted
Equisetum arvensis L. (Equisetaceae) Garcia 051	Cavalinha (MG1)□	Exotic (C)	Diuretic (leaves)	Infusion - ingestion	No data found
Eucalyptus globulus Labill. (Myrtaceae) Garcia 055	Eucalipto, vick (MG1□, PE1△, PE2△, SE1□)	Exotic (C)	Sinusitis* (leaves)	Infusion - inhalation	Antihyperglycemic actions (Gray & Flatt, 1998), analgesic and anti-inflammatory effects (Silva et al., 2003), antimicrobial activity (Takahashi et al., 2004) and antibacterial effects (Salari et al., 2006)
Euphorbia heterophylla L. (Euphorbiaceae) Garcia 047	Amendoim-bravo, burra-leiteira (MG1, SP1, SE1, PE1, PE2)□	Native - Americas (S)	Toxic* (whole plant)	Any oral dose is dangerous	Cytotoxic properties (De Almeida Barbosa et al., 2006)
Euphorbia tirucalli L (Euphorbiaceae) Garcia 046	Avelóz (PE1, PE2)□	Exotic - Brazilian territory (C)	Toxic* (whole plant) (latex) / Breast cancer* (latex)	Restricted use (reports of blindness) / Macerate - ingestion	Anti-tumour activity (Valadares et al., 2006), cause eye injury (Shlamovitz et al., 2007) and effect against arthritis diseases (Bani et al., 2007)
Fevillea passiflora Vell. (Cucurbitaceae) Garcia 022	Pucunã (SE1)□	Native - North and southeast Brazil (S)	Toxic - abortive (seeds)	In natura - ingestion	No data found
Foeniculum vulgare Mill. (Apiaceae) Garcia 064	Erva-doce, funcho (MG1, SP1, PE1, PE2)□	Exotic -Brazilian territory (C)	Sedative (whole plant) / Bronchitis* (whole plant) / Laxative (whole plant)	Infusion - Ingestion / Infusion - Inhalation / Infusion or macerate - ingestion	Antimicrobial activity (Aridoğan et al., 2002), antiinflammatory, analgesic and antioxidant activities (Choi et al., 2004), acaricidal activity (Lee, 2004), antifungal effect (Ozcan et al., 2006), antithrombotic activity (Tognolini et al., 2007) and larvicidal activity of the mosquito Aedes aegypti (Pitasawat et al., 2007)
Gossypium sp. (Malvaceae) Garcia 066	Algodão (MG1)□	No data (C)	Anti-inflammatory (leaves)	Infusion - inhalation	Not consulted
Hypochoeris sp. (Asteraceae) Garcia 009	Almeirão-boca-de- leão (SE1)△	No data (S)	pain (leaves)	In natura - ingestion	Not consulted
Hyptis sp. (Lamiaceae) Garcia 041	Samba-caitá (SE1)□	No data (S)	y ache (leaves)	In natura - ingestion	Not consulted

Specimen (family) Voucher code	Popular(s) name(s) (migrant) dynamic of use	Origin –geographical distribution - cultivated (C) or spontaneous (S)	Use (part)	Formula and route of administration	Pharmacological studies
Impatiens hawkeri W. Bull. (Balsaminaceae) Garcia 044	Impatiens (PE1)ᴬ	Exotic - Brazilian territory (C)	Toxic (whole plant)	In closed environment causes tearing, allergy and headache	No data found
Jacaranda sp. (Bignoniaceae) Garcia 011	Salsa-parreira (SE1)ᶜ	No data (S)	External allergies, wounds in the body and purifier (leaves)	Decoction - bath	Not consulted
Jatropha gossypiifolia L. (Euphorbiaceae) Garcia 017	Pinhão-roxo (SP1)ᶜ	Native - southeast to northeast Brazil (S)	Laxative (powder fruit)	In natura - ingestion	Antimalarial effects (Cbeassor et al., 1989), hypotensive and vasorelaxant effects (Abreu et al., 2003)
Leonurus sibiricus L. (Lamiaceae) Garcia 002	Rubim (MG1, SP1)ᶜ	Exotic - Brazilian territory (C)	Healing wounds* (aerial parts)	In natura - plaster	Stimulating action on the uterus (Shi et al., 1995), analgesic and anti-inflammatory activity (Islam et al., 2005) and antibacterial activity (Ahmed et al., 2006)
Lippia alba (Mill.) N. E. Br. (Verbenaceae) Garcia 005	Erva-cidreira (MG1, SE1, PE2)ᶜ	Native - almost all Brazilian territory (S)	Expectorant* (aerial parts) Sedative* (aerial parts)	Infusion - Inhalation Infusion or decoction - ingestion	Treatment of respiratory diseases (Cáceres et al., 1991), antiulcerogenic activity (Pascual et al., 2001), sedative and anticonvulsant effects (Zétola et al., 2002), antiviral and antiherpes (Andrighetti-Fröhner et al., 2005)
Ludwigia sp. (Onagraceae) Garcia 078	Erva-de-bicho (SE1)ᶜ	No data (S)	Hemorrhoid (whole plant)	Decoction - bath	Not consulted
Malva sylvestris L. (Malvaceae) Garcia 059	Malva-decheiro (MG1)ᶜ	Exotic - south and southeast Brazil (S)	Wounds in the body (roots)	Medicinal wine - ingestion	Skin anti-aging property (Talbourdet et al., 2007)
Manihot esculenta Crantz (Euphorbiaceae) Garcia 050	Mandioca (SE1)ᶜ	Native - Brazilian territory (C)	conjunctivitis/sty* (dew on the leaves)	In natura - topic	Analgesics and anti-inflammatory effects (Adeyemi et al., 2008)
Mentha arvensis L. (Lamiaceae) Garcia 031	Hortelã (MG1, PE1)ᶜ	Exotic - Brazilian territory (C)	Bronchitis* (leaves) Laxative (leaves)	Syrup - ingestion Infusion - ingestion	Antifungal property (Tiwari et al., 1998), vasodilatory actions (Runnie et al., 2004), antioxidative activity (Ka et al., 2005), antibacterial properties (Wannissorn et al., 2005) and insect repellents and fumigants (Moore et al., 2007)
Mentha pulegium L. (Lamiaceae) Garcia 029	Poejo (MG1, PE2)ᶜ	Exotic - Brazilian territory (C)	Bronchitis (leaves)	Syrup - ingestion	Larvicidal activity (Cetin et al., 2006), acaricidal effects (Rim et al., 2006) and insecticidal properties (Pavela, 2008)
Mikania glomerata Spreng. (Asteraceae) Garcia 032	Guaco (PE1ᶜ, PE2ᶜ, SE1ᴬ)	Native - northeast to southeast Brazil (S)	Bronchitis* (leaves)	Syrup - ingestion	Analgesic and anti-inflammatory activities (Ruppelt et al., 1991), bronchodilator activity (Soares et al., 2002) and antiophidian properties (Maiorano et al., 2005)
Mimosa pudica L. (Fabaceae s.l.) Garcia 069	Dormideira (SE1)ᶜ	Exotic - Brazilian territory (C)	Healing wounds (aerial parts)	In natura - plaster	Antidepressant activity (Molina et al., 2005), antitoxin of the snake Naja kaouthia (Mahanta et al., 2001), anticonvulsant (Ngo et al., 2004) and for reproductive problems (Lans, 2007)
Mirabilis jalapa L. (Nyctaginaceae) Garcia 065	Maravilha (SP1, PE2)ᶜ	Native - Brazilian territory (C)	Healing wounds* (aerial parts)	Infusion - plaster	Antibacterial effect (Kusamba et al., 1991) and antimicrobial (Shao et al., 1999)

Specimen (family) Voucher code	Popular(s) name(s) (migrant) dynamic of use	Origin -geographical distribution - cultivated (C) or spontaneous (S)	Use (part)	Formula and route of administration	Pharmacological studies
Ocimum basilicum L. (Lamiaceae) Garcia 061	Manjericão (MG1)□	Exotic - Brazilian territory (C)	Bronchitis* (leaves)	Syrup - ingestion	Antibacterial (Nguefack et al., 2004), mosquito repellent activity (Ntonifor et al., 2006), antimicrobial activity (Viyoch et al., 2006), antigiardial activity (De Almeida et al., 2007) and decreases cholesterol (Bravo et al., 2008)
Ocimum selloi Benth. (Lamiaceae) Garcia 033	Alfavaca (SP1)□	Native - northeast to south Brazil (C)	Soothing (aerial parts) Bronchitis (leaves)	Infusion - inhalation p - ingestion	Mosquito repellent activity (Padilha de Paula et al., 2003)
Petiveria alliaceae L. (Phytolaccaceae) Garcia 004	Guiné (SE1)△	Native - north Brazil (S)	Sedative (aerial parts) Muscle pain* (leaves)	Environment purifier - inhalation Decoction - massage	Antimicrobial substance (Von Szczepanski et al., 1972), antimitotic action (Malpezzi et al. 1994), anti-inflammatory and analgesic effects (Lopes-Martins et al., 2002), antibacterial and antifungal activity (Kim et al., 2006) and antioxidant (Okada et al., 2008)
Phyllanthus caroliniensis Walter (Euphorbiaceae) Garcia 024	Quebra-pedra (SP1, PE1, PE2, SE1)□	Native - USA to Brazil (S)	Kidney stone* (aerial parts)	Infusion or decoction - ingestion	Antinociceptive action (Cechinel Filho et al., 1996)
Piper umbellatum L. (Piperaceae) Garcia 072	Pariparoba (MG1)□	Native - Tropical America (S)	Belly ache and liver pain (leaves)	Infusion - ingestion	Antioxidant (Agbor et al., 2007) and antifungal activity (Tabopda et al., 2008)
Plantago sp. (Plantaginaceae) Garcia 008	Tanchagem (SP1, PE2)□	No data (S)	Anti-inflammatory - mouth and throat (leaves)	Decoction - gargling	Not consulted
Plectranthus amboinicus (Lour.) Spreng. (Lamiaceae) Garcia 073	Hortelã-grande (PE1)□	Exotic - Brazilian territory (C)	For digestion and urine with blood (leaves) Cough (leaves)	Infusion - Ingestion Syrup - ingestion	Scorpion venon antidote (Ka et al, 2005) and antimicrobial activity (Nogueira et al, 2008)
Pluchea sagittalis (Lam.) Cabrera (Asteraceae) Garcia 042	Quitoco (SE1)□	Native - south and southeast Brazil (S)	Diuretic (aerial parts)	Infusion - ingestion	Anti-inflammatory activity (Pérez-Garcia et al., 1996)
Porophyllum ruderale (Jacq.) Cass. (Asteraceae) Garcia 075	Arnica (PE1)□	Native - Brazilian territory (S)	Muscle pain* (aerial parts)	Decoction - massage	Anti-inflammatory (Souza et al., 2004)
Psidium guajava L. (Myrtaceae) Garcia 058	Goiaba (SE1)□	Native - Mexico to Brazil (S)	Heartburn (leaves) Diarrhea (fruit)	Infusion or in natura - ingestion In natura - ingestion	Antibacterial activity (Anas et al., 2008; Cheruiyot et al., 2009; Rahim et al., 2010) and hepatoprotective activity (Roy & Das, 2010)
Rhododendron simsii Planch. (Ericaceae) Garcia 043	Azaléia (PE1)△	Exotic - Brazilian territory (C)	Toxic (whole plant)	Any oral dose is dangerous	Antioxidative (Takahashi et al., 2001)
Rosmarinus officinalis L. (Lamiaceae) Garcia 060	Alecrim (MG1)□	Exotic - all countries with temperate climate (C)	Muscle pain* (leaves)	Decoction - massage	Antibacterial effects (Fu et al., 2007), antimicrobial effect (Weckesser et al., 2007), anti-inflammatory and antitumor effects (Peng et al., 2007), cause reduction of reproductive fertility in male rats (Nusier et al., 2007), antinociceptive effect (González-Trujano et al., 2007), mosquito repellent activity (Gillij et al., 2008), antidiabetic and antioxidant properties (Bakirel et al., 2008)

The Influence of Displacement by Human Groups Among Regions in the Medicinal Use of Natural Resource:
A Case Study in Diadema, São Paulo - Brazil

17

Specimen (family) Voucher code	Popular(s) name(s) (migrant) dynamic of use	Origin –geographical distribution - cultivated (C) or spontaneous (S)	Use (part)	Formula and route of administration	Pharmacological studies
Ruta graveolens L. (Rutaceae) Garcia 028	Arruda (MG1, PE1, PE2)□	Exotic – Brazilian territory (C)	Earache and conjunctivitis/sty* (leaves)	In natura – topic	Antifertility (Gandhi et al., 1991), fungicide (Oliva et al., 2003), cytotoxic (Ivanova et al., 2005), abortive (De Freitas et al., 2005), anti-tumour (Preethi et al., 2006), anti-inflammatory (Raghav et al., 2006), antiarrhythmic (Khori et al., 2008) and antimicrobial (Nogueira et al., 2008)
			Muscle pain (leaves)	Decoction – massage	
Sambucus canadensis L. (Caprifoliaceae) Garcia 025	Sabugueiro (MG1)□	Native – Brazilian territory (S)	Bronchitis* (flowers)	Syrup – ingestion	Infectious diseases and antioxidant activity (Holetz et al., 2002)
Schinus terebinthifolius Raddi (Anacardiaceae) Garcia 035	Aroeira (MG1)□	Native – northeast to south Brazil (S)	Diuretic (leaves)	Infusion – ingestion	Antifungal activity (Schmourlo et al., 2005) and antibacterial (De Lima et al., 2006)
Scoparia dulcis L. (Scrophulariaceae) Garcia 014	Vassourinha (SE1, PE2)□	Native – Brazilian territory (S)	Hip pain/kidneys (leaves	Decoction - bath	Antitumor-promoting activity (Nishino et al., 1993), antioxidant (Ratnasooriya et al., 2005), antimicrobial and antifungal activities (Latha et al., 2006)
Sedum sp. (Crassulaceae) Garcia 038	Bálsamo (MG1, SP1, PE1, SE1)□	No data (C)	Earache (leaves) Laxative (aerial parts)	In natura – topic In natura – ingestion	Not consulted
Senna pendula (Humb. & Bonpl. Ex Willd.) H.S. Irwin & Barneby (Fabaceae s. l.) Garcia 034	Fedegoso (MG1)□	Native – Brazilian territory (S)	Osteoporosis prevention (roots)	Medicinal wine - ingestion	No data found
Serjania sp. (Sapindaceae) Garcia 012	Cipó-cruz (SE1, PE2)▲	No data (S)	Reduces cholesterol and diarrhea (leaves) External allergies, wounds in the body and detoxifying (leaves)	Macerate - Ingestion Infusion - bath	Not consulted Not consulted
Sida rhombifolia L. (Malvaceae) Garcia 067	Guanxuma (SE1)▲	Exotic – Brazilian territory (S)	Sedative (aerial parts)	Infusion – ingestion or inhalation	Cytotoxicity, antibacterial activity (Islam et al., 2003) and antioxidant (Dhalwal et al., 2007)
Solanum americanum L. (Solanaceae) Garcia 070	Maria-pretinha (MG1)□	Native – Americas (S)	Sore throat* (aerial parts)	Infusion – gargle	Treatment of protozoal infections (American trypanosomes) (Cáceres et al., 1998) and moderate antioxidant activity (Iwalewa et al., 2005)
Solanum variabile Mart. (Solanaceae) Garcia 056	Jurubeba (MG1, SE1, PE2)□	Native – southeast and south Brazil (S)	Sedative (leaves) Laxative (powder fruit)	Infusion - Ingestion In natura – ingestion	Antiulcerogenic activity (Antonio et al., 2004)
Sonchus oleraceus L. (Asteraceae) Garcia 016	Serralha (PE1)▲	Exotic – Brazilian territory (S)	Diabetes (leaves)	In natura – ingestion	Larvicidal potential (Shama et al., 2006)
Stachytarpheta cayennensis (Rich.) Vahl (Verbenaceae) Garcia 054	Gervão (MG1)□	Native – Brazilian territory (S)	Laxative (aerial parts)	Infusion or decoction - ingestion	Anti-inflammatory and anti-ulcerogenic properties (Penido et al., 2006) and hypoglycaemic constituents (Adebajo et al., 2007)

Specimen (family) Voucher code	Popular(s) name(s) (migrant) dynamic of use	Origin –geographical distribution - cultivated (C) or spontaneous (S)	Use (part)	Formula and route of administration	Pharmacological studies
Synadenium grantii Hook. F. (Euphorbiaceae) Garcia 074	Jarnaúba (PE1)A	Exotic - southeast to northeast Brazil (C)	Toxic (whole plant) Stomach cancer (latex)	Restricted use Macerate - ingestion	Healing action and anti-hemorrhagic (Rajesh et al., 2007)
Tropaeolum majus L. (Tropaeolaceae) Garcia 057	Capuchinha (SP1, MG1)A	Exotic - south and southeast Brazil (C)	Ulcer and laxative (aerial parts)	Infusion or in natura - ingestion	Antitumor activity (Pintão et al., 1995)
Vernonia condensata Baker (Asteraceae) Garcia 001	Boldo-do-Chile, figatil (PE1□, SE1A)	Exotic - northeast to southeast Brazil (C)	Liver pain* (leaves)	Infusion - ingestion	Anti-ulcerogenic (Frutoso et al., 1994) and analgesic and anti-inflammatory (Valverde et al., 2001)
Vernonia sp. (Asteraceae) Garcia 048	Assa-peixe (MG1, SE1)□	No data (S)	Chitis (leaves) Expectorant (leaves) Healing wounds (leaves)	Infusion - Ingestion Infusion - Inhalation infusion - plaster	Not consulted
Waltheria indica L. (Sterculiaceae) Garcia 077	Malva-branca (SE1)□	Native - Brazilian territory (S)	Gingivitis* (leaves) Inflammation in the mouth and/or throat* (leaves)	Infusion - gargling	Anti-inflammatory activities (Rao et al., 2005)
Zea mays L. (Poaceae) Garcia 023	Milho (SE1)□	Exotic - Brazilian territory (C)	Bronchitis (flowers) Blood purifier and diuretic (flowers)	Syrup - ingestion Infusion - ingestion	No data found

* their popular and scientific names, geographical origin and distribution, if cultivated or spontaneous, uses, parts utilized, formula, route of administration and pharmacological studies. Marked by (□) the 68 plants whose use had been maintained by the respective migrant, while 14, marked by (A) are those whose applications have been incorporated by migrants, finally, 3 (#) are replacements. The matches between the uses proclaimed by the interviewees and pharmacological data have been posted by (*).

Table 1. The 78 plant specimens used by five Diadema's migrants (MG1, SP1, PE1, PE2, SE1)* (adapted of Garcia et al., 2010).

4.2.5 Replacement of use

Three plants used by migrants in their cities of origin were replaced because they were not available or were less effective than plants present in Diadema (highlighted with # in Table 1). Most of these replacements were made according to the criteria listed in the previous section. The interviewee MG1 explained that in his homelands, he used "quebra-pedra"* (*Phyllanthus* cf. *caroliniensis* Walter - Euphorbiaceae) for kidney stone disturbance, but when he arrived in Diadema, he found another plant, "sofre-do-rim-quem-qué" (*Cissus* sp.), that seemed to have a stronger effect.

Another interviewee, PE1, reported that the bark and seeds of "amburana-de-cheiro"* (*Amburana* cf. *cearensis* (Allemão) A.C. Sm. - Fabaceae s.l.) were widely used for anti-inflammatory therapy in Pernambuco state but had to be replaced by "mentruz" (*Chenopodium ambrosioides* L.) because the former was not found in Diadema. In addition, SE1 had to replace "pau-de-sapo"* (*Pouteria* cf. *melinoniana* Boehni - Sapotaceae), whose leaves were used for chronic wounds, with "carrapicho" (*Acanthospermum austrole* (Loefl.) Kuntze). The vernacular names of some plants are registered trademarks of allopathic medicines and active ingredients, e.g., Novalgina® (*Achillea millefolium*) and Vick® (*Eucalyptus globulus*) for sinusitis, and Anador® (*Alternanthera* sp.), which is used as a sedative and for general pain. Contact between migrants and allopathic medicine thus led to the 'baptisms' of these plants, following the observation that both, the commercially available products and herbal source have similar effects, as reported by Pires et al., (2009).

Biocultural adaptation, negotiation and cultural identity are key-issues for issues anthropological in the displacement of human groups between regions (Belliard & Ramírez-Johnson, 2005; Janes & Pawson, 1986). Research in culturally homogeneous places and/or non-urban has shown that to follow the pattern of changes in traditional knowledge and use of plant among migrants must involve the degree the process of acculturation (Bodeker et al., 2005; Nesheim et al., 2006 as cited in Pieroni & Vandebroek, 2007). This dynamic interaction between migrants and host societies may result in changes pharmacopeial adapted with plants exchanged(Pieroni & Vandebroek, 2007).

4.2.6 Discontinued use

According to MG1, the following plants used in his homeland fell into disuse because they were not found in Diadema, although he tried to acquire them from local commercial sources: "quina"* (*Strychnos* cf. *pseudoquina* A. St. Hil - Loganiaceae), whose root is used to combat pain in the stomach and intestine; bark oil of "jatobá"* (*Hymenaea* cf. *courbaril* L. - Fabaceae s.l.), used for combat wounds; "batata-de-purga"* (*Operculina* cf. *macrocarpa* (L.) Urb - Convolvulaceae), whose tuber is ingested as a purgative and to clean the blood; bark and leaf of "jalapa"* (*Mirabilis* cf *jalapa* L. - Nyctaginaceae), used to clean the blood; tea of "junco"* (*Cyperus* cf. *esculentus* L. - Cyperaceae), whose root is used for inflammation; bark or seed of "emburana"* (*Amburana* cf. *cearensis* - Fabaceae s.l.), used for migraine and sleeping; and bark of "angico"* (*Anadenanthera* cf. *colubrine* (Vell.) Brenan - Fabaceae s.l.), prepared as a tea for pain in the body and fever. These plants were not described in Table 1, since they could not be collected and identified as well.

In a study performed by Waldstein (2008), it became clear that there is great influence of the host culture (USA) on the lifestyles of immigrants (Mexicans). The study reports that immigrants go through an intense process of acculturation and loss of traditional knowledge over the years, adopting the lifestyle of the host country. One of the problems that can affect traditional knowledge is the possibility of loss due to migration of people to industrialized regions (Pieroni et al., 2005). Due to contact with a new routine of life and, often, different environments (flora, fauna, culture, food, language, religion) people moving between regions, usually adapt more to the new location (those more culturally flexible) or not (those culturally less flexible) variable which makes the loss or incorporation of traditional knowledge about medicinal use of natural resources. For newcomers to the host country, it seems that the adoption of values, language, beliefs, traditions of the dominant group are constant, but, alternatively, some groups reject this and maintain their traditional customs(Ceuterick et al., 2007). The use of traditional foods, for example, is often seen as a symbol of maintenance ethnic identity and a cultural trait very resistant to change (Nguyen, 2003 as cited in Ceuterick et al., 2007).

4.2.7 Plants used for therapeutic purposes

Of the 78 plants, 10 carry some restrictions, as they can be toxic depending on the dose, route or part utilized (Table 1). The uses described in Table 1 are written just as they were reported by the interviewees. The 68 plants used exclusively for medicinal purposes were cited for 41 complaints, which were grouped into 12 functional categories according to bodily system, as detailed in Table 3. Thus, gastrointestinal disturbances include the following complaints (numbers of medicinal plants reported): endoparasitosis (1), ulcer (1), diarrhoea (1), bellyache (2), heartburn (1), intestinal infections (1), liver pain (3). This category also includes plants used to improve digestion (1), to treat tables of haemorrhoid (1), as laxatives (10) and to purify the stomach (2), comprising a total of 24 plants employed in 44 formulas. The most relevant categories of use, measured by number of species employed, were gastrointestinal disturbances (30.8% of plants), inflammatory processes (24.4%) and respiratory problems (23.1%). As seen in Table 4, the group of illnesses representing immunological problems obtained the highest informant consensus factor value (Fic = 0.66), while the other categories presented Fic values lower than 0.5. These low values reflect the diversity of knowledge displayed by migrants, which can probably be attributed to different cultural influences during their migrations through Brazilian territory. Furthermore, the small number of interviewees may have resulted in low values of Fic. The parts of the plants most often used in the formulas were leaves (45.4%) and other aerial parts (22.7%). The most common formula was the infusion (37.8%), followed by in natura (17.6%) and syrup (10.1%). The most cited route of administration was ingestion (51.3%), followed by inhalation (8.4%) and topical (3.4%).

4.2.8 Plants with restrictions on use and/or toxic

Among the 10 specimens with restrictions on use, 6 were designated as only toxic: "alamanda-amarela" (*Allamanda cathartica*), "algodão-do-mato" (*Asclepias curassavica* L.), "amendoim-bravo/burra-leiteira" (*Euphorbia heterophylla* L.), "azaléa" (*Rhododendron simsii*), "comigo-ninguém-pode" (*Dieffenbachia* sp.) and "impatiens" (*Impatiens hawkeri*). The interviewees explained that depending on the dose, the latex of "alamanda- amarela" and "amendoim-bravo" can cause discomfort or even blindness. According to Oliveira et al. (2003), the leaves of *Dieffenbachia picta* Schott contain calcium oxalate, which damages the oral mucosa and provokes pain and oedema, while the leaves of *Allamanda cathartica* contain cardiotonic glycosides and induce intense gastrointestinal disturbances. Although reported as toxic, the latex of two other plants can be used at low doses to treat breast and stomach cancer: "avelóz" (*Euphorbia tirucalli* L.) and "jarnaúba" (*Synadenium grantii* Hook. F.), respectively. The sap of "embaúba" (*Cecropia pachystachya* Tréc.) was indicated as toxic, but its fruits are used to combat bronchitis. Finally, the seeds of "pucunã" (*Fevillea passiflora* Vell.) are toxic, being indicated as abortive. In a recent study, Rodrigues (2007) also described plants with restrictions of use as reported by three Brazilian cultures: the Krahô Indians use two plants as abortives in a single prescription: "aprytytti" (*Acosmium dasycarpum* (Vogel) Yakovlev) and "ahkryt" (*Anacardium occidentale* L.) (Anacardiaceae); their barks are boiled, and the beverage is ingested in at dawn. It is an extremely bitter beverage, rich in tannin and therefore extremely astringent.

4.2.9 Pharmacological data

As can be seen in Table 1, 57 species (73.1%) were featured in previous pharmacological studies. For 30 of these species (52.6%), the uses cited by the migrants showed some similarity to the investigated effects/actions, demonstrating concordance between popular knowledge and academic science (marked with an asterisk in Table 1).

4.2.10 Animals used for therapeutic purposes and dynamics of use

From the five interviewees, only one (PE2) offered knowledge on the medicinal uses of 12 animals. They belong to four taxonomic classes: Reptilia (6 species), Insects (3), Mammalia (2) and Amphibia (1). However, the interviewee has used only two animals since he arrived in Diadema, the other ten animals fell into disuse because they are not available in this city. The two animals were collected, identified and deposited in the Museum of Zoology-USP: ant (*Atta sexdens* L.) and cockroach (*Periplaneta americana* L.). These species belong to the maintenance of use category (highlighted with □ in Table 2). The other ten species therefore belong to the discontinued use category (highlighted with ○ in Table 2) which could not be collected. Their identifications were made by PE2 through consulting images from books (as described in Methodology). For three animals (snake, alligator and giant water bug) PE2 could only hesitantly confirm their identity, probably due to the great diversity of these animals in Brazil. Therefore, they are denoted in Table 2 as probably belonging to one of three possible genera. The animals were used in 14 different medicinal formulas, with the skin most commonly used (33.3%), followed by whole animal (20.0%), bone (13.4%), fat (6.7%), rattle (6.7%), tooth (6.7%), anthill (6.7%) and turtleshell (6.7%). Some studies conducted in Brazil show that concomitant data corroborate and sustain these uses (Alves, 2009; Costa-Neto, 2005; Ferreira et al., 2009; Santos-Fita & Costa-Neto, 2007; Torres et al., 2009). The formulas were cited for the treatment of nine complaints, which were grouped into six functional categories, as shown in Table 5. The most commonly cited formula was powder (66.7%), followed by in natura (20%). The most frequent route of administration was ingestion (78.6%). The most common complaint involved respiratory problems (58.4%; 7 animals) followed by central nervous system (8.3%), inflammatory processes (8.3%),

Scientific name or only genus (family/class) Voucher	Popular name dynamic of use	Complaint (part used) - formula - route of administration
Abedus sp., *Belostoma* sp. or *Diplonychus* sp. (Belostomatidae/Insecta)*	Water cockroach (barata d'água)°	Bronchitis and asthma (whole animal) - powder - ingested
Atta sexdens L. (Formicidae/Insecta) Garcia 001	Ant (formiga) ϒ	Epilepsy (anthill) - in natura - ingested
Chironius sp., *Liophs* sp. (Colubridae/Reptilia)* or *Bothops* sp. (Viperidae/Reptilia)*	Snake (cobra)°	Bronchitis (skin) - powder - ingested
Crocodilus sp., *Cayman* sp. or *Paleosuchus* sp. (Alligatoridae/Reptilia)*	Alligator (jacaré)°	Apoplexy (skin) - syrup of skin powder - ingested Bronchitis (bone) - powder - ingested
Crotalus cf. *durissus* L. (Viperidae/Reptilia)*	Rattlesnake (cascavel)°	Back pain (fat) - in natura - ingested Bronchitis (rattle) - tie it in the neck - topic Heart problems (tooth) - put it in the pocket of shirt
Geochelone sp. (Testudinidae/Reptilia)*	Turtle (tartaruga)°	Bronchitis and asthma - (turtleshell) - powder - ingested
Hydrochoerus cf. *hydrochaeris* L. (Hydrochaeridae/ Mammalia)*	Capybara (capivara)°	Bronchitis and asthma - (skin) - powder - ingested
Iguana cf. *iguana* L. (Iguanidae/Reptilia)*	Iguana (iguana)°	Osteoporosis and rheumatism (bone) - powder - ingested
Periplaneta americana L. (Blattidae/Insecta) Garcia 002	Cockroach (barata) ϒ	Bronchitis and asthma (whole animal) - powder - ingested
Placosoma sp. (Gymnophthalmidae/Reptilia)*	Lizard (calango)°	Wounds in the body (skin) - powder - ingested
Rhinella sp. (Bufonidae/ Amphibia)*	Cururu frog (sapocururu)°	Cancer of skin (whole animal) - in natura: tie it on the cancer for some time each day - topic
Tolypeutes sp. (Dasypodidae/Mammalia)*	Armadillo-ball (tatubola)°	Wounds in the body (skin) - powder - ingested

Marked by (ϒ) the two animals whose use had been maintained, while 10, marked by (°) are those whose uses have fallen into disuse. * Animals that couldn't be collected because were not available in Diadema.

Table 2. The 12 animals indicated by migrant PE2, their popular and scientific names, complaints (part used), formula and route of administration (adapted of Garcia et al., 2010).

Category of use	Complaints (number of plants cited)	Total number of plants
1- Gastrointestinal disturbances	To combat worms (1), ulcer (1), diarrhoea (1), bellyache (2), heartburn (1), intestinal infections (1), liver pain (3), to improve digestion (1), hemorrhoid (1), as laxative (10) and for stomach purify (2)	24
2- Inflammatory processes	As anti-inflammatory (3) and healing (6), to treat sty/conjunctivitis (2), inflammation in the mouth/throat (3), rheumatism (2), sinusitis (2) and gingivitis (1)	19
3- Respiratory problems	To combat cough (1), bronchitis (15) and as expectorant (2)	18
4- Anxiolytic/ hypnotics	As sedative (11)	11
5-Osteomuscular problems	To ease back pain (1), muscles pain (6), hip pain (1), prevent osteoporosis (1) and to treat lesions in bone (1)	10
6- Dermatological problems	To combat external allergies (2), wounds in the body (5) and inhibits the growth of skin stains (1)	8
7- Genitourinary disturbances	As diuretic (5), to combat kidney stone (2) and treating urine with blood (1)	8
8- Endocrine system	To reduce cholesterol (1) and diabetes (3)	4
9- Cardiovascular problems	Treat heart problems (1) and as blood purifier (2)	3
10- Immunological problems	To combat breast cancer (1) and stomach cancer (1)	2
11- Analgesics	Earache (2)	2
12- Fever	To combat fever (1)	1
Total		110*

*Some plants have been cited for more than one complaint, so the total number of plants above (110) is higher than the ones indicated by the interviewees.

Table 3. The 12 categories of use comprising the 41 complaints, their total and partial number of plants cited by the five migrants (adapted of Garcia et al., 2010).

dermatological problems (8.3%), analgesics (8.3%), cardiovascular problems (8.3%) as shown in Table 5. The high humidity of the region (with annual rainfall between 1.000 and 1750 mm) (IBAMA, 2011) is known to lead to bronchitis, cough and asthma. This may explain why so many plants and animals were used to treat respiratory disturbances in Diadema, which has been shown in studies of the Sistema Único de Saúde (2011) to be the second largest cause of death in Diadema - 14,4%. Many animals have been used for medical purposes since antiquity (Antonio, 1994; Conconi & Pino, 1988; Gudger, 1925; Weiss, 1947). Despite the existence of several ethnopharmacological studies suggesting the bioactive potential of Brazilian fauna (Alves & Delima, 2006; Alves & Dias, 2010; Alves & Rosa, 2005; Costa-Neto, 2002, 2006; Hanazaki et al., 2009; Rodrigues, 2006), only marine animals have been investigated by chemical and pharmacological methods (Berllink et al., 2004; Gray, 2006; Kossuga, 2009). No pharmacological data was found in the literature for the five animals identified in the present study: rattlesnake (*Crotalus* cf. *durissus* L.), capybara (*Hydrochoerus* cf. *hydrochaeris* L.), iguana (*Iguana* cf. *iguana* L.), ant (*Atta sexdens*) and cockroach (*Periplaneta americana*). The lack of information available on medicinal animal products leads us to conclude that this is a largely unexplored topic in Brazil and that future pharmacological studies should confirm the potential therapeutic value of these species.

SN	Category of use	Plant specimen	% All Species	Use citation	% All use citation	Fic
1	Gastrointestinal disturbances	24	30.77	44	25.29	0.46
2	Inflammatory processes	19	24.36	28	16.09	0.33
3	Respiratory problems	18	23.07	31	17.82	0.43
4	Anxiolytic/hypnotics	11	14.10	19	10.92	0.44
5	Osteomuscular problems	10	12.82	13	7.47	0.25
6	Dermatological problems	8	10.26	11	6.32	0.3
7	Genitourinary disturbances	8	10.26	13	7.47	0.41
8	Endocrine system	4	5.13	5	2.87	0.25
9	Immunological problems	2	2.56	4	2.30	0.66
10	Cardiovascular problems	3	3.84	3	1.72	0
11	Analgesics	2	2.56	2	1.15	0
12	Fever	1	1.28	1	0.57	0

Table 4. Values of Informant consensus factor (Fic) for each category of use, considering the plants cited by the five Diadema's migrants (adapted of Garcia et al., 2010).

Category of use	Complaints (number of animals)
1-Respiratory problems	bronchitis (7), asthma (4)
2-Central nervous system	epilepsy (1)
3-Inflammatory processes	rheumatism (1)
4-Dermatological problems	wounds in the body (1), skin cancer (1)
5-Analgesics	back pain (1)
6-Cardiovascular problems	treat heart problems (1), hemorrhage (1)
Total	18*

* some animals have been cited for more than one complaint, so their total number above (18) is higher than the number of animals indicated: 12.

Table 5. The 6 categories of use comprising the 9 complaints, their respective number of animals mentioned by the migrant PE2 (adapted of Garcia et al., 2010).

5. Conclusion

The ethnobotanical/ethnopharmacological survey among migrants becomes important in that it rescues the knowledge and values that are rapidly disappearing with the death of older migrants and destruction of biomes around the world (Ososki et al. 2007; Reyes-Garcia et al. 2005).

The studies that rescue a large number of uses for different categories (for exemple: gastrointestinal disorders, inflammation, fever and others), can expand several lines of pharmacological and phytochemical investigations. In addition, it may be more important for the development of new drugs with large pharmacological/phytochemicals effects and safer, as well some therapeutic uses mentioned by the migrants were confirmed by previous studies in the literature.

The study of case in Diadema (São Paulo – Brazil) the migrant interviewees demonstrated a large knowledge about the toxic and medicinal properties of some plants and animals. Migration contributed to increase of knowledge regarding the use of natural resources, mainly through the processes of incorporation and/or resource replacement.

The seven plants [*Impatiens hawkeri* W. Bull., *Artemisia canphorata* Vill., *Zea mays* L., *Equisetum arvensis* L., *Senna pendula* (Humb. & Bonpl. ex Willd.) H.S. Irwin & Barneby, *Fevillea passiflora* Vell. and *Croton fuscescens* Spreng] showed maintenance of use among migrants and have not been studied by pharmacologists yet. These species should be highlighted in further investigations because the maintenance of use during human migrations can be indicative of bioactive potential.

The interviewed migrants had passed through several Brazilian cities and were exposed to distinct vegetation and cultures. In this migration, they have passed on and incorporated knowledge in an intensive exchange where formulas and uses are mixed and re-invented as a result of contact between cultures.

This chapter is an attempt to demonstrate based on some scientific papers, the importance of the field (ethnobotanical/ethnopharmacological) in search of new bioactive molecules and how the information about the use of natural resources for health promotion may be more diverse and enriched when human groups displace among regions. We hope this text can assist as a basis for future multidisciplinary research to development new drugs.

6. Acknowledgment

We thank the interviewees for their hospitality, help, and mainly for providing us with information for the purpose of this study in the city of Diadema – São Paulo - Brazil. We are grateful to Julino Assunção Rodrigues Soares Neto and Valéria Basti. We also appreciate the help of FAPESP (Fundação de Amparo à Pesquisa do Estado de São Paulo), FIC (Faculdade Integral Cantareira), AFIP (Associação Fundo de Incentivo à Psicofarmacologia), FUNDUNESP (Fundação para o Desenvolvimento da UNESP) and Herbário Municipal de São Paulo (PMSP), which provided financial support which made this research possible. We thank Dr. Lúcia Rossi and Prof. Dr. Hussam El Dine Zaher, for conducting the botanical and animal identification, respectively. Finally, we really like to thank Prof. Eliana Rodrigues and Prof. Marcus Vinicius Domingues for their participation and orientation.

7. References

Abreu, I.C.; Marinho, A.S.; Paes, A.M.; Freire, S.M.; Olea, R.S.; Borges, M.O. & Borges, A.C. (2003). Hypotensive and vasorelaxant effects of ethanolic extract from Jatropha gossypiifolia L. in rats. *Fitoterapia*, vol.74, pp.650-657.

Adebajo, A.C.; Olawode, E.O.; Omobuwajo, O.R.; Adesanya, S.A.; Begrow, F.; Elkhawad, A.; Akanmu, M.A.; Edrada, R.; Proksch, P.; Klaes, M. & Verspohl, E.J. (2007). Hypoglycaemic constituents of Stachytarpheta cayennensis leaf. *Planta Med*, vol. 7, pp. 3241-3250.

Adeneye, A.A. & Agbaje, E.O. (2007). Hypoglycemic and hypolipidemic effects of fresh leaf aqueous extract of Cymbopogon citratus Stapf. in rats. *J Ethnopharmacol*, vol. 25, pp.440-444.

Adeyemi, O.O.; Yemitan, O.K. & Afolabi, L. (2008). Inhibition of chemically induced inflammation and pain by orally and topically administered leaf extract of Manihot esculenta Crantz in rodents. *J Ethnopharmacol*, vol. 2, pp. 6-11.

Agbor, G.A.; Vinson, J.A.; Oben, J.E. & Ngogang, J.Y. (2007). In vitro antioxidant activity of three Piper species. *J Herb Pharmacother*, vol. 7, pp. 49-64.

Ahmed, F.; Islam, M.A. & Rahman, M.M. (2006). Antibacterial activity of Leonurus sibiricus aerial parts. *Fitoterapia*, vol. 77, pp.316-317.

Akinpelu, D.A. (2000). Antimicrobial activity of Bryophyllum pinnatum leaves. *Fitoterapia*, vol. 71, pp.193-194.

Alcorn, J.B. (1995). The scope and aims of ethnobotany in a developing world. In: R.E. Schultes & S.V. Reis (eds.). Ethnobotany: evolution of a discipline. Timber Press, Cambridge, pp. 23-39.

Almeida, C. & Albuquerque, U.P. (2002). Uso e conservação de plantas e animais medicinais no estado de Pernambuco (nordeste do Brasil): um estudo de caso. *Interciencia*, vol. 27 pp.276-285.

Alves, R.R.N. (2009). Fauna used in popular medicine in Northeast Brazil. *J Ethnobiol Ethnomed*, vol. 5.

Alves, R.R.N. & Delima, Y.C.C. (2006). Snakes used in ethnomedicine in northeast Brazil environment, development and sustainability. *CAB Abstr Lite*, vol.9, pp.455-464.

Alves, R.R.N. & Dias, T.L.P. (2010). Usos de invertebrados na medicina popular no Brasil e suas implicações para conservação. *Tropical Conservation Science*, vol. 2, pp.159-174.

Alves, R.R.N. & Rosa, I.L. (2005). Why study the use of animal products in traditional medicines? *J Ethnobiol Ethnomed*, vol. 30, pp.1-5.

Anas, K. Jayasree, P.R.; Vijayakumar, T. & Manish Kumar, P.R. (2008). In vitro antibacterial activity of Psidium guajava Linn. leaf extract on clinical isolates of multidrug resistant Staphylococcus aureus. *Indian J Exp Biol*, vol.46, pp.41-46.

Andrighetti-Fröhner, C.R.; Sincero, T.C.; da Silva, A.C.; Savi, L.A.; Gaido, C.M.; Bettega, J.M.; Mancini, M.; de Almeida, M.T.; Barbosa, R.A.; Farias, M.R.; Barardi, C.R. & Simões, C.M. (2005). Antiviral evaluation of plants from Brazilian Atlantic Tropical Forest. *Fitoterapia*, vol.76, pp.374-378.

Antonio, J.M.; Gracioso, J.S.; Toma, W.; Lopez, L.C.; Oliveira, F. & Brito, A.R. (2004). Antiulcerogenic activity of ethanol extract of Solanum variabile (false "jurubeba"). *J Ethnopharmacol*, vol.93, pp.83-88.

Antonio, T.M.F. (1994). Insects as remedies for illnesses in Zaire. *The Food Insects Newsletter*, vol.7, pp. 4-5.

Anuar, N.S.; Zahari, S.S.; Taib, I.A. & Rahman, M.T. (2008). Effect of green and ripe
    Caricapapaya epicarp extracts on wound healing and during pregnancy. *Food Chem
    Toxicol*, vol.46, pp.2384-2389.
Araújo, V.T.; Diogo, D.C.; da Silva, M.A.P.; Riggio, L.M.T.; Lapa, A.J. & Souccar, C. (1999).
    Evaluation of the antiurolithiatic activity of the extract of Costus spiralis Roscoe in
    rats. *J Ethnopharmacol*, vol.66, pp.193-198.
Aridoğan, B.C.; Baydar, H.; Kaya, S.; Demirci, M.; Ozbaşar, D. & Mumcu, E. (2002).
    Antimicrobial activity and chemical composition of some essential oils. *Arch Pharm
    Res*, vol.25, pp.860-864.
Atlas de Desenvolvimento Humano/PNUD, 2011, Avaiable from:
    <http://www.pnud.org.br/atlas/>.
Bakirel, T.; Bakirel, U.; Keles, O.U.; Ulgen, S.G. & Yardibi, H. (2008). In vivo assessment of
    antidiabetic and antioxidant activities of rosemary (Rosmarinus officinalis) in
    alloxan-diabetic rabbits. *J Ethnopharmacol*, vol. 28, pp.64-73.
Balick, M. J. (1990). Ethnobotany and the identification of therapeutic agents from the
    rainforest. In: CIBA Foundation Symposium on Bioactive Compounds from Plants.
    Bangkok: CIBA, pp. 22-39,
Balick, M.J. & Cox, P.A. (1997). Plants, people and culture. New York: Scientific American
    Library.
Bani, S.; Kaul, A.; Khan, B.; Gupta, V.K.; Satti, N.K.; Suri, K.A. & Qazi, G.N. (2007). Anti-
    arthritic activity of a biopolymeric fraction from Euphorbia tirucalli. *J
    Ethnopharmacol*, vol.1, pp.92-98.
Begossi, A.; Leitão-Filho, H.F. & Richerson, P.J. (1993). Plant uses a Brazilian coastal fishing
    community (Búzios Island). *J Ethnobiol Ethnomed*, vol.13, pp.233-256.
Belliard, J.C. & Ramirez-Jhonson, J. (2005). Medical pluralism in the life of Mexican
    immigrant woman. *Hispanic Journal of Behavioral Science*, vol. 27, pp.267-285.
Berlink, R.G.S.; Hajdu, E.; Rocha, R.M.; Oliveira, J.H.L.L.; Hernandez, I.L.C.; Seleghim,
    M.H.R.; Granato, A.C.; Almeida, E.V.R.; Nunnez, C.V.; Muricy, G.; Peixinho, S.;
    Pessoa, C.; Moraes, M.O.; Cavalcanti B.C.; Nascimento, G.G.F.; Thiemann. O;H. &
    Silva, M. (2004). Challenges and Rewards of Research in Marine Natural Products
    Chemistry in Brazil. *J Nat Prod*, vol.67, pp.510-522.
Bernard, R.H. (1988). Research methods in cultural anthropology, Sage publications:
    London.
Berson, D.S. (2008). Natural antioxidants. *J Drugs Dermatol*, vol.7, pp.7-12.
Bharat, K. P. & Badola, K.H. (2008). Ethnomedicinal plant use by Lepcha tribe of Dzongu
    valley, bordering Khangchendzonga Biosphere Reserve, in North Sikkim, India.
    Journal of Ethnobiology and Ethnomedicine, vol. 4.
Biavatti, M.W.; Farias, C.; Curtius, F.; Brasil, L.M.; Hort, S.; Schuster, L.; Leite, S.N. & Prado,
    S.R. (2004). Preliminary studies on Campomanesia xanthocarpa (Berg.) and Cuphea
    carthagenensis (Jacq.) J.F. Macbr. aqueous extract: weight   control   and
    biochemical parameters. *J Ethnopharmacol*, vol.93, pp.385-389.
Bodeker, G.C.; Neumann, P.; Lall, Z. & Min, O.O. (2005). Tradicional medicine use and
    health worker training in a refugee setting at the Thai-Burma border. *Journal of
    Refugee Studies*, vol.18, pp. 76-99.

Braga, F.G.; Bouzada, M.L.; Fabri, R.L. de O.; Matos, M.; Moreira, F.O.; Scio, E. & Coimbra, E.S. (2007). Antileishmanial and antifungal activity of plants used in traditional medicine in Brazil. *J Ethnopharmacol*, vol. 4, pp.396-402.

Bravo, E.; Amrani, S. & Aziz, M. (2008). Ocimum basilicum ethanolic extract decreases cholesterol synthesis and lipid accumulation in human macrophages. *Fitoterapia*, vol.79, pp.515-523.

Cáceres, A.; Alvarez, A.V.; Ovando, A.E. & Samayoa, B.E. (1991). Plants used in Guatemala for the treatment of respiratory diseases. Screening of 68 plants against gram-positive bacteria. *J Ethnopharmacol*, vol. 31, pp.193-208.

Cáceres, A.; López, B.; González, S.; Berger, I.; Tada, I. & Maki, J. (1998). Plants used in Guatemala for the treatment of protozoal infections. I. Screening of activity to bacteria, fungi and (protozoário) American trypanosomes of 13 native plants. *J Ethnopharmaco*, vol. 62, pp.195-202.

Camargo, M.T.L. de A. (2000). Trabalhos de Antropologia e Etnologia. vol.15, pp.179-187.

Candan, F.; Unlu, M.; Tepe, B.; Daferera, D.; Polissiou, M.; Sökmen, A. & Akpulat, H.A. (2003). Antioxidant and antimicrobial activity of the essential oil and methanol extracts of Achillea millefolium subsp. millefolium Afan. (Asteraceae). *J Ethnopharmacol*, vol. 87, pp.215-220.

Cano, J.H. & Volpato, G. (2004). Herbal mixtures in the traditional medicine of Eastern Cuba. *J Ethnopharmacol*, vol. 90, pp. 293-316.

Carney, J. A. (2001). African Plants in the Columbian Exchange. *Journal of African History*, vol.42, pp.377-396.

Carney, J. & Voeks, R.A. (2003). Landscape legades of the African Diaspora in Brazil. *Prog Hum Geogr*, pp.27-6.

Carrier, N. (2007). In Pieroni, A., and Vandebroek, I. (eds.), A Strange Drug in a Strange Land. Traveling Plants and Cultures. The Ethnobiology and Ethnopharmacy of Migrations. Berghahn, Oxford, pp. 186–203.

Carvalho, L.H. & Krettli, A.U. (1991). Antimalarial chemotherapy with natural products and chemically defined molecules. *Mem Inst Oswaldo Cruz*, vol. 2, pp.181-184.

Cavalcanti, E.S.; Morais, S.M.; Lima, M.A. & Santana, E.W. (2004). Larvicidal activity of essential oils from Brazilian plants against Aedes aegypti L. *Mem Inst Oswaldo Cruz*, vol. 99, pp.541-544.

Cechinel Filho, V.; Santos, A.R.; De Campos, R.O.; Miguel, O.G.; Yunes, R.A.; Ferrari, F.; Messana, I. & Calixto, J.B. (1996). Chemical and pharmacological studies of Phyllanthus caroliniensis in mice. *J Pharm Pharmacol*, vol. 48, pp.1231-1236.

Cetin, H.; Cinbilgel, I.; Yanikoglu, A. & Gokceoglu, M. (2006). Larvicidal activity of some Labiatae (Lamiaceae) plant extracts from Turkey. *Phytother Res*, vol. 20, pp.1088-1090.

Ceuterick, M.; Vandebroek, I.; Torry, B. & Pieroni, A. (2007). The use of home remedies for health care and well-being by Spanish-speaking latino immigrants in London: a reflection on acculturation, pp.145-165.

Ceuterick, M.; Vandebroek, I.; Torry, B. & Pieroni, A. (2008). Cross-cultural adaptation in urban ethnobotany: the Colombian folk pharmacopoeia in London. *J Ethnopharmacol*, vol.120, pp.342-359.

The Influence of Displacement by Human Groups Among Regionsin the Medicinal Use of Natural Resource:
A Case Study in Diadema, São Paulo - Brazil

29

Chah, K.F.; Eze, C.A.; Emuelosi, C.E. & Esimone, C.O. (2006). Antibacterial and wound healing properties of methanolic extracts of some Nigerian medicinal plants. J Ethnopharmacol, vol. 8, pp.164-167.

Chang, C.L.; Kuo, H.K.; Chang, S.L.; Chiang, Y.M.; Lee, T.H.; Wu, W.M.; Shyur, L.F. & Yang, W.C. (2005). The distinct effects of a butanol fraction of Bidens pilosa plant extract on the development of Th1-mediated diabetes and Th2-mediated airway inflammation in mice. J Biomed Sci, vol.12, pp.79-89.

Cheruiyot, K.R.; Olila, D. & Kateregga, J. (2009). In-vitro antibacterial activity of selected medicinal plants from Longisa region of Bomet district, Kenya. Afr Health Sci, vol.1, pp.42-46.

Chiasson, H.; Bélanger, A.; Bostanian, N.; Vincent, C. & Poliquin, A. (2001). Acaricidal properties of Artemisia absinthium and Tanacetum vulgare (Asteraceae) essential oils obtained by three methods of extraction. J Econ Entomol, vol.94, pp.167-171.

Chiasson, H.; Bostanian, N.J. & Vincent, C. (2004). Insecticidal properties of a Chenopodium-based botanical. J Econ Entomol, vol.97, pp.1373-1377.

Choi, E.M. & Hwang, J.K. (2004). Antiinflammatory, analgesic and antioxidant activities of the fruit of Foeniculum vulgare. Fitoterapia, vol.75, pp.557-565.

Conconi, J.R. & Pino, J.M. (1988). The utilization of insects in the empirical medicine of ancient Mexicans. J Ethnobiol Ethnomed, vol.8, pp.195-202.

Consolini, A.E.; Ragone, M.I.; Migliori, G.N.; Conforti, P. & Volonté, M.G. (2006). Cardiotonic and sedative effects of Cecropia pachystachya Mart. (ambay) on isolated rat hearts and conscious mice. J Ethnopharmacol, vol.15, pp.90-96.

Costa-Neto, E.M. (2002). The use of insects in folk medicine in the state of Bahia, northeastern Brazil, with notes on insects reported elsewhere in Brazilian folk medicine. Hum Ecol, vol. 30, pp.245-263.

Costa-Neto, E.M. (2005). Animal-based medicines: biological prospection and the sustainable use of zootherapeutic resources. Annals of the Brazilian Academy of Sciences, vol. 77, pp.33-43.

Costa-Neto, E.M. (2006). Os moluscos na zooterapia: medicina tradicional e importância clínico-farmacológica. Biotemas, vol. 19, pp.71-78.

Da Silva Filho, A.A.; de Sousa, J.P.; Soares, S.; Furtado, N.A.; Andrade e Silva, M.L.; Cunha, W.R.; Gregório, L.E.; Nanayakkara, N.P. & Bastos, J.K. (2008). Antimicrobial activity of the extract and isolated compounds from Baccharis dracunculifolia D. C. (Asteraceae). Z Naturforsch C J Biosci, vol. 63, pp.40-46.

Das, N.G.; Baruah, I.; Talukdar, P.K. & Das, S.C. (2003). Evaluation of botanicals as repellents against mosquitoes. J Vector Borne Dis, vol.40, pp.49-53.

Davis, E.W. (1995). Ethnobotany: an old practice, a new discipline. In: Schultes, R.E. & von Reis, S. (eds.). Ethnobotany: evolution of a discipline. Dioscorides Press, Portland.

De Almeida Barbosa, L.C.; de Alvarenga, E.S.; Demuner, A.J.; Virtuoso, L.S. & Silva, A.A. (2006). Synthesis of new phytogrowth-inhibitory substituted aryl-pbenzoquinones. Chem Biodivers, vol.3, pp.553-567.

De Almeida, I.; Alviano, D.S.; Vieira, D.P.; Alves, P.B.; Blank, A.F.; Lopes, A.H.; Alviano, C.S. & Rosa, M.S. (2007). Antigiardial activity of Ocimum basilicum essential oil. Parasitol Res, vol. 101, pp.443-452.

De Araújo, P.F.; Coelho-de-Souza, A.N.; Morais, S.M.; Ferreira, S.C. & Leal-Cardoso, J.H. (2005). Antinociceptive effects of the essential oil of Alpinia zerumbet on mice. *Phytomedicine*, vol.12, pp.482-486.

De Freitas, T.G.; Augusto, P.M. & Montanari, T. (2005). Effect of Ruta graveolens L. on pregnant mice. *Contraception*, vol.71, pp.74-77.

De Lima, M.R.; de Souza Luna, J.; dos Santos, A.F.; de Andrade, M.C.; Sant'Ana, A.E.; Genet, J.P.; Marquez, B.; Neuville, L. & Moreau, N. (2006). Anti-bacterial activity of some Brazilian medicinal plants. *J Ethnopharmacol*, vol.21, pp.137-147.

De Moura, R.S.; Emiliano, A.F.; de Carvalho, L.C.; Souza, M.A.; Guedes, D.C.; Tano, T. & Resende, A.C. (2005). Antihypertensive and endothelium-dependent vasodilator effects of Alpinia zerumbet, a medicinal plant. *J Cardiovasc Pharmacol*, vol. 46, pp. 288-294.

Dhalwal, K.; Deshpazde, Y.S. & Purohit, A.P. (2007). Evaluation of in vitro antioxidant activity of Sida rhombifolia (L.) ssp. retusa (L.). *J Med Food*, vol.10, pp.683-688

Di Stasi, L.C.; Oliveira, G.P.; Carvalhares, M.A.; Queiroz-Junior, M.; Tien, O.S.; Kakinami, S.H.; & Reis, M.S. (2002). Medicinal plants popularly used in the Brazilian Tropical Atlantic Forest. *Fitoterapia*, vol. 73, pp.69-91.

Díaz, J.L. (1977). Ethnopharmacology of sacred psychoactive plants used by the Indians of Mexico. *Pharmacol Toxicol*, vol.17, pp.647-675.

Dickel, M.L.; Rates, S.M. & Ritter, M.R. (2007). Plants popularly used for loosing weight purposes in Porto Alegre, South Brazil. *J Ethnopharmacol*, vol. 3, pp.60-71.

Dimo, T.; Nguelefack, T.B.; Kamtchouing, P.; Dongo, E.; Rakotonirina, A. & Rakotonirina, S.V. (1999). Hypotensive effects of a methanol extract of Bidens pilosa Linn on hypertensive rats. *C R Acad Sci Gen*, vol. 322, pp.323-329.

Emeruwa, A.C. (1982). Antibacterial substance from Carica papaya fruit extract. *J Nat Prod*, vol. 45, pp.123-127.

FAPESP (2011). Avaiable from: <http://agencia.fapesp.br/14176>.

Ferreira, F.S.; Brito, S.V.; Ribeiro, S.C; Saraiva, A.A.F.; Almeida, W.O. & Alves, R.R.N. (2009). Animal-based folk remedies sold in public markets in Crato and Juazeiro do Norte, Ceará, Brazil. *BMC Complement Altern Med*, vol. 9.

Findley, S. E, De Jong G.F. (1985). Community and family factors influencing family migration in Ilocos Norte. *Philippine Population Journal*, vol.1 pp.18-44.

Freitas, M.A. & Silva, T.F.S. (2005). A herpetofauna da Mata Atlântica nordestina. USEB, Pelotas.

Freitas, M.A. & Silva, T.F.S. (2007). A herpetofauna das caatingas e áreas de altitudes do nordeste Brasileiro. USEB, Pelotas.

Frutuoso, V.S.; Gurjão, M.R.; Cordeiro, R.S. & Martins, M.A. (1994). Analgesic and antiulcerogenic effects of a polar extract from leaves of Vernonia condensata. *Planta Med*, vol. 60, pp. 21-25.

Fu, Y.; Zu, Y.; Chen, L.; Efferth, T.; Liang, H.; Liu, Z. & Liu, W. (2007). Investigation of antibacterial activity of rosemary essential oil against Propionibacterium acnes with atomic force microscopy. *Planta Med*, vol.73, pp.1275-1280.

Fukuda, M.; Ohkoshi, E.; Makino, M. & Fujimoto, Y. (2006). Studies on the constituents of the leaves of Baccharis dracunculifolia (Asteraceae) and their cytotoxic activity. *Chem Pharm Bull*, vol. 54, pp.1465-1468.

Fundação Cultural Palmares (2011). Avaiable from: <http://palmares.gov.br/>.

The Influence of Displacement by Human Groups Among Regionsin the Medicinal Use of Natural Resource:
A Case Study in Diadema, São Paulo - Brazil

31

Gandhi, M.; Lal, R.; Sankaranarayanan, A. & Sharma, P.L. (1991). Post-coital antifertility action of Ruta graveolens in female rats and hamsters. *J Ethnopharmacol,* vol.34, pp.49-59.

Garcia, D.; Domingues, M.V. & Rodrigues, E. (2010). Ethnopharmacological survey among migrants living in the Southeast Atlantic Forest of Diadema, São Paulo, Brazil. *J Ethnobiol Ethnomed,* vol. 6, pp. 29-48.

Gbeassor, M.; Kossou, Y.; Amegbo, K.; de Souza, C.; Koumaglo, K. & Denke, A. (1989). Antimalarial effects of eight African medicinal plants. *J Ethnopharmacol,* vol.25, pp.115-118.

Gené, R.M.; Cartaña, C.; Adzet, T.; Marín, E.; Parella, T. & Cañigueral, S. (1996). Antiinflammatory and analgesic activity of Baccharis trimera: identification of its active constituents. *Planta Med,* vol. 62, pp.232-235.

Gillij, Y.G.; Gleiser, R.M. & Zygadlo, J.A. (2008). Mosquito repellent activity of essential oils of aromatic plants growing in Argentina. *Bioresour Technol,* vol.99, pp.2507-2415.

Giorgetti, M.; Negri, G. & Rodrigues, E. (2007). Brazilian plants with possible action on the central nervous system—A study of historical sources from the 16th to 19th century. *Journal of Ethnopharmacology,* vol.109, pp.338–347.

Giulietti, A.M.; Harley, R.M.; Queiroz, L.P. de.; Wanderley, M. das G. & van den Berg, C. (2005). Biodiversidade e conservação das plantas no Brasil. *Megadiversidade,* vol.1, pp. 52-61.

González-Trujano, M.E.; Peña, E.I.; Martínez, A.L.; Moreno, J.; Guevara-Fefer, P.; Déciga-Campos, M. & López-Muñoz, F.J. (2007). Evaluation of the antinociceptive effect of Rosmarinus officinalis L. using three different experimental models in rodents. *J Ethnopharmacol,* vol. 22, pp.476-482.

Gopalakrishnan, M. & Rajasekharasetty, M.R. (1978). Effect of papaya (Carica papaya Linn) on pregnancy and estrous cycle in albino rats of Wistar strain. *Indian J Physiol Pharmacol,* vol.22, pp.66-70.

Gray, A.M. & Flatt, P.R. (1998). Antihyperglycemic actions of Eucalyptus globulus (Eucalyptus) are associated with pancreatic and extra-pancreatic effects in mice. *J Nutr,* vol.128, pp.2319-2323.

Gray, C.A.; Lira, S.P.; Silva, M.; Pimenta, E.F.; Thiemann, O.H.; Oliva, A.G.; Hajdu, E.; Andersen, R.J. & Berlink, R.G.S. (2006). Sulfated Meroterpenoids from the Brazilian Sponge Callyspongia sp. are Inhibitors of the Antileishmaniasis Target Adenosine Phosphoribosyl Transferase. *J Org Chem,* vol. 71, pp.8685-8690.

Gudger, E.W. (1925). Stitching wounds with the mandibles of ants and beetles. *J Am Med Assoc,* vol. 84, pp.1861-1864.

Han, G. S. & Ballis, H. (2007). Ethnomedicine and dominant medicine in multicultural Australia: a critical realist reflection on the case of Korean-Australian immigrants in Sydney. *Journal of Ethnobiology and Ethnomedicine,* vol. 3.

Hanazaki, N.; Alves, R.R.N. & Begossi, A. (2009). Hunting and use of terrestrial fauna used by Caiçaras from the Atlantic Forest coast (Brazil). *J Ethnobiol Ethnomed,* vol. 5, pp. 5-36.

Heinrich, M. (2000). Ethnobotany and its role in drug development. *Phytother Res,* vol.14, pp.479-488.

Holetz, F.B.; Pessini, G.L.; Sanches, N.R.; Cortez, D.A.; Nakamura, C.V. & Filho, B.P. (2002). Screening of some plants used in the Brazilian folk medicine for the treatment of infectious diseases. *Mem Inst Oswaldo Cruz*, vol.97, pp.1027-1031.

IBAMA (2011). Avaiable from: <http://ibama.gov.br/ecossistemas/mata_atlantica.htm>.

IBGE (2011). Avaiable from: <http://www.ibge.gov.br/home/>.

Instituto Socioambiental (2011). Avaiable from: <http://www.socioambiental.org/>.

Islam, M.A.; Ahmed, F.; Das, A.K. & Bachar, S.C. (2005). Analgesic and anti-inflammatory activity of Leonurus sibiricus. *Fitoterapia*, vol.76, pp.359-362.

Islam, M.E.; Haque, M.E. & Mosaddik, M.A. (2003): Cytotoxicity and antibacterial activity of Sida rhombifolia (Malvaceae) grown in Bangladesh. *Phytother Res*, vol. 17, pp. 973-975.

Ivanova, A.; Mikhova, B.; Najdenski, H.; Tsvetkova, I. & Kostova, I. (2005). Antimicrobial and cytotoxic activity of Ruta graveolens. *Fitoterapia*, vol. 3, pp.344-347.

Iwalewa, E.O.; Adewunmi, C.O.; Omisore, N.O.; Adebanji, O.A.; Azike, C.K.; Adigun, A.O.; Adesina, O.A. & Olowoyo, O.G. (2005). Pro- and antioxidant effects and cytoprotective potentials of nine edible vegetables in southwest Nigeria. *J Med Food*, vol. 8, pp.539-544.

Janes, C. R. & Pawson, I.G. (1986). Migration and biocultural adaptation: Samoans in California. *Social Science & Medicine*, vol. 22, pp. 821-834.

Januário, A.H.; Santos, S.L.; Marcussi, S.; Mazzi, M.V.; Pietro, R.C.; Sato, D.N.; Ellena, J.; Sampaio, S.V.; França, S.C. & Soares, A.M. (2004). Neo-clerodane diterpenoid, a new metalloprotease snake venom inhibitor from Baccharis trimera (Asteraceae): anti-proteolytic and anti-hemorrhagic properties. *Chem Biol Interact*, vol.7, pp.243-251.

Ka, M.H.; Choi, E.H.; Chun, H.S. & Lee, K.G. (2005). Antioxidative activity of volatile extracts isolated from Angelica tenuissimae roots, peppermint leaves, pine needles, and sweet flag leaves. *J Agric Food Chem*, vol. 18, pp.4124-4129.

Khori, V.; Nayebpour, M.; Semnani, S.; Golalipour, M.J. & Marjani, A. (2008). Prolongation of AV nodal refractoriness by Ruta graveolens in isolated rat hearts. Potential role as an anti-arrhythmic agent. *Saudi Med J*, vol.29, pp.357-363.

Kim, S.; Kubec, R. & Musah, R.A. (2006). Antibacterial and antifungal activity of sulfurcontaining compounds from Petiveria alliacea L. *J Ethnopharmacol*, vol. 8, pp.188-192.

Klopell, F.C.; Lemos, M.; Sousa, J.P.; Comunello, E.; Maistro, E.L.; Bastos, J.K. & de Andrade, S.F. (2007). Nerolidol, an antiulcer constituent from the essential oil of Baccharis dracunculifolia DC (Asteraceae). *Z Naturforsch C J Biosci*, vol. 62 pp.537-542.

Kordali, S.; Kotan, R.; Mavi, A.; Cakir, A.; Ala, A. & Yildirim, A. (2005). Determination of the chemical composition and antioxidant activity of the essential oil of Artemisia dracunculus and of the antifungal and antibacterial activities of Turkish Artemisia absinthium, A. dracunculus, A. santonicum, and A. spicigera essential oils. *J Agric Food Chem*, vol. 30, pp.9452-9458.

Kossuga, M.H.; Lira, S.P.; Mchugh, S.; Torres, Y.R.; Lima, B.A.; Veloso, K.; Ferreira Antonio, G.; Rocha, R.M. & Berlink, R.G.S. (2009). Antibacterial Modified Diketopiperazines from two Ascidians of the Genus Didemnum. *J Braz Chem Soc*, vol. 20, pp.704-711.

Kumar, R.; Mishra, A.K.; Dubey, N.K. & Tripathi, Y.B. (2007). Evaluation of Chenopodium ambrosioides oil as a potential source of antifungal, antiaflatoxigenic and antioxidant activity. *Int J Food Microbiol*, vol.10, pp.159-164.

Kupchan, S.M.; Knox, J.R.; Kelsey, J.E. & Saenzrenauld, J.A. (1964). Calotropin, a cytotoxic principle isolated from Asclepias curassavica L. *Science*, vol. 25, pp.1685-1686.

Kury, L. (2001). Viajantes-naturalitas no Brasil oitocentista: experiencia, relato e imagem. *História, Ciência, Saúde-Manguinhos*, vol. 8, pp. 863–880.

Kusamba, C.; Byamana, K. & Mbuyi, W.M. (1991). Antibacterial activity of Mirabilis jalapa seed powder. *J Ethnopharmacol*, vol. 35, pp.197-199.

Kviecinski, M.R.; Felipe, K.B.; Schoenfelder, T.; de Lemos Wiese, L.P.; Rossi, M.H.; Gonçalez, E.; Felicio, J.D.; Filho, D.W. & Pedrosa, R.C. (2008). Study of the antitumor potential of Bidens pilosa (Asteraceae) used in Brazilian folk medicine. *J Ethnopharmacol*, vol.17, pp.69-75.

Lacuna-Richman, C. (2006). The use of non-wood forest products by grants in a new settlement: experiences of a Visayan community in Palawan, Philippines. *Journal of Ethnobiology and Ethnomedicine*, pp. 2:36.

Lans, C. (2007). Ethnomedicines used in Trinidad and Tobago for reproductive problems. *J Ethnobiol Ethnomed*, vol.15, pp.3-13.

Latha, M.; Ramkumar, K.M.; Pari, L.; Damodaran, P.N.; Rajeshkannan, V. & Suresh, T. (2006). Phytochemical and antimicrobial study of an antidiabetic plant: Scoparia dulcis L. *J Med Food*, vol.9, pp. 391-394.

Lee, H.S. (2004). Acaricidal activity of constituents identified in Foeniculum vulgare fruit oil against Dermatophagoides spp. (Acari: Pyroglyphidae). *J Agric Food Chem*, vol.19, pp.2887-2889.

Lee, R.A.; Balick, M.J.; Ling, D.L.; Sohl, F.; Brosi, B.J. & Raynor, W. (2001). Cultural dynamism and change in Micronesia. *Economic Botany*, vol. 55, pp.9-13.

Lin, L.Y.; Peng, C.C.; Yeh, W.T.; Wang, H.E.; Yu, T.H. & Peng, R.Y. (2008). Alpinia zerumbet potentially elevates high- density lipoprotein cholesterol level in hamsters. *J Agric Food Chem*, vol. 25, pp. 4435-4443.

Lipp, F.J. (1989). Methods for ethnopharmacological field work. *J Ethnopharmacol*, vol. 25, pp.139-150.

Lopes-Lutz, D.; Alviano, D.S.; Alviano, C.S. & Kolodziejczyk, P.P. (2008). Screening of chemical composition, antimicrobial and antioxidant activities of Artemisia essential oils. *Phytochemistry*, vol.69, pp.1732-1738.

Lopes-Martins, R.A.; Pegoraro, D.H.; Woisky, R.; Penna, S.C. & Sertié, J.A. (2002). The anti-inflammatory and analgesic effects of a crude extract of Petiveria alliacea L. (Phytolaccaceae). *Phytomedicine*, vol. 9, pp. 245-248.

Lorenzi, H. & Matos, de A. F.J. (2008). Plantas medicinais do Brasil: nativas e exóticas cultivadas. Instituto Plantarum: São Paulo.

Luo, Q.F.; Sun, L.; Si, J.Y.; Chen, D.H. & Du, G.H. (2008). Hypocholesterolemic effect of stilbene extract from Cajanus cajan L. on serum and hepatic lipid in diet-induced hyperlipidemic mice. *Yao Xue Xue Bao*, vol. 43, pp.145-149.

Mahanta, M. & Mukherjee, A.K. (2001). Neutralisation of lethality, myotoxicity and toxic enzymes of Naja kaouthia venom by Mimosa pudica root extracts. *J Ethnopharmacol*, vol.75, pp.55-60.

Maiorano, V.A.; Marcussi, S.; Daher, M.A.; Oliveira, C.Z.; Couto, L.B.; Gomes, O.A.; França, S.C.; Soares, A.M. & Pereira, O.S. (2005). Antiophidian properties of the aqueous extract of Mikania glomerata. *J Ethnopharmacol*, vol. 1, pp. 364-370.

Malpezzi, E.L.; Davino, S.C.; Costa, L.V.; Freitas, J.C.; Giesbrecht, A.M. & Roque, N.F. (1994). Antimitotic action of extracts of Petiveria alliacea on sea urchin egg development. *Braz J Med Biol Res*, vol. 27, pp.749-754.

Manila University Press, Quezon City, Philippines. pp. 38-48.

Ming, L.C. (2006). Levantamento de plantas medicinais na Reserva Extrativista "Chico Mendes". UNESP-Botucatu, pp.160.

Molina, M.; Contreras, C.M. & Tellez-Alcantara, P. (1999). Mimosa pudica may possess antidepressant actions in the rat. *Phytomedicine*, vol. 6, pp.319-323.

Moore, S.J.; Hill, N.; Ruiz, C. & Cameron, M.M. (2007). Field evaluation of traditionally used plant-based insect repellents and fumigants against the malaria vector Anopheles darlingi in Riberalta, Bolivian Amazon. *J Med Entomol*, vol.44, pp.624-630.

Moreira, M.D.; Picanço, M.C.; Barbosa, L.C.; Guedes, R.N.; Barros, E.C. & Campos, M.R. (2007). Compounds from Ageratum conyzoides: isolation, structural elucidation and insecticidal activity. *Pest Manag Sci*, vol.63, pp.615-621.

Moura, A.C.; Silva, E.L.; Fraga, M.C.; Wanderley, A.G.; Afiatpour, P. & Maia, M.B. (2005). Antiinflammatory and chronic toxicity study of the leaves of Ageratum conyzoides L. in rats. *Phytomedicine*, vol.12, pp.138-142.

Nayak, S.; Nalabothu, P.; Sandiford, S.; Bhogadi, V. & Adogwa, A. (2006). Evaluation of wound healing activity of Allamanda cathartica. L. and Laurus nobilis. L. extracts on rats. *BMC Complement Altern Med*, vol.12, pp.138-142.

Nesheim, I.; Dhillion, S.S. & Stolen, K.A. (2006). What happens to traditional knowledge and use of natural resourceswhen people migrate? *Human Ecology*, vol. 34, pp. 99-131.

Ngo Bum, E.; Dawack, D.L.; Schmutz, M.; Rakotonirina, A.; Rakotonirina, S.V.; Portet, C.; Jeker, A.; Olpe, H.R. & Herrling, P. (2004). Anticonvulsant activity of Mimosa pudica decoction. *Fitoterapia*, vol. 75, pp.309-314.

Nguefack, J.; Budde, B.B. & Jakobsen, M. (2004). Five essential oils from aromatic plants of Cameroon: their antibacterial activity and ability to permeabilize the cytoplasmic membrane of Listeria innocua examined by flow cytometry. *Lett Appl Microbiol*, vol. 39, pp.395-400.

Nguyen, M. (2003). Comparison of food plant knowledge between urban Vietnamese living in Vietnam and in Hawai'i. *Economic Botany*, vol.57, pp. 47-80.

Niñez, V. K. (1987). Household gardens: theoretical and policy considerations. *Agricultural Systems*, vol.23, pp.167-186.

Nishino, H.; Hayashi, T.; Arisawa, M.; Satomi, Y. & Iwashima, A. (1993). Antitumorpromoting activity of scopadulcic acid B, isolated from the medicinal plant Scoparia dulcis L. *Oncology*, vol.50, pp.100-103.

Nogueira, J.C.; Diniz, M. de F. & Lima, E.O. (2008). In vitro antimicrobial activity of plants in Acute Otitis Externa. *Braz J Otorhinolaryngo*, vol.74, pp.118-124.

Ntonifor, N.N.; Ngufor, C.A.; Kimbi, H.K. & Oben, B.O. (2006). Traditional use of indigenous mosquito-repellents to protect humans against mosquitoes and other insect bites in a rural community of Cameroon. *East Afr Med J*, vol.83, pp.553-558.

Nusier, M.K.; Bataineh, H.N. & Daradkah, H.M. (2007). Adverse effects of Rosemary (Rosmarinus officinalis L.) on reproductive function in adult male rats. *Exp Biol Med*, vol.232, pp.809-813.

Obaseiki-Ebor, E.E. (1985). Preliminary report on the in vitro antibacterial activity of Bryophyllum pinnatum leaf juice. *Afr J Med Med Sci*, vol.14, pp.199-202.

Ojewole, J.A. (2005). Antinociceptive, anti-inflammatory and antidiabetic effects of Bryophyllum pinnatum (Crassulaceae) leaf aqueous extract. *J Ethnopharmacol*, vol. 13, pp.13-19.

Okada, Y.; Tanaka, K.; Sato, E. & Okajima, H. (2008). Antioxidant activity of the new thiosulfinate derivative, S-benzyl phenylmethanethiosulfinate, from Petiveria alliacea L. *Org Biomol Chem*, vol.21, pp.1097-1102.

Oliva, A.; Meepagala, K.M.; Wedge, D.E.; Harries, D.; Hale, A.L.; Aliotta, G. & Duke, S.O. (2003). Natural fungicides from Ruta graveolens L. leaves, including a new quinolone alkaloid. *J Agri Food Chem*, vol. 12, pp.890-896.

Oliveira, A.C.; Endringer, D.C.; Amorim, L.A.; das Graças, L.; Brandão, M. & Coelho, M.M. (2005). Effect of the extracts and fractions of Baccharis trimera and Syzygium cumini on glycaemia of diabetic and non-diabetic mice. J Ethnopharmacol, vol. 1, pp. 465-169.

Oliveira, R.B.; Godoy, S.A.P. & Costa, F.B. (2003). Plantas Tóxicas: Conhecimento e prevenção de acidentes Holos. São Paulo.

Orsi, R.O.; Sforcin, J.M.; Funari, S.R.; & Bankova, V. (2005). Effects of Brazilian and Bulgarian propolis on bactericidal activity of macrophages against Salmonella typhimurium. *Int Immunopharmacol*, vol. 5, pp.359-368.

Ososki, A.L.; Balick, M.J & Daly, D.C. (2007). Medicinal plants and cultural variation across dominican rural, urban, and transnational landscapes. In. Pieroni, A. & Vandebroek, I. *Traveling cultures and plants: the ethnobiology and ethnopharmacy of human migrations* (Berghahn Books), ISBN-13: 978-1-84545-373-2, New York.

Ozcan, M.M.; Chalchat, J.C.; Arslan, D.; Ates, A. & Unver, A. (2006). Comparative essential oil composition and antifungal effect of bitter fennel (Foeniculum vulgare ssp. piperitum) fruit oils obtained during different vegetation. *J Med Food*, vol.9, pp.552-561.

Padilha de Paula, J.; Gomes-Carneiro, M.R. & Paumgartten, F.J. (2003). Chemical composition, toxicity and mosquito repellency of Ocimum selloi oil. *J Ethnopharmacol*, vol. 88, pp.253-260.

Pal, S. & Nag Chaudhuri, A.K.(1991). Studies on the anti-ulcer activity of a Bryophyllum pinnatum leaf extract in experimental animals. *J Ethnopharmacol*, vol.33, pp. 97-102.

Palmieri MMB: Efeitos sobre o Sistema Nervoso Central de extratos de plantas popularmente citadas como anticonvulsivantes. MsD thesis Universidade Estadual Paulista, Ribeirão Preto; 2000.

Pascual, M.E.; Slowing, K.; Carretero, M.E. & Villar, A. (2001). Antiulcerogenic activity of Lippia alba (Mill.) N. E. Brown (Verbenaceae). *Farmaco*, vol. 56, pp.501-504.

Paulino, N.; Abreu, S.R.; Uto, Y. Koyama, D.; Nagasawa, H.; Hori, H.; Dirsch, V.M.; Vollmar, A.M.; Scremin, A. & Bretz, W.A. (2008). Anti-inflammatory effects of a bioavailable compound, Artepillin C, in Brazilian propolis. *Eur J Pharmacol*, vol.10, pp.296-301.

Pavela, R. (2008). Insecticidal properties of several essential oils on the house fly (Musca domestica L.). *Phytother Res*, vol. 22, pp. 274-278.

Peng, C.H.; Su, J.D.; Chyau, C.C.; Sung, T.Y.; Ho, S.S.; Peng, C.C. & Peng, R.Y. (2007). Supercritical fluid extracts of rosemary leaves exhibit potent antiinflammation and anti-tumor effects. *Biosci Biotechnol Biochem*, vol. 71, pp.2223-2232.

Penido, C.; Costa, K.A.; Futuro, D.O.; Paiva, S.R.; Kaplan, M.A.; Figueiredo, M.R. & Henriques, M.G. (2006). Anti-inflammatory and anti-ulcerogenic properties of Stachytarpheta cayennensis (L.C. Rich) Vahl. *J Ethnopharmacol*, vol. 8, pp.225-233.

Pérez-García, F.; Marín, E.; Cañigueral, S. & Adzet, T. (1996). Anti-inflammatory action of Pluchea sagittalis: involvement   of an antioxidant mechanism. *Life Sci*, vol. 59, pp.2033-2040.

Pieroni, A., Nebel, C., Quave, C.L., Münz, H. & Heinrich, M. (2002a). Ethnopharmacology of Liakra, traditional weedy vegetables of the Arbëreshë of the Vulture área in southern Italy. *J Ethnopharmacol*, vol. 81, pp.165-185.

Pieroni, A.; Quave, C.L.; Nebel, S. & Heinrich, M. (2002b). Ethnopharmacy of ethnic Albanians (Arbëreshë) in northern Basilicata (southern Italy). *Fitoterapia*, vol.73, pp.217-241.

Pieroni, A.; Quave, C.L.; Villanelli, M.L.; Mangino, P.; Sabbatini, G. & Santini, L. (2004). Ethnopharmacognostic survey on the natural ingredients used in folk cosmetics, cosmeceuticals and remedies for healing skin diseases in the   inland   Marches, Central-Eastern Italy. *J Ethnopharmacol*, vol 91, pp. 331-344.

Pieroni, A. & Quave, C.L. (2005a). Traditional pharmacopoeias and medicines among Albanians and Italians in southern Italy: a comparison. *J Ethnopharmacol*, vol.101, pp.258-270.

Pieroni, A.; Münz, H.; Akbulut, M.; Baser, K.H.C. & Durmuskahya, C. (2005b). Traditional phytotherapy and transcultural pharmacy among Turkish immigrants living in Cologne, Germany. *Journal of Ethnopharmacology*, vol.102, pp. 69-88.

Pieroni, A. & Vandebroek, I. (2007). *Traveling cultures and plants: the ethnobiology and ethnopharmacy of human migrations* (Berghahn Books), ISBN-13: 978-1-84545-373-2, New York.

Pintão, A.M.; Pais, M.S.; Coley, H.; Kelland, L.R. & Judson, I.R. (1995). In vitro and in vivo antitumor activity of benzyl isothiocyanate: a natural product from Tropaeolum majus. *Planta Med*, vol. 61, pp.233-236.

Pio Corrêa, M. (1926). Dicionário das plantas úteis do Brasil e das exóticas cultivadas. Imprensa Nacional, pp. 747, Rio de Janeiro.

Pires, J.M.; Mendes, F.R.; Negri, G.; Duarte-Almeida, J.M. & Carlini, E.A. (2009). Antinociceptive peripheral effect of Achillea millefolium L. and Artemisia vulgaris L.: Both plants known popularly by Brand Names of analgesic drugs. *Phytother Res*, vol. 23, pp.212-219.

Pitasawat, B.; Champakaew, D.; Choochote, W.; Jitpakdi, A.; Chaithong, U.; Kanjanapothi, D.; Rattanachanpichai, E.; Tippawangkosol, P.; Riyong, D.; Tuetun, B. & Chaiyasit, D. (2007). Aromatic plant-derived essential oil: an alternative larvicide for mosquito control. *Fitoterapia*, vol.78, pp.205-210.

Portillo, A.; Vila, R.; Freixa, B.; Adzet, T. & Cañigueral, S. (2001). Antifungal activity of Paraguayan plants used in traditional medicine. *J Ethnopharmacol*, vol. 76, pp.93-98.

Preethi, K.C.; Kuttan, G. & Kuttan, R. (2006). Anti-tumour activity of Ruta graveolens extract. *Asian Pac J Cancer Prev*, vol. 7, pp. 439-443.

Prefeitura de Diadema (2011). Avaiable from: <http://www.diadema.sp.gov.br/apache2-default/>.

PUBMED (2010). Avaiable from: <http://www.ncbi.nlm.nih.gov/pubmed>.

Radford, D.J.; Gillies, A.D.; Hinds, J.A. & Duffy, P. (1986). Naturally occurring cardiac glycosides. *Med J Aust*, vol.12, pp.540-544.

Raghav, S.K.; Gupta, B.; Agrawal, C.; Goswami, K. & Das, H.R. (2006). Anti-inflammatory effect of Ruta graveolens L. in murine macrophage cells. *J Ethnopharmacol*, vol. 8, pp.234-239.

Rahim, N.; Gomes, D.J.; Watanabe, H.; Rahman, S.R.; Chomvarin, C.; Endtz, H.P. & Alam, M. (2010). Antibacterial activity of Psidium guajava leaf and bark against multidrug-resistant Vibrio cholerae: implication for cholera control. *Jpn J Infect Dis*, vol.63, pp.271-274.

Rajesh, R.; Shivaprasad, H.V.; Gowda, C.D.; Nataraju, A.; Dhananjaya, B.L. & Vishwanath, B.S. (2007). Comparative study on plant latex proteases and their involvement in hemostasis: a special emphasis on clot inducing and dissolving properties. *Planta Med*, vol. 73, pp.1061-1067.

Rao, Y.K.; Fang, S.H. & Tzeng, Y.M. (2005). Inhibitory effects of the flavonoids isolated from Waltheria indica on the production of NO, TNF-alpha and IL-12 in activated macrophages. *Bio Pharm Bull*, vol. 28, pp. 912-915.

Ratnasooriya, W.D.; Jayakody, J.R.; Premakumara, G.A. & Ediriweera, E.R. (2005). Antioxidant activity of water extract of Scoparia dulcis. *Fitoterapia*, vol. 76, pp. 220-222.

Ribeiro, D. (1996). O povo brasileiro: A formação e o sentido do Brasil. *Companhia das Letras*, São Paulo, Brasil.

Rim, I.S. & Jee, C.H. (2006). Acaricidal effects of herb essential oils against Dermatophagoides farinae and D. pteronyssinus (Acari: Pyroglyphidae) and qualitative analysis of a herb Mentha pulegium (pennyroyal). Korean J Parasitol, vol. 44, pp.133-138.

Rizzini, C.T. (1968). Problemas relacionados com o estudo da distribuição geográfica e identificação das plantas medicinais brasileiras. *Arquivos do Instituto Biológico*, vol. 35, pp. 10-14.

Rodrigues, E. & Carlini, E.A. (2003). Possíveis Efeitos sobre o Sistema Nervoso Central de Plantas Utilizadas por Duas Culturas Brasileiras (quilombolas e índios). *Arquivos Brasileiros de Fitomedicina Científica*, vol.1.

Rodrigues, E. & Carlini, E.A. (2004). Plants used by a Quilombola group in Brazil with potential central nervous system effects. *Phytother Res*, vol.18, pp.748-753.

Rodrigues, E. (2005). A parceria Universidade – Empresa privada na produção de fitoterápicos no Brasil. *Revisa Fármacos e Medicamentos*, Vol. 37, year IV, pp. 30-39.

Rodrigues, E. & Carlini, E.A. (2005). Ritual use of plants with possible action on the central nervous system by the Kraho indians, Brazil. *Phytother Res*, vol.19, pp.129-135.

Rodrigues, E.; Mendes, F.R. & Negri, G. (2005). Plants indicated by Brazilian Indians to Central Nervous System disturbances: a bibliographical approach. *Curr Med Chem*, vol.6, pp.211-244.

Rodrigues, E. (2006). Ethnopharmacology in the Jaú National Park (JNP), state of Amazonas, Brazil. *Phytother Res*, vol. 5, pp.378-391.

Rodrigues, E.; Mendes, F. R. & Negri, G. (2006). Plants indicated by Brazilian Indians to Central Nervous System disturbances: A bibliographical approach. *Current Medicinal Chemistry* – Central Nervous System Agents, Vol. 6, pp. 211-244.

Rodrigues, E and Carlini, E.A. (2006). Use of South American plants for the treatment of neuropsychiatric disorders. *Bulletin of the Board of International Affairs of the Royal College of Psychiatrists,* vol. 3.

Rodrigues, E. (2007). Plants of restricted use indicated by three cultures in Brazil (Caboclo-river dweller, Indian and Quilombola). *Journal of Ethnopharmacology,* Vol. 111, pp. 295–302.

Rodrigues, E.; Tabach, R.; Galduroz, J.C.F. & Negri, G. (2008). Plants with possible anxiolytic and/or hypnotic effects indicated by three Brazilian cultures - Indians, Afrobrazilians, and River-dwellers. *Studies in Natural Products Chemistry,* vol. 35, 549-595.

Rojas, J.J.; Ochoa, V.J.; Ocampo, A.S. & Muñoz, J.F. (2006). Screening for antimicrobial activity of ten medicinal plants used in Colombian folkloric medicine: a possible alternative in the treatment of non-nosocomial infections. *BMC Complement Altern Med,* vol.6.

Roy, C.K. & Das, A.K. (2010). Comparative evaluation of different extracts of leaves of Psidium guajava Linn. for hepatoprotective activity. *Pak J Pharm Sci,* vol. 23, pp.15-20.

Runnie, I.; Salleh, M.N.; Mohamed, S.; Head, R.J. & Abeywardena, M.Y. (2004). Vasorelaxation induced by common edible tropical plant extracts in isolated rat aorta and mesenteric vascular bed. *J Ethnopharmacol,* vol. 92, pp.311-316.

Ruppelt, B.M.; Pereira, E.F.; Gonçalves, L.C. & Pereira, N.A. (1991). Pharmacological screening of plants recommended by folk medicine as anti-snake venom-I. Analgesic and anti-inflammatory activities. *Mem Inst Oswaldo Cruz,* vol. 2, pp.203-205.

Salari, M.H.; Amine, G.; Shirazi, M.H.; Hafezi, R. & Mohammadypour, M. (2006). Antibacterial effects of Eucalyptus globulus leaf extract on pathogenic bacteria isolated from specimens of patients with respiratory tract disorders. *Clin Microbiol Infect,* vol.12, pp.194-196.

Santos-Fita, D. & Costa-Neto, E.M. (2007). As interações entre os seres humanos e os animais: a contribuição da etnozoologia. *Biotemas,* vol.20, pp.99-110.

Sawangjaroen, N.; Phongpaichit, S.; Subhadhirasakul, S.; Visutthi, M.; Srisuwan, N. & Thammapalerd, N. (2006). The anti-amoebic activity of some medicinal plants used by AIDS patients in southern Thailand. *Parasitol Res,* vol. 98, pp. 588-592.

Schapoval, E.E.; Vargas, M.R.; Chaves, C.G.; Bridi, R.; Zuanazzi, J.A. & Henriques, A.T. (1998). Antiinflammatory and antinociceptive activities of extracts and isolated compounds from Stachytarpheta cayennensis. *J Ethnopharmacol,* vol. 60, pp.53-59.

Schinella, G.; Aquila, S.; Dade, M.; Giner, R.; Recio Mdel, C.; Spegazzini, E.; de Buschiazzo, P.; Tournier, H. & Ríos, J.L. (2008). Anti-inflammatory and apoptotic activities of pomolic acid isolated from Cecropia pachystachya. *Planta Med,* vol.74, pp.215-220.

Schmourlo, G.; Mendonça-Filho, R.R.; Alviano, C.S. & Costa, S.S. (2005). Screening of antifungal agents using ethanol precipitation and bioautography of medicinal and food plants. *J Ethnopharmacol,* vol. 15, pp.563-568.

Schuldt, E.Z.; Ckless, K.; Simas, M.E.; Farias, M.R. & Ribeiro-Do-Valle, R.M. (2000). Butanolic fraction from Cuphea carthagenensis Jacq McBride relaxes rat thoracic aorta through endothelium-dependent and endothelium- independent mechanisms. *J Cardiovasc Pharmacol,* vol.35, pp.234-239.

Schultes, R.E. & Raffaulf, R.F. (1990). In The Healing Forest. Medicinal and Toxic Plants of the Nortwest Amazonia. vol. 2. Dioscorides Press: Oregon.

Schultes, R.E. (1988). Ethnopharmacological conservation: a key to progress in medicine. *Acta Botanica*, vol.18, pp. 393-406.

SCIFINDER (2011) Avaiable from: <http://www.cas.org/products/sfacad/index.html>.

Shao, F.; Hu, Z.; Xiong, Y.M.; Huang, Q.Z.; Wang, C.G.; Zhu, R.H. & Wang, D.C. (1999). A new antifungal peptide from the seeds of Phytolacca americana: characterization, amino acid sequence and cDNA cloning. *Biochim Biophys Acta*, vol.19, pp.262-268.

Sharma, P.; Mohan, L. & Srivastava, C.N. (2006). Phytoextract-induced developmental deformities in malaria vector. *Bioresour Technol*, vol. 97, pp.1599-1604.

Shi, M.; Chang, L. & He, G. (1995). Stimulating action of Carthamus tinctorius L., Angelica sinensis (Oliv.) Diels and Leonurus sibiricus L. on the uterus. *Zhongguo Zhong Yao Za Zhi*, vol.20, pp.173-175.

Shlamovitz, G.Z.; Gupta, M. & Diaz, J.A. (2007). A case of acute keratoconjunctivitis from exposure to latex of Euphorbia tirucalli (Pencil Cactus). *J Emerg Med*, vol. 36, pp. 239-241.

Silva, J.; Abebeb, W.; Sousa, S.M.; Duarte, V.G.; Machado, M.I.L. & Matos, F.J.A. (2003). Analgesic and anti-inflammatory effects of essential oils of Eucalyptus. *J Ethnopharmacol*, vol.89, pp. 277-283.

Simões, L.L. & Lino, C.F. (2004). Sustentável Mata Atlântica: a exploração de seus recursos florestais. *SENAC*, São Paulo.

Simões-Pires, C.A.; Queiroz, E.F.; Henriques, A.T. & Hostettmann, K. (2005): Isolation and on-line identification of antioxidant compounds from three Baccharis species by HPLC-UV-MS/MS with post-column derivatisation. *Phytochem Anal*, vol.16, pp.307-314.

Singh, H.P.; Batish, D.R.; Kaur, S.; Kohli, R.K. & Arora, K. (2006). Phytotoxicity of the volatile monoterpene citronellal against some weeds. *Z Naturforsch*, vol. 61, pp.334-340.

Sistema Único de Saúde (2010). Avaiable from: <http://tabnet.datasus.gov.br/tabdata/cadernos/ cadernosmap.htm>.

Soares de Moura, R.; Costa, S.S.; Jansen, J.M.; Silva, C.A.; Lopes, C.S.; Bernardo-Filho, M.; Nascimento da Silva, V.; Criddle, D.N.; Portela, B.N.; Rubenich, L.M.; Araujo, R.G. & Carvalho, L.C. (2002). Bronchodilator activity of Mikania glomerata Sprengel on human bronchi and guinea-pig trachea. *J Pharm Pharmacol*, vol. 54, pp.249-256.

Soicke, H. & Leng-Peschlow, E. (1987). Characterisation of flavonoids from Baccharis trimera and their antihepatotoxic properties. *Planta Med*, vol. 53, pp.37-39.

Souza, M.C.; Siani, A.C.; Ramos, M.F.; Menezes-de-Lima, O.J. & Henriques, M.G. (2004). Evaluation of anti-inflammatory activity of essential oils from two Asteraceae species. *Pharmazie*, vol. 58, pp.582-586.

Spjut, R.W. & Perdue, J.R. (1976). Plant folcklore: a tool for predicting sources of antitumor activity? *Cancer Treatment Reports*, Vol. 60, pp. 979-985.

Sripanidkulchai, B.; Wongpanich, V.; Laupattarakasem, P.; Suwansaksri, J. & Jirakulsomchok. (2001). Diuretic effects of selected Thai indigenous medicinal plants in rats. *J Ethnopharmacol*, vol.75, pp.185-190.

Sundararajan, P.; Dey, A.; Smith, A.; Doss, A.G.; Rajappan, M. & Natarajan, S. (2006). Studies of anticancer and antipyretic activity of Bidens pilosa whole plant. *Afr Health Sci*, vol.6, pp.27-30.

Suzuki, N. (1996). Investing for the future: education, migration and intergenerational conflict in South Cotabato, the Philippines. In Binisaya nga kinabuhi (Visayan life). Edited by Ushijima, Iwao, Cynthia Neri Zayas. Visayas Maritime Anthropological Studies, College of Social Sciences and Philosophy, University of the Philippines, pp. 43-58, Quezon City, Philippines.

Tabopda, T.K.; Ngoupayo, J.; Liu, J.; Mitaine-Offer, A.C.; Tanoli, S.A.; Khan, S.N.; Ali, M.S.; Ngadjui, B.T.; Tsamo, E.; Lacaille-Dubois, M.A. & Luu, B. (2008). Bioactive aristolactams from Piper umbellatum. *Phytochemistry*, vol.69, pp.1726-1731.

Takahashi, H.; Hirata, S.; Minami, H. & Fukuyama, Y. (2001). Triterpene and flavanone glycoside from Rhododendron simsii. *Phytochemistry*, vol. 56, pp.875-879.

Takahashi, T.; Kokubo, R. & Sakaino, M. (2004): Antimicrobial activities of eucalyptus leaf extracts and flavonoids from Eucalyptus maculata. *Lett Appl Microbiol*, vol.39, pp.60-64.

Talbourdet, S.; Sadick, N.S.; Lazou, K.; Bonnet-Duquennoy, M.; Kurfurst, R.; Neveu, M.; Heusèle, C.; André, P.; Schnebert, S.; Draelos, Z.D. & Perrier, E. (2007). Modulation of gene expression as a new skin anti-aging strategy. *J Drugs Dermatol*, vol.6, pp.25-33.

Tchoumbougnang, F.; Zollo, P.H.; Dagne, E. & Mekonnen, Y. (2005). In vivo antimalarial activity of essential oils from Cymbopogon citratus and Ocimum gratissimum on mice infected with Plasmodium berghei. *Planta Med*, vol.7, pp.20-23.

Thomas, E.; Vandebroek, I.; Sanca, S. & Van Damme, P. (2009). Cultural significance of medicinal plant families and species among Quechua farmers in Apillapampa, Bolivia. *Journal of Ethnopharmacology*, vol. 122, pp.60-67.

Tiwari, T.N.; Varma, J.; Dubey, N.K.; Chansouria, J.P. & Ali, Z. (1998). Pharmacological evaluation of some bioactive plant products on albino rats. *Hindustan Antibiot Bull*, vol.40, pp.38-41.

Tognolini, M.; Ballabeni, V.; Bertoni, S.; Bruni, R.; Impicciatore, M. & Barocelli, E. (2007). Protective effect of Foeniculum vulgare essential oil and anethole in na experimental model of thrombosis. *Pharmacol Res*, vol. 56, pp.254-260.

Torres, D.F.; de Oliveira, E.S.; Alves, R.R.N. & Vasconcellos, A. (2009). Etnobotânica e etnozoologia em unidades de conservação: uso da biodiversidade na APA de Genipabu, Rio Grande do Norte, Brasil. *Interciencia*, vol. 34, p.623-629.

Torres, L.M.; Gamberini, M.T.; Roque, N.F.; Lima-Landman, M.T.; Souccar, C. & Lapa, A.J. (2000). Diterpene from Baccharis trimera with a relaxant effect on rat vascular smooth muscle. *Phytochemistry*, vol. 55, pp.617-619.

Trotter, R.T. & Logan, M.H. (1986). Informant consensus: a new approach for identifying potentially effective medicinal plants. In Plants in indigenous medicine and diet: biobehavioral approachs. Edited by: Etkin NL. New York: Redgrave Publishing, pp.91-112.

Valadares, M.C.; Carrucha, S.G.; Accorsi, W. & Queiroz, M.L. (2006). Euphorbia tirucalli L. modulates myelopoiesis and enhances the resistance of tumour-bearing mice. *Int Immunopharmacol*, vol.6, pp.294-299.

Valverde, A.L.; Cardoso, G.L.; Pereira, N.A.; Silva, A.J. & Kuster, R.M. (2001). Analgesic and antiinflammatory activities of vernonioside B2 from Vernonia condensata. *Phytother Res*, vol. 15, pp. 263-264.

van Andel, T.R. & Westers P. (2010). Why Surinamese migrants in the Netherlands continue to use medicinal herbs from their home country. *J Ethnopharmacol*, vol.127pp.694-701.

Velázquez, E.; Tournier, H.A.; de Buschiazzo, P.; Saavedra, G. & Schinella, G.R. (2003). Antioxidant activity of Paraguayan plant extracts. *Fitoterapia*, vol.74, pp.91-97.

Viyoch, J.; Pisutthanan, N.; Faikreua, A.; Nupangta, K.; Wangtorpol, K. & Ngokkuen, J. (2006). Evaluation of in vitro antimicrobial activity of Thai basil oils and their micro-emulsion formulas against Propionibacterium acnes. *Int J Cosmet Sci*, vol. 28, pp.125-133.

Voeks, R.A. & Leony, A. (2004). Foegetting the forest: Assessing medicinal plant erosion in Eastern Brazil. *Economic Botany*, vol. 58.

Voeks, R.A. (2009). Traditions in transition: African diaspora ethnobotany in lowland South America. In Mobility and Migration in Indigenous Amazonia: Contemporary Ethnoecological Perspectives. Edited by: Alexiades, M., pp.275-294, London: Berghahn.

Volpato, G.; Ahmadi, A.; Lamin, S.M.; Broglia, A. & Di Lello, S. (2007). Procurement of traditional remedies and transmission of medicinal knowledge among Sahrawi people displaced in Southwestern Algerian refugee camps. In Traveling Plants and Cultures The Ethnobiology and Ethnopharmacy of Migrations Edited by: Pieroni A, Vandebroek I.; pp. 245-269 Oxford: Berghahn

Volpato, G.; Godínez, D. & Beyra, A. (2008). Migration and Ethnobotanical Practices: The Case of *Tifey* Among Haitian Immigrants in Cuba. *Human Ecology*, vol.37, pp. 43–53.

Volpato, G.; Godínez, D.; Beyra, A. & Barreto, A. (2009). Uses of medicinal plants by Haitian immigrants and their descendants in the Province of Camagüey, Cuba. *Journal of Ethnobiology and Ethnomedicine*, pp.5-16.

Von Szczepanski, C.; Zgorzelak, P. & Hoyer, G.A. (1972). Isolation, structural analysis Arzneimittelforschung vol. 22, pp.1975-1976.

Waldstein, A. (2006): Mexican migrant ethnopharmacology: pharmacopoeia, classification of medicines and explanations of efficacy. *J Ethnopharmacol*, vol. 108, pp.299-310.

Waldstein, A. (2008). Diaspora and Health? Traditional Medicine and Culture in a Mexican Migrant Community. *International Migration*, vol. 46, pp.95-117.

Wannissorn, B.; Jarikasem, S.; Siriwangchai, T. & Thubthimthed, S. (2005). Antibacterial properties of essential oils from Thai medicinal plants. *Fitoterapia*, vol.76, pp. 233-236.

Weckesser, S.; Engel, K.; Simon-Haarhaus, B.; Wittmer, A.; Pelz, K. & Schempp, C.M. (2007). Screening of plant extracts for antimicrobial activity against bacteria and yeasts with dermatological relevance. *Phytomedicine*, vol.14, pp. 508-516.

Weiss, H.B. (1947). Entomological medicaments of the past. *Journal of the New York Entomological Society*, vol.55, pp.155-168.

Woodland, D.W. (1997). Contemporary plant systematics Andrews University Press, London.

Yemitan, O.K. & Salahdeen, H.M. (2005). Neurosedative and muscle relaxant activities of aqueous extract of Bryophyllum pinnatum. *Fitoterapia*, vol. 76, pp.187-193.

Zétola, M.; De Lima, T.C.; Sonaglio, D.; González-Ortega, G.; Limberger, R.P.; Petrovick, R. & Bassani, V.L. (2002) CNS activities of liquid and spray-dried extracts from Lippia alba-Verbenaceae (Brazilian false melissa). *J Ethnopharmacol*, vol. 82, pp.207-215.

Zheng, Y.Y.; Yang, J.; Chen, D.H. & Sun, L. (2007). Effects of the stilbene extracts from Cajanus cajan L. on ovariectomy-induced bone loss in rats. *Yao Xue Xue Bao*, vol. 42, pp.562-565.

2

Elucidating the Role of Biliverdin Reductase in the Expression of Heme Oxygenase-1 as a Cytoprotective Response to Stress

James R. Reed
Department of Pharmacology,
Louisiana State University Health Sciences Center, New Orleans, LA,
USA

1. Introduction

Hemin is a cofactor in which an atom of iron is coordinated to the nitrogens of four pyrrole groups that make up the protoporphyrin IX ring (see figure below).

Hemin

Many types of enzymes in living systems use hemin as a prosthetic group to catalyze oxidation/reduction reactions or for the binding/transport of reactive molecules (e.g. oxygen). For instance, several cytochromes of the mitochondrial electron transport chain are "heme" enzymes as are the major drug/xenobiotic-metabolizing enzymes of the endoplasmic reticulum, the cytochromes P450 (CYP or P450). The heme group of the P450s allows these enzymes to use redox chemistry to bind molecular oxygen and cleave the O-O bond, thus forming a reactive, high-valent oxygen species that can insert oxygen into otherwise stable carbon-hydrogen bonds of drugs/xenobiotics (White and Coon, 1980). The unfavorable thermodynamics of this type of reaction has caused the P450s to be likened to "catalytic blowtorches" (Schlichting et al., 2000), and the process is essential for the elimination and clearance of many lipophilic compounds ingested from the environment. Catalase is an important protective heme enzyme that is responsible for degrading hydrogen peroxide. Furthermore, the heme enzymes, nitric oxide synthase and cyclooxygenase, have important signaling roles in the regulation of various cellular processes such as inflammation. However, in terms of the sheer abundance in higher living systems, hemoglobin is the most important heme enzyme as it uses the cofactor to transport oxygen in blood circulation to facilitate oxidative/phosphorylation and energy generation in distal tissues. Because the heme proteins interact with reactive oxygen species (ROS), they are susceptible to ROS-mediated damage, which in turn, results in the accumulation of free or unused heme.

1.1 The toxicity of heme

The reactive nature of hemin does not come without a cost. The free (not enzyme bound) form of the cofactor has been shown *in vitro* to increase the peroxidation of lipids and the fragmentation and cross-linking of DNA and protein resulting from oxidative stress (Kumar and Bandyopadhyay, 2005;Vincent, 1989). One likely explanation for these findings can be drawn from two of the basic reactions of reactive oxygen chemistry, the Fenton reaction and the Haber-Weiss reaction. In the Fenton reaction (below), superoxide anion reduces free molecular iron.

$$O_2^- + Fe^{+3} \longrightarrow O_2 + Fe^{+2} \qquad \text{(Fenton Reaction)}$$

In the Haber-Weiss reaction, the reduced iron can interact with hydrogen peroxide, resulting in cleavage of the O-O bond to form hydroxyl anion and hydroxyl radical (Vincent, 1989).

$$Fe^{+2} + H_2O_2 \longrightarrow Fe^{+3} + HO^- + HO \quad \text{(Haber-Weiss Reaction)}$$

Using the Haber-Weiss system as an analogy, it is likely that the free hemin functions in a manner similar to that of free iron as a means to produce hydroxyl radical. The hydroxyl radical has been shown to be much more destructive to proteins and DNA than both hydrogen peroxide and superoxide (Davies et al., 1987;Jackson et al., 1987).

It also has been proposed that hemin interacts with hydrogen peroxide to form a putative, hypervalent iron-oxygen species analogous to the reactive intermediate of peroxidase enzymes referred to as Compound I (Vincent, 1989).

$$Fe^{+2} + H_2O_2 \longrightarrow Fe^{+3}:O \cdot + H_2O \quad \text{(Peroxidase-like Reaction)}$$

Because hemin is much more lipophilic than free iron, the oxidative stress associated with free hemin is more destructive to membrane lipids and organelles (Balla et al., 1991). In this respect, the putative iron-oxo species resulting from the reaction of hemin and hydrogen peroxide could be even more deleterious than hydroxyl radical as suggested by the fact that free radical scavengers of hydroxyl radical (e.g. dimethyl sulfoxide) did not protect lipids and proteins from damage when incubated with hemin and hydrogen peroxide (Vincent, 1989). Understandably, the propensity of hemin to damage lipid mixtures causes it to be extremely harmful to cellular membranes and organelles. Free hemin also has been shown to promote inflammatory reactions that have been associated with hepatic, renal, neuronal, and vascular injury (Kumar and Bandyopadhyay, 2005). In particular, several studies have demonstrated the contribution of hemin to the pathogenesis associated with atherosclerosis and ischemia/reperfusion (Wagener et al., 2001).

1.2 The regulation of cellular heme levels

Because of the harmful effects of free heme accumulation, the synthesis and catabolism of heme in living systems is highly regulated. The rate-limiting enzyme for heme synthesis is α-aminolevulinic acid synthetase, and its expression and activity is highly regulated by a variety of agents and stress signals (Ponka, 1997). Heme catabolism is carried out by two enzymatic reactions. The rate-limiting step of heme catabolism is catalyzed by heme oxygenase (HO). This enzyme catalyzes a complicated, multi-step reaction that uses molecular oxygen and electrons (received from a separate redox partner, the cytochrome P450 reductase) to cleave the α-meso bridge of the protoporphyrin IX ring and form ferrous iron, CO, and biliverdin in the process (Kikuchi et al., 2005;Liu et al., 1997;Liu and Ortiz de Montellano, 2000) (see figure below).

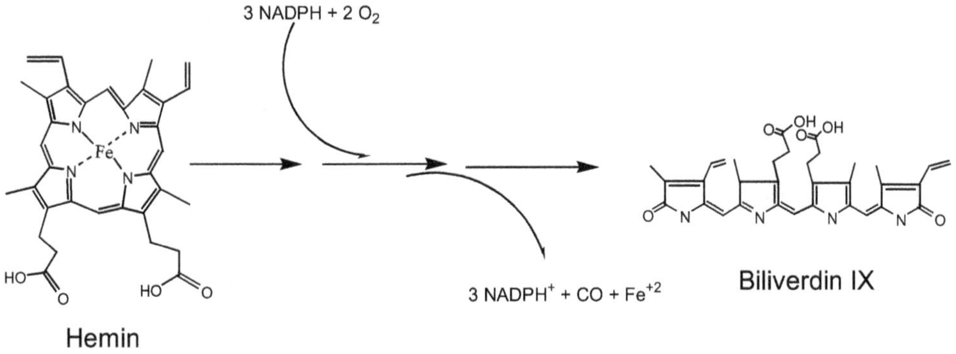

3 NADPH + 2 O_2

3 NADPH$^+$ + CO + Fe^{+2}

Biliverdin IX

Hemin

(HO Reaction)

The final step of heme catabolism involves the reduction of the biliverdin formed by HO to bilirubin. This enzymatic step (below) is catalyzed by the biliverdin reductase (BVR). BVR has dual cofactor specificity as both NADH and NADPH can provide electrons to the enzyme. NADPH is the preferred cofactor under basic conditions, whereas NADH is more favorable at lower pH (< 7.0) (Noguchi et al., 1979). The activities of both HO and BVR are highly regulated to effectively coordinate heme catabolism with its synthesis under different conditions.

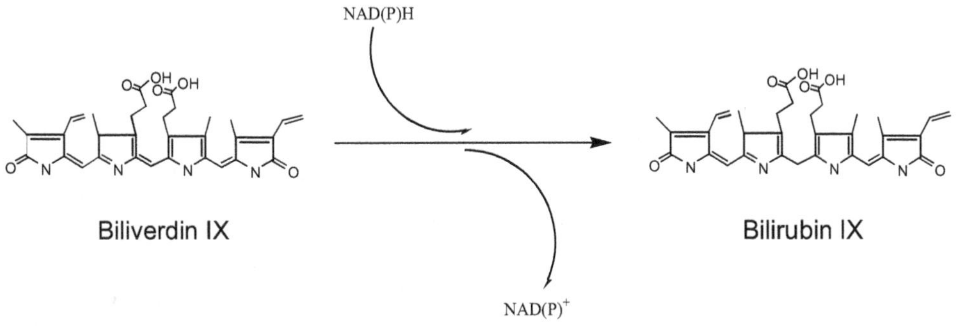

NAD(P)H

Biliverdin IX

Bilirubin IX

NAD(P)$^+$

(BVR Reaction)

2. Cellular functions of HO-1 and HO-2

There are two isoforms of HO, known as HO-1 and HO-2 that are expressed through two different genes and are immunologically distinct (Maines et al., 1986;Maines, 1988). The two enzymes are approximately 40% homologous as both have in common a catalytic region of about 24 amino acids (Rotenberg and Maines, 1991) and a hydrophobic, C-terminal tail that serves to anchor the enzymes to the endoplasmic reticulum. HO-1, which is 33 kDa, is highly inducible by a multitude of stimuli and compounds and is constitutively expressed in liver and spleen. HO-2 is constitutively expressed in most tissues, and is highly expressed in brain, kidney, and testes. The HO-2 protein is 36 kDa as it contains additional regulatory sequences (e.g. extra heme-binding sites) which affect its activity in a tissue-specific manner and which might also be regulated by CO and NO binding (Ryter et al., 2006).

2.1 Functions of HO-2

It is generally believed that the main role of HO-2 might be to maintain homeostatic levels of heme during normal cellular metabolism. In one study, HO-2 knockout mice only displayed mild phenotypes and did not show evidence of altered iron maintenance (Poss et al., 1995). The study did show that the mice displayed ejaculation abnormalities (in males) and increased susceptibility to hyperoxic lung damage. Illustrating the importance of HO-2 to brain heme metabolism, these mice also showed dramatically reduced levels of HO activity in the brain. In addition, another study did demonstrate oxygen toxicity and iron accumulation in the lungs of HO-2 knockout mice (Dennery et al., 1998). Thus, HO-1 cannot completely compensate for the absence of HO-2 in terms of cellular function and the regulation of heme levels.

In brain, testes, and cardiovascular tissue, HO-2 activity plays a critical role in function by generating CO which functions as a tissue-specific signaling messenger that acts mainly through activation of guanylyl cyclase. In smooth muscle and endothelial tissue, CO mimics the effects of NO by causing relaxation and vasodilatation, respectively (Hangai-Hoger et al., 2007;Patel et al., 1993). CO also has anti-apoptotic and anti-inflammatory effects mediated through mitogen-activated protein kinases (MAPK) and not guanylyl cyclase (Piantadosi and Zhang, 1996). These signaling relationships will be discussed in more detail below in the chapter. CO also has been postulated to play a role in inhibiting P450 enzymes since the ferrous form of this type of heme protein forms a tight-binding complex with CO.

2.2 Functions of HO-1

Whereas HO-2 seems to be important in managing heme levels during normal cellular metabolism, HO-1 serves to maintain homeostatic levels of heme under conditions of cellular stress. Oxidative stress is associated with increased rates of heme protein damage and in turn, free heme accumulation.   Early studies with HO-1 speculated on a cytoprotective role for this enzyme given the following: 1) It was identified as a 32 kDa heat shock protein (Keyse and Tyrrell, 1989) induced by a variety of stressors that included direct oxidative stress; 2) it metabolized a compound (hemin) that was known to be harmful to cells at high concentrations (Kutty and Maines, 1984); and 3) it was induced (greater than 40-fold in some instances (Wright et al., 2006)) in virtually all tissues following exposure to a variety of cellular stressors including oxidative stress, UV radiation, hyperoxia, hypoxia, hyperthermia, heavy metals, metal porphyrins, tumor factors, insulin, endotoxin, and sulfhydryl-reactive compounds (Keyse and Tyrrell, 1989) (reviewed in (Ryter et al., 2006)). Because most of the HO-1-inducing agents also cause elevated levels of oxidative stress, it has been postulated that HO-1 induction represents an early, "sentinel-type" response by the cell to counteract the deleterious effects of oxidative stress (Otterbein et al., 2000;Poss and Tonegawa, 1997b).

3. Experimental evidence for the cytoprotective role of HO-1

3.1 In vitro evidence for the cytoprotective role of HO-1

Most of the in vitro/in vivo evidence for HO-1 playing a cytoprotective role has examined the effects of inducers and inhibitors of HO-1 when cells/animals are dosed with a stressor. These types of studies are described in the paragraphs below. More sophisticated lines of in vivo evidence using gene knockout/therapy to modulate HO-1 levels will be referred to separately. Metal porphyrins and heavy metals are often used alternately in studies to implicate a function of HO in a cellular process. Whereas in most cases, both types of compounds induce the HO-1 gene (a major exception is tin mesoporphyrin which inhibits HO-1 induction) and elevate protein expression, the metal porphyrins will often bind to the HO active site resulting in the inhibition of enzyme activity.

Both in vitro and in vivo studies have demonstrated that the elevated expression and activity of HO-1 is associated with a greater tolerance to various types of stress. It was already mentioned how an in vitro study was used to demonstrate that HO-1 was a 32 kDa heat shock protein which was induced by cellular stress and protected cells from toxicities related to these stressors (Keyse and Tyrrell, 1989). Another interesting in vitro study used HepG2 cells that were transfected to constitutively express CYP2E1 to demonstrate the protective role of HO-1 during CYP2E1-mediated metabolism and oxidative stress (Gong et al., 2004). Of the P450 enzymes, CYP2E1 is especially prone to the breakdown of its monoxygenase catalytic cycle with the concomitant release of superoxide, hydrogen peroxide, and excess water (Gorsky et al., 1984). A previous study by the same lab used these cells to show that the oxidative stress associated with CYP2E1-mediated metabolism could be cytotoxic, especially after prior cellular depletion of glutathione by treatment with L-buthionine-(S,R)-sulfoximine (Chen and Cederbaum, 1998). In the study examining the role of HO-1, the cytotoxicity associated with the CYP2E1-mediated metabolism of arachidonic acid was not observed when HO-1 expression was up-regulated by transfection of the cells with an adenovirus containing the cDNA for human HO-1 (Gong et al., 2004). Furthermore, when the cells were treated with chromium mesoporphyrin, which acts as an inhibitor of HO-1, the CYP2E1-related toxicity was potentiated. The in vitro study also implicated CO but not bilirubin in the protective effects of HO-1, probably through the CO-related inhibition of P450 activity (discussed below).

In another in vitro study, the protective effect of the flavonoid, quercetin, on the hepatotoxicity of ethanol was attributed to its induction of HO-1 in hepatocytes because the effects of quercetin were abrogated by treatment with zinc mesoporphyrin (Yao et al., 2009). Addition of free iron increased the damage caused by ethanol, whereas CO treatment protected the cells from ethanol-induced toxicity. Thus, it was thought that the protection afforded by HO-1 induction was in part caused by the inhibition of P450-mediated activation of ethanol by CO. Another study by this group indicated that HO-1 was induced through the MAPK/Nrf2 pathways of signal transduction (Yao et al., 2007). The in vitro studies of course are critical in elucidating the signaling pathways involved in heme metabolism. These pathways are discussed more completely below. Interestingly, the second enzyme responsible for heme metabolism, BVR has a very active role in the signaling required to modulate HO-1 levels with the ever-changing levels of heme in the cell.

3.2 In vivo evidence for the cytoprotective role of HO-1

Many in vivo studies have also tested for the protective role of HO-1 after exposure to toxins. Acetominophen is a widely-used analgesic that unfortunately has a narrow therapeutic index, and overdosing results in liver failure. Cytochrome P450-mediated metabolism is responsible for the harmful effects of acetaminophen as it converts the compound to a reactive quinone-imine that alkylates cellular protein and DNA. Interestingly, cellular glutathione effectively scavenges the reactive intermediate and protects against cytotoxicity. However, when an overdose occurs, the intracellular glutathione gets depleted resulting in the destruction of critical proteins that are necessary for cell function (Gibson et al., 1996). Several studies have tested for the ability of HO-1 to protect against acetaminophen toxicity in rats. In one of these studies, acetaminophen treatment resulted in HO-1 induction. To test whether the HO-1 expression was cytoprotective, the rats were treated with hemin to induce HO-1 prior to exposure to acetaminophen. These rats were indeed protected from acetaminophen hepatotoxicity compared to animals that were not pretreated with hemin. The study also found that biliverdin pretreatment was able to protect the rats from acetaminophen-induced hepatotoxicity (Chiu et al., 2002).

HO-1 induction was also shown to be protective from liver damage caused by carbon tetrachloride (Nakahira et al., 2003) and halothane (Odaka et al., 2000). Both of these compounds can be activated to free radical species by P450-mediated metabolism. Treatment with hepatotoxic doses of these compounds resulted in the rapid accumulation of intracellular free heme which was followed by HO-1 induction. It was found that when the rats were pre-treated with hemin (to induce HO-1) before halothane administration, hepatotoxicity was not observed. Similarly, when rats were treated with tin porphyrin 1 hour before administration of carbon tetrachloride to inhibit HO-1 activity, the carbon tetrachloride-induced liver injury was exacerbated (Nakahira et al., 2003). The findings of these studies suggest that free heme accumulation, presumably derived from the destruction of P450 enzymes, may be the main source of toxicity by these compounds. Thus, HO-1 induction was proposed to be an adaptive response that was critical for recovery from the toxic insults.

Many studies have investigated the ability of HO-1 to protect against endotoxin exposure. Endotoxin is a lipopolysaccharide produced by gram negative bacteria. Tissue exposure to endotoxin results in inflammatory injury and oxidative stress (Murphy et al., 1998) (McCord, 1993). In two separate studies, HO-1 induction in rats by hemin (Wen et al., 2007) and hemoglobin (Otterbein et al., 1995) pretreatment was protective against the deleterious effects of a subsequent (otherwise lethal) dose of endotoxin. In contrast, the rats were more susceptible to endotoxin toxicity, and the protective effects of HO-1 induction were ablated when the animals were treated with metal porphyrins that inhibited the HO-1 activity.

Elucidating the Role of Biliverdin Reductase in the Expression of Heme Oxygenase-1 as a Cytoprotective
Response to Stress

49

In vivo studies also demonstrated the ability of HO-1 induction to protect against acute renal failure in rats following ischemia/reperfusion (Toda et al., 2002) and exposure to mercuric chloride (Yoneya et al., 2000). Ischemia/reperfusion involves exposing the tissue to a sequence of oxygen deprivation followed by reoxygenation. Reoxygenation is associated with high levels of oxidative stress. Thus, it is a good model to examine the protective role of HO-1. The kidney ischemia/reperfusion study used tin chloride to induce the HO-1. Tin chloride induces HO-1 in a tissue-specific manner and does not induce HO-1 in the liver but does induce it in the kidney, demonstrating the complicated regulation of the HO-1 gene (discussed below). The fundamental role of HO-1 in mediating renal protection was demonstrated by showing that treatment with tin mesoporphyrin, an inhibitor of HO-1, did not prevent renal injury in the rats (Toda et al., 1995).

3.3 Gene knockout/therapy evidence for the cytoprotective role of HO-1

Over the last 10-15 years, novel research studies and interesting clinical findings have confirmed the cytoprotective role for HO-1. One of the seminal studies to demonstrate the protective role of HO-1 examined embryonic fibroblasts from HO-1 knockout mice and compared their attributes to those from normal wild-type animals (Poss and Tonegawa, 1997b). The cells from the knockout mice produced higher levels of ROS and also were less resistant to toxicity caused by hydrogen peroxide, paraquat, heavy metals, and heme exposure. The effects of HO-1 in the protection from free hemin exposure were quite dramatic offering 50% survival at a hemin concentration (200 µM) that was completely toxic to the cells from knockout mice. Another study from the same group, also compared the response of wild-type and HO-1 knockout mice to an intraperitoneal injection of endotoxin (Poss and Tonegawa, 1997a). Because the adult HO-1 knockout mice had a variety of health issues including anemia, iron-overloading, and chronic inflammation, younger mice (6 to 9 weeks) that did not display these phenotypes were used to study the effects of endotoxin. In terms of survival, the knockout mice were significantly more sensitive to endotoxin treatment and demonstrated higher levels of hepatic injury including increased serum liver enzyme levels and liver vacuolization. Interestingly, the hepatic injury seemed to be spatially and temporally related to iron loading malfunctions in both Kupffer cells and hepatocytes. Iron also accumulated in renal proximal cortical tubules.

Gene therapy studies to upregulate HO-1 have also been instrumental in proving that HO-1 is protective against cellular stress. In a study to demonstrate the role of HO-1 in vascular protection, a retroviral vector was used to transfect the human HO-1 gene into rat lung microvessel endothelium (Yang et al., 1999). Cells transfected with the retrovirus had over a 2-fold increase in HO-1 expression and activity. Furthermore, cGMP levels (probably regulated by CO activation of guanyly cyclase was almost 3-fold higher. These endothelial cells were significantly more resistant than untransfected cells to toxicity resulting from hydrogen peroxide and heme exposure. This protection was abolished upon treatment with stannic mesoporphyrin indicating the role of HO-1.

In another gene therapy study to investigate the ability of HO-1 to protect against the exposure of endotoxin in lung, an adenovirus encoding HO-1 was directly inoculated into rat trachea (Inoue et al., 2001). As a result, HO-1 was upregulated in both airway epithelium and alveolar macrophages. This therapy was found to be as effective as HO-1 induction by hemin pretreatment in preventing the inflammatory reaction caused by aerosolized endotoxin exposure. Furthermore, the protection conferred by increased HO-1 expression seemed to be related to higher endogenous levels of Interleukin-10 production by the macrophages.

Gene therapy was also used to compare the oxidative stress resistance of cerebellar granular neurons isolated from wild type and transgenic, homozygous mice that were engineered to overexpress HO-1 (Chen et al., 2000) The transgenic mice overexpressing HO-1 generated lower levels of ROS and were more resistant to oxidative stress resulting from either glutamate or hydrogen peroxide treatment.

3.4 Clinical evidence for the cytoprotective role of HO-1

Finally, in a tragic clinical example, the protective role of HO-1 was profoundly demonstrated by an individual who did not have a functional HO-1 gene (Kawashima et al., 2002). The six-year old male patient presented with growth retardation, anemia, elevated levels of ferritin and heme in serum, low serum bilirubin, intravascular hemolysis, and hyperlipidemia. In contrast to the HO-1 knockout mice showing toxicity from iron overloading, the endothelial tissue of the human patient was more severely affected causing a spectrum of cardiovascular maladies. A lymphoblastoid-derived cell line from this patient was also extremely sensitive to hemin-induced oxidative stress (Yachie et al., 1999).

3.5 Therapeutic potential of HO-1 modulation

On the basis of these scientific and clinical findings, the role of HO-1 in maintaining homeostasis and protecting against cellular stress is now well established. In conjunction, the enzyme has been shown to be protective in various types of disease/injury models including the following: 1) inflammation (sepsis, atherosclerosis), 2) lung injury (pulmonary fibrosis, ventilator-induced injury), 3) cardiovascular injury/disease (myocardial infarction, hypertension), 4) ischemia/reperfusion, and 5) organ transplantation/rejection. There are now several excellent reviews that discuss the pharmacologic potential of HO-1 induction (Abraham and Kappas, 2008;Mancuso and Barone, 2009;Ryter et al., 2006). Unfortunately, this type of therapy is not straightforward as it has been observed that over-expression of HO-1 can be harmful from the accumulation of reactive iron (Suttner and Dennery, 1999) and the bilirubin that results from HO-1-mediated heme catabolism (Claireaux et al., 1953). Thus, HO-1 expression in this type of therapeutic treatment would need to be highly regulated to prevent over-expression of the enzyme.

4. Mechanisms of cellular protection by HO-1

Originally, it was thought that the sole mechanism by which HO-1 protected cells was through the catabolism of free heme and the elimination of its prooxidant activities (discussed at the beginning of the chapter). Ironically, it was originally thought that the other products of the HO-1 reaction were useless (or even toxic) by-products. Now, it is known that CO and biliverdin play multiple roles in protection and that there are actually several mechanisms by which HO-1 performs its cytoprotective functions. It is very likely that there are more mechanisms yet to be identified.

4.1 Protective roles of CO: Cell signaling mediated by CO

The most definitive proof for the protective effects of CO has been derived from studies using CO-releasing molecules (Motterlini et al., 2003) as a surrogate for HO-1-derived CO. As indicated above, the CO formed by HO-1 has been shown to activate guanylyl cyclase to mediate the relaxation and dilation responses of smooth muscle and vascular endothelial cells, respectively (Cardell et al., 1998;Christodoulides et al., 1995). In vascular tissue, CO has also been shown to stimulate relaxation of endothelial smooth muscle cells by activation of calcium-dependent potassium channels (Williams et al., 2004) via a poorly-understood mechanism that does not involve guanylyl cyclase. CO has been shown to serve as a partial agonist to nitric oxide synthetase (NOS) and thus, may down-regulate the level of NOS-dependent signaling (Hangai-Hoger et al., 2007;Ishikawa et al., 2005).

Interestingly, it also was reported that cGMP-dependent signaling was able to induce HO-1 through the cAMP responsive element in its promoter by a mechanism that was not elucidated (Immenschuh et al., 1998a). Logically, these cGMP-related effects may be initiated by HO-1-generated CO. Of course, the cAMP promoter element also allows HO-1 to be induced directly through cAMP-dependent signaling and activation of protein kinase A (Immenschuh et al., 1998b).

Many of the details about other types of signaling involving CO are poorly understood as it appears to be both cell type- and stressor-specific (Song et al., 2003a){Song, 2003 2563 /id}. Most studies have implicated the ability of CO (and CO-releasing molecules) to activate the P38 MAPK pathway in carrying out its anti-apoptotic and anti-inflammatory effects (Brouard et al., 2000;Dérijard et al., 1995;Keum et al., 2006;Otterbein et al., 2000).

The MAPK pathways have been shown to regulate processes such as inflammation, differentiation, tumor promotion, proliferation, apoptosis, stress response, and ion channels (reviewed in (Shen et al., 2005;Wada and Penninger, 2004)). Two of the three arms of the MAPK pathway (JNK and p38) have been implicated in the cellular stress response. Downstream activation of the MAPK pathway, and specifically the JNK arm, leads to the dimerization and DNA binding of the stress response factors, c-Jun and c-fos. CO dramatically inhibited JNK MAPK signaling in murine macrophages exposed to endotoxin which resulted in lower production of inflammatory cytokine, IL-6 (Morse et al., 2003). Furthermore, c-Jun activation has been linked to cellular proliferation (Yoshioka et al., 1995) so this would explain part of the role of CO in mediating proliferation/transformation.

The p38 arm of the MAPK kinase activates ATF-2 which competes with c-fos for binding to c-Jun. This heterodimer binds with greater affinity to the HO-1 promoter than the c-fos/c-Jun heterodimer (Kravets et al., 2004). Furthermore, ATF-2 dimers can bind and directly activate the cyclic AMP responsive element (CRE) in the promoter region of HO-1 (Lee et al., 2002). ATF-2 activation may play a role in the activation of transcription factor, NFκB (Kaszubska et al., 1993). NFκB plays an essential role in the response to both apoptotic and inflammatory stimuli and regulates the expression of cytokines, growth factors, and cell cycle effector proteins (reviewed in (Bonizzi and Karin, 2004;Shen et al., 2005)). ATF-2 involvement in the activation of NFκB could explain the anti-apoptotic/anti-inflammatory affects of CO (see below for more details). In support of the idea that ATF-2 and c-Jun oppose one another in the protective gene expression associated with HO-1 induction, c-Jun has been shown to inhibit activation of NFκB (Tan et al., 2009).

The ERK 1/2 MAPK regulates cellular growth and differentiation. Stimulation of the pathway has been shown to be protective against apoptosis (Wada and Penninger, 2004). However, overstimulation of ERK appears to be the major mechanism by which some oncogenes transforms cells (e.g. Ha-Ras (Hibi et al., 1993)). In one study of human airway smooth muscle cells, CO-mediated affects on guanylyl cyclase led to inhibition of ERK1/2 MAPK (Song et al., 2003b). Thus, this effect of CO on ERK 1/2 MAPK would serve to prevent overstimulation of this pathway and in turn, the uncontrolled proliferation of cells. ERK has been shown to phosphorylate the inhibitory protein of NFκB and thus facilitate activation of the transcription factor (Chun et al., 2003).

It has also been postulated that CO can activate transcription factors indirectly by mitochondrial-driven ROS production (Piantadosi, 2008). More specifically, it is known that CO is a potent inhibitor of the complex III-mediated terminal step of oxidative phosphorylation. The inhibition of this step of the mitochondrial electron transport chain results in excess ROS production which in turn, reacts with critical thiol groups of the phosphatases that turn off activated transcription factors. In this regard, CO-mediated, mitochondrial ROS production has been implicated in the prolonged activation of the phosphoinositide-3-kinase (PI3 kinase)/Akt pathway (Piantadosi, 2008;Pischke et al., 2005). Numerous studies have implicated this pathway in the protective effects of plant-derived antioxidants (that include induction of HO-1) by ultimately leading to the activation of the transcription factors, Nrf2 (Martin et al., 2004;Park et al., 2011;Pugazhenthi et al., 2007). Nrf2 is a member of the Cap-N-Collar/basic leucine zipper family of transcription factor that responds directly and indirectly to oxidative stress to mediate cytoprotective gene transcription through the antioxidant response elements (ARE) of gene promoters (reviewed in (Itoh et al., 1997;Itoh et al., 2003;Kwak et al., 2004)). Thus, CO-mediated activation of PI3 kinase/Akt provides anti-oxidative protection.

4.2 Regulation of important enzymes by HO-1

It was also discussed how the CO released from HO-1 can inhibit various enzyme activities. The ability of the molecule to inhibit cyclooxygenase may provide an anti-inflammatory effect by preventing the synthesis of inflammatory prostaglandins from arachidonic acid. CO also inhibits cytochromes P450. This action could be cytoprotective because unproductive P450-mediated metabolism results in the release of hydrogen peroxide and/or superoxide from the P450 active site. This activity is an unavoidable consequence of metabolism by these enzymes, and the amount of ROS produced in this manner is dependent on the substrate being metabolized and the specific type of P450 carrying out the reaction (Gorsky et al., 1984;Gruenke et al., 1995;Reed and Hollenberg, 2003). Furthermore, it has been reported that P450-mediated metabolism can generate destructive hydroxyl radicals under certain circumstances (Paller and Jacob, 1994;Terelius and Ingelman-Sundberg, 1988). The oxidative stress generated by P450-mediated metabolism is significant as it has been estimated that the rate of ROS formation by the endoplasmic reticulum can be as much as 30% of that by mitochondria during oxidative phosphorylation (Zangar et al., 2004).

In an idea originally proposed at the turn of the century, HO-1 may provide cytoprotection by indirectly inhibiting P450 activity (and its associated production of ROS) through its competition with P450 for binding to the P450 reductase (Emerson and LeVine, 2000). Both P450s and HO-1 obtain electrons needed for their respective reactions by binding to the P450

Elucidating the Role of Biliverdin Reductase in the Expression of Heme Oxygenase-1 as a Cytoprotective
Response to Stress

53

reductase. One of the odd aspects of the stoichiometry of these enzymes in the endoplasmic reticulum is that the amount of P450 enzymes far outnumber the amount of P450 reductase (with estimates as high as 25 P450s for every P450 reductase (Peterson et al., 1976). Thus, P450-mediated metabolism in the liver endoplasmic reticulum is extremely limited by the amount of available P450 reductase. Although the level of HO-1 in unstressed liver is very low, it can be induced to an amount that is comparable to that of P450s (Reed et al., 2011). Therefore, it seems likely that the induction of HO-1 would attenuate the rate of P450-mediated metabolism by limiting the ability of P450 to interact with P450 reductase. A preliminary investigation from our lab has provided support for this effect of HO-1 induction (Reed et al., 2011). Furthermore, recent studies in which cells were protected from oxidative stress by the transfection and induction of a mutant HO-1 which was not able to catalyze heme degradation also provides support for this type of indirect mechanism of cytoprotection (Lin et al., 2007;Lin et al., 2008). However as discussed below, the results with the shortened, inactive mutant could be explained if the mutant serves as a heme-carrier to shuttle heme to the nucleus in order to directly modulate gene transcription.

Although far from proven, HO-1 also might actually interact with P450 enzymes to accelerate the degradation of the P450s. Several studies, including a few that were cited above (Nakahira et al., 2003;Odaka et al., 2000), have postulated that HO-1 induction following a stress event coincides with a rapid accumulation of free heme which presumably originates from damaged P450 enzymes. Evidence also was derived by observing a dramatic increase in the rate of degradation of labeled heme from P450 enzymes after HO-1 was induced by either hemin or endotoxin treatment (Bissell and Hammaker, 1976). More specifically, the data suggested that HO-1 increased the degradation of the P450 and not just the catabolism of the heme released from the P450. Again, it is not possible to ascertain whether the damaged P450 releases the heme or the HO-1 binds to the P450 to scavenge and catabolize its heme group. More direct evidence of this putative effect of HO-1 was reported in a study finding that the incubation of purified P450s with either HO-1 and HO-2 caused the heme of the P450 enzymes to be degraded to biliverdin in essentially a 1 to 1 ratio (Kutty et al., 1988). The results also were consistent with the interaction of HO-1 and P450 causing one P450 (two were studied in the publication) to degrade to an inactive form.

Surprisingly, the research supporting the idea that HO-1 facilitates degradation of P450s is decades old but has not been followed up on and confirmed. One reason for this is the fact that the full-length HO-1 is very unstable and susceptible to truncation that generates an inactive, soluble form (28 kDa). The C-terminal part of the protein that is cleaved causes the HO-1 to interact with membrane lipids, and its removal alters the manner by which the enzyme interacts with potential membrane binding partners (Huber, III et al., 2009;Huber, III and Backes, 2007). Most in vitro studies of HO-1 have expressed and purified a modified, but active, 30 kDa form of the enzyme that lacks the C-terminal membrane-binding sequence and is soluble as a result. Our lab has recently modified the amino acid sequence of full-length HO-1 to remove a thrombin cleavage site in the C-terminal tale of HO-1 (Huber, III and Backes, 2007). This mutant is full-length and binds to lipid vesicles. The full-length HO-1 mutant also binds much tighter to the P450 reductase and has much higher catalytic efficiency than the active, soluble form of the enzyme (Huber, III et al., 2009). Thus, studies with this mutant will finally enable researchers to understand the enzymatic capability of HO-1 with respect to those of the other potential binding partners in the endoplasmic reticulum. The putative interaction of HO-1 with P450 may allow for very efficient inhibition of the P450 by the HO-1-generated CO, providing a cytoprotective role by effectively removing the P450 as a contributor to cellular, oxidative stress.

4.3 Protective role of biliverdin/bilirubin

Originally biliverdin and the bilirubin formed by the BVR-catalyzed reduction of biliverdin were thought to be cellular waste products. However, it is apparent that both compounds have antioxidant properties and elicit various cytoprotective effects. Early studies implicated the antioxidant effects of these compounds by showing that they reacted with enzymatically generated superoxide in vitro (Galliani et al., 1985;Robertson, Jr. and Fridovich, 1982). Subsequent studies showed bilirubin to be a more potent antioxidant than α-tocopherol with respect to scavenging lipid peroxides (Neuzil and Stocker, 1993). In fact, both biliverdin and bilirubin were found to interact synergistically with vitamin E to prevent lipid peroxidation by an azo compound (Stocker and Peterhans, 1989). The fact that both of these bile pigments are lipophilic, especially bilirubin, makes them typically more effective than water soluble antioxidants in preventing the damage of membranes and organelles. Bilirubin bound to albumin was also shown to be an effective antioxidant in plasma by protecting the oxidation of low density lipoproteins (Stocker et al., 1987). In addition to its ability to scavenge ROS, bilirubin also inhibits the superoxide-generating NADPH oxidase (Kwak et al., 1991).

Evidence for cytoprotection mediated by the bile pigments comes from several studies. Bilirubin was shown to protect both neuronal cultures (Dore et al., 1999) and HeLa cells (Baranano et al., 2002) from hydrogen peroxide-induced toxicity. Furthermore, when cellular bilirubin was depleted by incubation of the cells with short antisense RNA to BVR, preventing the expression of BVR and in turn, its catalyzed conversion of biliverdin to bilirubin, intracellular levels of ROS increased and promoted apoptotic death of neuronal and HeLa cells (Baranano et al., 2002). It was found that the effects of bilirubin depletion had a greater pro-oxidant effect than depletion of cellular glutathione. In another study, pretreatment of cultured endothelial cells with bilirubin also protected cultured endothelial cells from pro-inflammatory responses after challenge by oxidized LDL and TNF-α (Kawamura et al., 2005). The level of protection of the endothelial cells was comparable to that achieved by preinduction of HO-1 with hemin. Interestingly, CO treatment of the cells did not protect them from these responses.

Bilirubin and biliverdin have also been shown to be protective in animal studies. Injection of bilirubin into rats prevented glutathione depletion following administration of cadmium chloride (Ossola and Tomaro, 1995). The two bile pigments also have been shown to be effective in various models of ischemia/reperfusion injury (Clark et al., 2000;Fondevila et al., 2004). Biliverdin treatment was as effective as hemin-mediated HO-1 induction in protecting rats from acetaminophen toxicity (Chiu et al., 2002). Bilirubin treatment also protected rats challenged with endotoxin by preventing an inflammatory response in the animals (Wang et al., 2004). Biliverdin and bilirubin also react with reactive nitrogen species such as nitric oxide and peroxynitrite. Thus, the compounds can attenuate NO signaling, and this was believed to be the cause of the anti-inflammatory effect in the endotoxin study (Wang et al., 2004). Another anti-nitrosative effect of HO-1 recently discovered is the finding that increased HO-1 expression was associated with induction of endothelial cell superoxide dismutase (Kruger et al., 2005). This, in turn, would lower the amount of superoxide available to react with NO to form peroxynitrite.

Biliverdin also inhibits activation of NF-κB in HEK293 cells (Gibbs and Maines, 2007). The effect was observed to be specific for biliverdin and not bilirubin. In fact, overexpression of BVR, which converts the biliverdin to bilirubin, overcame the biliverdin-mediated inhibition of NF-κB. Thus, part of the anti-inflammatory effect of biliverdin may be caused by preventing activation of NF-κB. Biliverdin has also been shown to be a potent inhibitor of c-Jun N-terminal kinase and AP-1 pathway (Tang et al., 2007), and this effect has been associated with pro-inflammatory and pro-apoptotic responses. Bilirubin has been shown to modulate ERK1/2 signaling pathways (Taillé et al., 2003). Furthermore, it has now been shown that both biliverdin and bilirubin activate the aryl hydrocarbon receptor to induce expression of a spectrum of genes including CYP1A1 (Phelan et al., 1998). At this point, it is not fully appreciated how these cell-signaling effects mediated by biliverdin and bilirubin relate to cytoprotection.

In summary, the effects of biliverdin and bilirubin are complex and are poorly understood. Protection by these compounds seems to derive from antioxidant properties of the compounds as well as anti-nitrosative effects from scavenging NO. However, many more mechanisms may be involved to explain their effects. In fact, the effects of these compounds on cell signaling pathways are only beginning to be elucidated. It should also be mentioned that the balance between cytoprotection and toxicity is delicate in the case of bilirubin. High concentrations of this compound are neurotoxic and pro-oxidative (Claireaux et al., 1953;Stocker and Ames, 1987) adding to the complexity and importance of cellular heme regulation.

4.4 Ferrous iron release: The participation of ferritin and HO-1

You can put a rose on a herring, but it will still stink and be red. The same analogy can be used when trying to argue the protective "benefits" of HO-1-mediated ferrous iron production. Free ferrous iron will be a "smelly, red herring" with regards to oxidative/reductive homeostasis in the cell. As mentioned at the beginning of the chapter, the metal is prone to generating highly destructive hydroxyl radicals. Thus, it is a powerful pro-oxidant which would cause it to potentiate oxidative stress. In fact, a study which over-expressed HO-1 through a tetracycline-inducible vector found that the mutant cells were much more prone to deleterious iron-overload (Suttner and Dennery, 1999). Thus, HO-1 expression had a negative effect on cell survival in this instance. Presumably, HO-1 over-expression also could have a negative health impact from the potential build-up of bilirubin levels, as described above.

On the other hand, the metal is essential for the synthesis of heme and in turn, for all of the functions carried out by the heme proteins. Thus, HO-1 does provide a way for the iron in free heme or heme attached to damaged enzymes (which may act as even more potent pro-oxidants than free iron) to be recycled for future heme synthesis in the cell, so its activity does have a net positive effect on cellular health. Furthermore, heme induction also activates expression of the iron-storage protein, ferritin (Eisenstein et al., 1991). Thus, during heme-related stress, both ferritin and HO-1 are coordinately regulated (Tsuji et al., 2000). Ferritin is an iron storage protein that allows for the controlled release of iron to coincide with the metabolic needs of the cell (Ponka, 1997).

Interestingly, it has been suggested that there are *at least* two types of HO-1 inducing agents, heme-dependent and heme-independent (Bauer and Bauer, 2002). Subsequently, it was shown that heme-independent HO-1 induction did not necessarily induce ferritin (Sheftel et al., 2007). However, HO-1 will only produce excess free iron when there is an abundant supply of heme, so the ferritin will be induced in the cell when it is needed. In the study cited above (Suttner and Dennery, 1999) indicating iron over-load in cells overexpressing HO-1, the cells were transfected with an expression vector. Thus, hemin was not involved in the induction of HO-1 and consequently, ferritin was not induced enough to protect against iron overload from catalytically active HO-1.

Although it has not been proven definitively, it has been speculated that the location of HO-1 in the endoplasmic reticulum may facilitate the migration of free iron to the extracellular space and in turn, help maintain iron blood levels (Poss and Tonegawa, 1997a). Whether or not this putative role of HO-1 exists, the activity of the enzyme and the co-ordinate regulation of ferritin when HO-1 is induced through its cognate promoter give the cell a protective way to recycle iron and manage its levels in the cell.

5. Mechanisms of cellular protection by BVR

5.1 BVR-catalyzed redox cycle with lipid peroxides

The anti-oxidant effects and other positive health benefits of bilirubin, that are attributable to catalysis by BVR, are obviously important means of BVR-mediated cytoprotection. The antioxidant effects of this compound were discussed above, but the reason for its potency involves metabolism by BVR. In a study examining the cytoprotective effects of bilirubin in neuronal cells, it was found that as little as 10 nM bilirubin (physiologic levels) protected against 10,000-fold higher concentrations of hydrogen peroxide (Baranano et al., 2002). From these results, it was postulated that BVR participates in a redox cycle with lipid peroxides in which bilirubin is oxidized by the lipid peroxides to biliverdin which, in turn, is reduced by BVR to reform bilirubin (Figure 1). Thus, BVR may have an important role in extending the antioxidant potency of bilirubin. It should be noted that a recent study concluded that the cytoprotective role of this redox cycle was limited as BVR overexpression and inhibition of BVR expression with antisense RNA did not seem to influence hydrogen peroxide-mediated cytotoxicity (Maghzal et al., 2009).

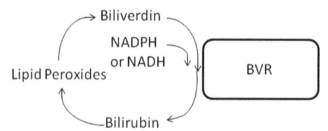

Fig. 1. BVR-catalyzed redox cycle with lipid peroxides. See text for details

5.2 BVR-mediated modulation of cell signaling

BVR may be the most versatile protein known. Research over the last decade has revealed new functions for the enzyme that have broadened its role in the cytoprotective response to cellular stress signals. It is now known that BVR also functions as a dual-specific kinase of serine/threonine and tyrosine residues in proteins, and in this capacity, BVR affects the signaling and cellular responses to a variety of stimuli (Reviewed in (Kapitulnik and Maines, 2009)). Kinases capable of phosphorylating both threonine and tyrosine residues have been identified as those regulating upstream events in signal transduction pathways (Pawson and Scott, 2005). The discovery of this function of BVR was preceded by finding that its ability to metabolize biliverdin was dependent on protein phosphorylation and that the enzyme could catalyze autophosphorylation of this residue (Salim et al., 2001).

Subsequently, it was shown that BVR is regulated by insulin/insulin growth factor stimulation through receptor-mediated tyrosine phosphorylation (Lerner-Marmarosh et al., 2005). BVR binding to this receptor competes with insulin receptor substrates (IRS) 1 and 2 for binding to the receptor. BVR phosphorylates serine residues of the IRS which attenuates their affinity for the insulin receptor kinase, essentially inactivating them. Phosphorylated BVR can activate two protein kinase C proteins, βII and ζ, which are involved in cross-talk between the upstream components of the MAPK and phosphatidylinositol 3-kinase pathways, respectively. Protein kinase C βII also can activate BVR which partly contributes to the activation of BVR by stress signals (Maines et al., 2007). The activation of protein kinase C βII by BVR leads to activation of all three arms of the MAPK signaling. Thus, all of the effects of CO caused by its activation of the P38 MAPK (discussed above) also apply to the activation of this pathway by BVR.

BVR-mediated signaling appears to play a critical role in the recruiting transcription factor, NFκB to the HO-1 promoter (Gibbs and Maines, 2007). Furthermore, NFκB has been shown to be activated by protein kinase Cζ which in turn, is directly activated by BVR (Lerner-Marmarosh et al., 2007). As described in detail below, the involvement of NFκB appears to be important in mediating the anti-apoptotic, anti-inflammatory, and anti-proliferative effects associated with expression of HO-1.

BVR has the ability to form protein complexes with itself and other proteins, and serves to shuttle activated transcription factors to the nucleus. The ability of BVR to function as a dual cofactor enzyme with different pH optima expands its range of function in the cell (Kapitulnik and Maines, 2009). In addition to the activation of the ERK MAPK pathway by BVR through protein kinase C βII, BVR has been shown to play a critical role in shuttling the activated ERK to the nucleus to influence gene transcription (Lerner-Marmarosh et al., 2008).

Interestingly, BVR also binds to NFκB (Gibbs and Maines, 2007). This is intriguing because the HO-1 promoter does not have a prototypical response element for NFκB, and it has been conjectured that it must be recruited to the promoter by other transcription factors (Alam and Cook, 2007). Thus, through this interaction, BVR also may play a role in allowing NFκB to influence HO-1 gene transcription.

In another transport capacity, BVR also complexes with heme and shuttles it to the nucleus where the heme can bind to regulatory elements that influence gene transcription. In fact, heme-mediated gene induction has been shown to be dependent on BVR in renal cells (Tudor et al., 2008). Interestingly, although HO-1 is most typically observed in the endoplasmic reticulum, instances of it being located in other parts of the cell including the plasma membrane (where it localizes to caveolae rafts (Kim et al., 2004)), mitochondria

(Converso et al., 2006), and even as a shortened, soluble component in the nucleus have been reported (Lin et al., 2007). The significance of these findings has yet to be elucidated, but they may indicate that HO-1 also can transport heme to the nucleus (discussed below) and may be involved in targeting BVR to different organelles to mediate signaling or the biliverdin/BVR redox cycle to scavenge ROS from the mitochondria (discussed above).

5.3 BVR-mediated modulation of gene transcription through DNA binding

Although the kinase-dependent activity described above ultimately results in the modulation of gene transcription, BVR also has the capacity to bind to DNA and directly influence gene expression through a basic leucine zipper-binding motif. BVR binds to AP-1/CRE sites in DNA which are typically bound by c-Jun/fos heterodimers to mediate the stress response (Ahmad et al., 2002). In this capacity, BVR binds as homo- and hetero-dimers to recruit or block the binding of other transcription factors and thus, BVR can enhance or inhibit gene expression directly. At this point, BVR-mediated gene transcription has been shown to induce ATF-2 (Kravets et al., 2004). ATF-2 has also been shown to be capable of binding to and activating NFκB (Kaszubska et al., 1993).

Thus, with regards to the role of BVR in recruiting NFκB to the HO-1 promoter, BVR can facilitate its binding directly or through the upregulation and activation of ATF-2. However, it is likely that NFκB would bind to the promoter in different 5′-flanking regions when bound to BVR and ATF-2. Most of the specific effects of BVR-DNA binding on gene expression have not been elucidated. But the enzyme has been shown to translocate to the nucleus of HeLa cells (Tudor et al., 2008) after hemin induction and in rat kidney after exposure of animals to nephrotoxins (Maines et al., 2001). In fact, HeLa, heme-mediated induction of HO-1 expression was shown to be dependent on BVR expression (Tudor et al., 2008).

6. Assessing the dependence of HO-1-mediated cytoprotection on BVR

Given the diverse abilities of BVR to regulate cellular processes, it has been postulated that the HO-1 cytoprotective response is completely dependent on BVR. The hypothesis proposes that the increased expression of HO-1 caused by the wide variety of inducing agents is mediated by the signaling and DNA binding activities of BVR. Furthermore, in a study examining the catalytic steps of the HO-1 reaction, it was determined that binding of BVR and HO-1 was required to increase the rate of release of biliverdin from the HO-1 active site. The study found that in the absence of BVR, biliverdin release was the rate-limiting step of the HO-1 reaction, and its presence dramatically increased turnover by HO-1. In showing that even the catalytic activity of the enzyme was dependent on BVR, the study supported the idea that the HO-1 cytoprotective response was totally dependent on BVR. However, finding that HO-1 activity was dependent on BVR was counter-intuitive because the level of HO-1 can be induced many-fold by cellular exposure to stress signals (Wright et al., 2006). In contrast, the expression level of BVR is typically unchanged after stress (although it may be inducible in kidney (Maines et al., 2001)). Thus, it would seem to be unproductive for the cell to induce HO-1 and have its activity be limited by the supply of BVR. Such a situation also would allow little opportunity for biliverdin to accumulate in cells. Yet, studies show that biliverdin has completely different cytoprotective roles than bilirubin (see above). Thus, the enzymatic data showing that BVR regulated HO-1 enzymatic activity were baffling.

More recent enzymatic studies measuring steady state metabolism by HO-1 showed that BVR had no effect on the rate of HO-1-mediated catalysis (Reed et al., 2010). In fact, this study showed that the rates of HO-1-mediated heme catabolism measured by the formation of both biliverdin and a ferrozene:ferrous iron complex in the absence of BVR were slightly higher than that measured by bilirubin formation in the presence of BVR. The earlier results finding that HO-1 activity was dependent on BVR were attributed to the unusual conditions required to monitor the individual catalytic steps (namely anaerobic with limiting concentrations of NADPH).

The question still remains whether the HO-1-related gene response following exposure to stress signals is completely dependent on BVR. The HO-1 promoter contains a variety of responsive elements that includes two AP-1 sites, a CRE, a Maf recognition domain (binding partner to Nrf2), and a partial site for NFκB binding (Alam and Cook, 2007). Understanding how these responsive elements recruit transcription factors to influence gene transcription is complicated by the fact that many of the response elements overlap and thus, may inhibit or enhance DNA binding by factors to adjacent elements. The transcription factors that activate the HO-1 promoter will vary with the types of stress to which the cell is exposed (reviewed in (Alam and Cook, 2007). Furthermore, studies have shown that the signaling pathways activated by the same stress signals also can vary in different cell types (Ryter et al., 2006). As a result, the transcription factors mediating a specific cytoprotective response can vary in different cell types. Thus, a type of HO-1-mediated cytoprotection may depend on BVR in some cell types but not others. Because of these considerations, the discussion pertaining to the dependence of HO-1 expression on BVR will be a generalization based on the typical roles of the implicated transcription factors in cellular processes.

6.1 Anti-oxidant protection

With this perspective in mind, the various protective roles of cell signaling and gene transcription associated with HO-1 induction are mediated largely through activation of either Nrf2 or NFκB. Certainly one of the first evolutionary roles needed for survival of a cell would have been to develop a defense system for the oxidative stress associated with the activity of heme enzymes. Heme oxygenase is the only enzyme that uses its heme cofactor as a substrate. Furthermore, as discussed below, HO-1 can be induced directly by heme interaction with the HO-1 gene repressor Bach-1. Therefore, it is the only known eukaryotic enzyme that has a substrate that regulates a transcription factor needed for its expression. This scenario would suggest that heme oxygenase represents a very old link in the evolutionary chain. By the same line of reasoning used above to rationalize the evolutionary role of HO-1 function, Nrf2/anti-oxidant response must represent an early evolutionary adaptation to allow living organisms to survive oxidative stress. Interestingly, Bach-1 is an effective repressor of the HO-1 gene because it blocks Nrf2 from binding to the HO-1 promoter. Because heme metabolism is intimately connected to reductive/oxidative homeostasis in the cell, it seems plausible that Nrf2 can mediate HO-1 expression independently from BVR as a response (initially at least) to oxidative stress.

One caveat to the hypothesis that the anti-oxidative response is independent of BVR is dictated by whether or not the shuttling of heme to the nucleus by BVR is the only mechanism by which this can occur (discussed above). As alluded to above, Bach 1 blocks the binding of Nrf2 to the antioxidant response element when Bach 1 is not bound to heme

(Sun et al., 2002). In support of the idea that an anti-oxidant response can be mediated directly by Nrf2 without involvement of BVR, HO-1 was found to be constitutively expressed in Bach 1 knockout mice (Sun et al., 2002). Thus, it is proposed that nuclear heme localization and functional Nrf2 are the essential components of the initial gene response to oxidative stress. In some instances, BVR has been shown to be critical for heme translocation to the nucleus. However, the results are mixed and may be cell type-specific. For instance, the same laboratory has shown that inhibition of BVR expression with small interference (antisense) RNA blocked the hemin-mediated induction of HO-1 cells in HeLa cells (Tudor et al., 2008) but had no effect in COS cells (Ahmad et al., 2002).

Recent studies showing that shortened HO-1 also translocates to the nucleus may serve as another mechanism by which hemin is transported to the nucleus to directly influence gene transcription (Lin et al., 2007). This would allow the shuttling role of BVR to be bypassed in some cells and would explain results showing that increased expression of a catalytically inactive mutant was also able to up-regulate HO-1 expression (Lin et al., 2008). Another way that cells could possibly bypass BVR-mediated heme shuttling can be postulated from the results of a study showing that heme bound to and stabilized Nrf2 (Alam et al., 2003). This led to activation of Nrf2 and the heme-responsive element in the HO-1 promoter. Thus, Nrf2 could also transport heme to the nucleus to influence gene transcription during oxidative stress. Therefore, it does seem necessary to require BVR to transport heme to the nucleus for most cell types.

There also are several general experimental findings that support this intuitive argument. First, Nrf2 is believed to be the primary transcription factor activated directly by oxidative stress, and its activation is associated with induction of phase II and antioxidant enzymes (Bellezza et al., 2010;Ishii et al., 2002;Shen et al., 2005). A multitude of studies have implicated Nrf2 in the induction of HO-1 during oxidative stress (Alam et al., 2003;Gong and Cederbaum, 2006a;Gong and Cederbaum, 2006b;Sun Jang et al., 2009). Finally, in two studies looking at the effects of oxidative stress (by hydrogen peroxide treatment), it was found that cell viability was only marginally affected (Baranano et al., 2002) or not affected at all (Maghzal et al., 2009) by silencing BVR (with interference RNA). The latter study also showed that BVR induction and over-expression also did not provide protection to the cells exposed to hydrogen peroxide. Thus, it may not be a coincidence that studies have not yet implicated a connection between BVR actions and Nrf2. In fact, the binding site for Nrf2 in the HO-1 promoter overlaps with one of the AP-1 sites to which BVR can bind (Alam and Cook, 2007). Differences between antioxidant response elements and AP-1 binding sites have been distinguished previously (Yoshioka et al., 1995). Thus, it appears Nrf2 binding and AP-1 binding by BVR might be somewhat competitive with Nrf2 binding occurring initially after oxidative stress and BVR replacing the transcription factor from the antioxidant response element after prolonged oxidative stress.

In addition, to the demonstration of constitutive HO-1 expression in Bach-1 knockout mice, there appears to be a unique aspect of the HO-1 promoter which allows Nrf2 to initiate transcription without recruitment of other transcription factors. It has been found that the chromatin remodeling protein, BRG1, interacts with Nrf2 to form a Z-DNA structure which permits access for RNA polymerase II to initiate transcription of the HO-1 gene (Zhang et al., 2006). This interaction between BRG-1 and Nrf2 was exclusive to the HO-1 gene (but not other Nrf2–regulated genes) by virtue of a series of TG repeats that are present in the HO-1 promoter. In fact, genetic polymorphisms affecting this region have been shown to correspond to susceptibility to oxidative stress-related diseases (Ishii et al., 2000).

Thus, the right panel of Figure 2 is drawn to indicate the BVR-independent activation of HO-1 gene transcription after exposure to oxidative stress. ROS can activate Nrf2 directly by oxidizing Keap-1 which is responsible for binding Nrf2 in the cytoplasm and facilitating its degradation (Itoh et al., 2003). Oxidation of critical cysteine residues in Keap-1 releases Nrf2, allowing it to translocate to the nucleus and activate gene transcription (reviewed in (Kwak et al., 2004)). In addition, CO inhibits mitochondrial electron transport resulting in ROS production which inhibit phosphatases needed to inactivate PI3K. Prolonged activation of PI3K results in stimulation of Akt which can phosphorylate Nrf2 (Piantadosi, 2008). Phosphorylation causes Keap-1 to release and activate Nrf2. ROS can also lead to activation of JNK MAPK. It has been shown that JNK target, c-Jun, can bind to Nrf2 (Shen et al., 2005). Thus, c-Jun/fos dimers binding to the AP-1 site facilitate the recruitment of Nrf2 to bind to the overlapping Maf-recognition element and induce HO-1 transcription. Previous binding by the c-Jun/fos dimer may help facilitate the binding of Nrf2 if Nrf2 can exchange with fos for binding to c-Jun. BVR is shown in this panel to serve as a heme transporter to the nucleus. That putative role is also indicated for the shortened form of HO-1 that has been identified in the nucleus (Lin et al., 2007) and for Nrf2. One additional role that BVR could play in the prolonged anti-oxidant response is to modulate the initial response by increasing or decreasing the anti-oxidant response depending on the needs of the cell.

6.2 Anti-apoptotic/proliferation protection

For the reasons below, it is postulated that BVR plays an integral role in the signaling responsible for anti-proliferative, anti-inflammatory, and anti-apoptotic responses by facilitating the interaction of NFκB with the HO-1 promoter and by modulating the activity of the transcription factor. As mentioned above, NFκB regulates the expression of cytokines, growth factors, and cell cycle effector proteins (Du et al., 1993;Hayden and Ghosh, 2011;Peng et al., 1995). As a result, the factor regulates important physiological processes such as immune response and apoptosis, and overstimulation or dysregulation of this factor is associated with inflammation, transformation, and proliferation of cells (Bubici et al., 2006). Thus, the cytoprotective role of HO-1 induction for processes such as inflammation, apoptosis, and proliferation would logically involve mechanisms affecting NFκB function. Scientific studies have shown that NFκB and Nrf2 are oppositely and variably regulated by different types of cellular stress (Bellezza et al., 2010). Nrf2 is typically activated by low or moderate levels oxidative stress, whereas NFκB is turned on by inflammatory signals or very high levels of oxidative stress. Thus, with regards to the HO-1 promoter and various cytoprotective responses mediated by enzyme induction, stress signals will specifically alter the relative levels of cellular transcription factors and in turn, will determine whether Nrf2 or NFκB binds to activate transcription of the HO-1 gene. The JNK MAPK target, c-Jun has been shown to bind to Nrf2 (Shen et al., 2005), and inhibit NFκB (Tan et al., 2009). However, the P38 MAPK target, ATF-2 has been shown to bind to NFκB (Kaszubska et al., 1993). The model below proposes that the relative levels of c-Jun and ATF-2 play a major role in different cytoprotective responses mediated by HO-1 induction.

One essential role that BVR may play in modulating cytoprotective gene expression associated with HO-1 induction is the activation and recruitment of NFκB to the HO-1 promoter (Gibbs and Maines, 2007). It is proposed that this function is the main determinant in mediating the anti-apoptotic response associated with HO-1 induction. NFκB activation has been associated with prevention of apoptosis following treatment with cytokines and tumor promoters (Papa et al., 2006;Sen et al., 1996). Biliverdin inhibits activation of NFκB (Gibbs and Maines, 2007), and BVR reverses this affect by metabolizing biliverdin to bilirubin and by promoting PKCζ-mediated phosphorylation and activation of the transcription factor (Lerner-Marmarosh et al., 2007).

The importance of BVR in mediating the apoptotic response has been demonstrated repeatedly. When BVR was over-expressed in HEK 293 and MCF-7 cells, the cells were arrested in G_1/G_0 stage (Gibbs and Maines, 2007). Furthermore, over-expression of BVR also protected cells from NFκB-mediated proliferation after stimulation with TNF-α (Gibbs et al., 2010). These findings are consistent with a number of studies that have used various cell types (HEK293 (Miralem et al., 2005), HeLa (Ahmad et al., 2002), cardiomyocytes (Pachori et al., 2007) and renal epithelial cells (Young et al., 2009)) to show that the inhibition of BVR expression using interference RNA resulted in apoptosis after the cells were challenged with arsenite, hydrogen peroxide, hypoxia/reoxygenation, and angiotensin II, respectively. Thus, repression of BVR expression consistently leads to apoptosis after cells are challenged with various types of stressors. Most importantly, with regards to protection from apoptosis, NFκB has been shown to be a necessary factor for the activation of the tumor suppressor protein, P53 (Ryan et al., 2000). Consistent with the role of BVR in preventing apoptosis, bilirubin also has been shown to have anti-apoptotic effects in a variety of studies (Bulmer et al., 2008;Kim et al., 2006;Parfenova et al., 2006). In addition, activation of ERK MAP kinases (mediated by BVR (Lerner-Marmarosh et al., 2008)) has been shown to favor anti-apoptotic responses (Wada and Penninger, 2004) which would also be consistent with the anti-apoptotic role of BVR. For these reasons, it seems probable that the BVR-mediated recruitment and activation of NFκB are essential for anti-apoptotic HO-1 induction.

It is speculated that BVR also plays another important role in the anti-apoptotic signal. Studies have shown that BVR induces expression of P38 MAPK target, ATF-2 (Kravets et al., 2004). ATF-2 is constitutively expressed and not induced by environmental stimuli (unlike c-Jun) (Angel and Karin, 1991;Herdegen and Leah, 1998). Furthermore, it can form mixed dimers with c-Jun, and this hetero-dimer binds with much tighter affinity to AP-1 sites than c-Jun/fos dimers (Benbrook and Jones, 1990). Furthermore, ATF-2 dimerizes with itself and binds to the CRE response element instead of the AP-1 stress response element. Most importantly with respect to anti-proliferative, anti-inflammatory, and anti-apoptotic cytoprotection, ATF-2 also has been shown to dimerize with NFκB (Kaszubska et al., 1993). It is proposed in the mechanism below that these functions of ATF-2 along with the participation of BVR mediate HO-1-related cytoprotection from apoptotic, inflammatory, and hyper-proliferative stimuli.

The left panel of Figure 2 shows cell signaling cascades that may mediate the general anti-apoptotic HO-1 response. It seems likely that apoptotic/anti-apoptotic specificity involves a change in gene expression mediated by c-Jun/fos dimerization to one mediated by ATF-2 homo-dimerization. The critical events in this transition are BVR-mediated activation of NFκB (by direct phosphorylation and metabolism of biliverdin (BV in figure) to bilirubin (BR) and amplification of P38 MAPK relative to the c-Jun arm of MAPK). As mentioned above, biliverdin has been shown to be an inhibitor of NFκB (Gibbs and Maines, 2007). The amplification of P38 MAPK relative to JNK and ERK MAPKs would be consistent with the effects of CO as the molecule activates P38 but inhibits JNK/ERK MAPKs (summarized above). In addition, biliverdin has been shown to be a potent inhibitor of JNK MAPK (Tang et al., 2007). Furthermore, c-Jun activation has been linked to cellular proliferation (Yoshioka et al., 1995) so switching from c-Jun-driven to ATF-2-driven transcription would be protective against proliferation/transformation. To show attenuation of the JNK MAPK pathway, the JNK arm of MAPK is shown as a dashed arrow in the figure panel to show that its activation is attenuated relative to that of P38 kinase. Because BVR has been shown to activate ERK MAPK (Lerner-Marmarosh et al., 2008), the arrow from ERK is a mixed dash/dot symbol to show moderate activation. Activation of ERK MAPK has been shown to facilitate anti-apoptotic responses (Wada and Penninger, 2004), and this might be related to the ability of ERK proteins to catalyze phosphorylation of the NFκB-inhibitory protein that keeps NFκB in the cytosol (for review of NFκB activation see (Shen et al., 2005)). As described above, signaling and DNA transcription mediated by BVR also lead to activation and increased expression of the P38 target, ATF-2, so this is another factor that increases the relative activation and concentration of ATF-2 (note the arrow from BVR to ATF-2 in the panel). Furthermore, BVR activates PKCβII (the latter can also activate BVR so a double headed arrow connects the two kinases in the panel) which serves to activate all three arms of MAPK signaling.

As ATF-2 concentrations and its level of activation increases relative to c-Jun and fos, c-Jun/fos hetero-dimerization would be replaced with c-Jun/ATF-2 dimerization at the AP-1 site. Because a P38-mediated pathway leading to activation of Nrf2 has been reported as a cytoprotective response in a cell line derived from human bronchial epithelial cells that were exposed to CeO2 nanoparticles, it is possible that the c-Jun/ATF-2 dimer serves as a more potent transcription factor in the recruitment of Nrf2 to the HO-1 promoter (Eom and Choi, 2009). Further increases in the concentration of ATF-2 would favor homo-dimerization of the transcription factor at the CRE site instead of the AP-1 site. ATF-2 has been shown to bind to NFκB (Kaszubska et al., 1993), and it has been shown that P38-mediated phosphorylation of Nrf2 promotes its association with the inhibitory protein, Keap1 (Keum et al., 2006). Both of these aspects of P38 pathway activation would favor activation of NFκB over Nrf2. Thus, it is proposed that the ATF-2 dimerization is the key signal that recruits NFκB to bind to the HO-1 promoter to induce expression of the gene. As proposed in the anti-oxidant response with the c-Jun/fos dimer facilitating recruitment of Nrf2 to the promoter, the ATF-2 dimer would allow NFκB to bind to the promoter as it exchanges with one of the ATF-2 units of the dimer. Another consistent aspect of the transition from the binding of c-Jun to that of ATF-2 in the recruitment of NFκB is the finding that c-Jun has been shown to inhibit NFκB activation (Tan et al., 2009).Thus, in the left panel of figure 2, the role of ATF-2 is represented by having its arrow point towards that for NFκB in the nucleus. Consistent with studies showing that Nrf2 and NFκB are co-regulated in opposite directions in response to stress signals (Bellezza et al., 2010), binding by NFκB is proposed to displace Nrf2 from the HO-1 promoter. The change in binding to the CRE site also may be critical in this regard because the AP-1 site overlaps more with the Nrf2 binding site than the CRE site. Thus, there would be less competition between Nrf2 and NFκB for binding to the HO-1 promoter. Because BVR can bind to both CRE and NFκB (Gibbs and Maines, 2007;Kravets et al., 2004), it may also serve to recruit NFκB to bind near the CRE.

In addition to activating NFκB, BVR also binds to the transcription factor in a manner that modulates its activity to favor protective gene expression relative to harmful pro-apoptotic, pro-inflammatory and pro-proliferative targets (Gibbs et al., 2010). Consistent with the possibility that BVR regulates the activity of NFĸB, TNF-α-mediated stimulation caused NFĸB to act as a repressor of BVR expression which demonstrates that BVR is competitive with the inflammation process mediated by TNF-α through activation of NFĸB. Because of the BVR-mediated modulation of NFĸB, the arrow from NFĸB is drawn as a dash in the panel.

6.3 Anti-inflammatory protection

It appears that the anti-inflammatory effects associated with HO-1 induction (middle panel of figure 2) might be mediated by both BVR-dependent and BVR-independent processes. ROS formation (produced by immune cells) is a big component of inflammation. Thus, it seems unlikely that the anti-inflammatory response is totally regulated by BVR (middle panel of figure 2). Thus, for the reasons given in the preceding paragraph, Nrf2 will be activated independently of BVR, probably as an initial response to inflammatory stimuli. Another implication of the role of Nrf2 in the HO-1-related anti-inflammatory response has come from studies with plant-derived, phenolic diterpenes that elicit both anti-oxidant and anti-inflammatory responses. Not coincidentally, these compounds also mediate HO-1 induction through Nrf2 following stimulation of phosphatidylinositol 3-kinase (PI3-kinase)/Akt signaling (Martin et al., 2004;Pugazhenthi et al., 2007). The Akt protein kinase activated by PI3K is distinct from the PKCζ that is known to be activated by BVR (Lerner-Marmarosh et al., 2007). As described above, CO has been implicated in mediating signaling through Akt (Piantadosi and Zhang, 1996). Thus, this pathway of Nrf2 activation appears to be related directly to the catalytic activity of HO-1. These mechanisms activating Nrf2 contribute to the anti-inflammatory effects associated with HO-1 induction.

An appealing hypothesis, that seems consistent with research findings, proposes that BVR-independent processes activate Nrf2 at the early stages of inflammation, whereas BVR-mediated MAPK and NFĸB activation play critical roles in the cellular response at later stages of inflammation. In support of this idea, NFĸB signaling typically opposes Nrf2 mediated signaling as a later event in response to many stress events (Bellezza et al., 2010). The putative ability of BVR to bind and modulate the activity of NFĸB is important in the latter response because agonist binding to immune receptors cause potent activation of NFĸB. It is important to emphasize that this modulating role is not the only way BVR would protect cells from NFĸB-mediated stress. By replacing NFĸB with Nrf2 at the HO-1 promoter, BVR would be diverting NFĸB from promoting harmful gene expression while freeing up Nrf2 to activate protective gene expression. The anti-inflammatory effects of CO generated by HO-1 activity also would act independently of BVR (described above). A recent study demonstrated that HO-1 activity (as opposed to merely BVR-related cell signaling and DNA binding) was essential for the anti-inflammatory effects following treatment with endotoxin (Tamion et al., 2006). The anti-inflammatory response demonstrated by the treated animals was explained by both the inhibition of tumor necrosis factor-α production and the elevation of interleukin-10. Because the anti-inflammatory effects required catalytic activity by the induced HO-1 (activity was inhibited by treatment with tin mesoporphyrin), it can be assumed that either BVR-mediated signaling/DNA-binding was dependent on HO-1 activity or the effects were caused by bilirubin/CO. Either premise dictates that BVR effects occurred secondary to those mediated by HO-1 activity. For these reasons, it seems that the anti-inflammatory response is pleiotropic and depends on both BVR-dependent and BVR-independent signaling and gene transcription.

In the middle panel, the anti-inflammatory signaling that results in the later-staged recruitment of NFκB to the HO-1 promoter is represented. The scheme for Nrf2 activation preceding NFκB activation is shown in the far right panel. In the anti-inflammatory response, CO formed by HO-1 inhibits the JNK and ERK MAPK pathways. The CO-mediated inhibition of c-Jun protects against uncontrolled proliferation. However, BVR modulates ERK to protect against apoptosis through activation of NFκB. Initially, c-Jun inhibits NFκB activation which is shown as the red block line. Eventually, ERK activity and ATF-2 dimerization at the HO-1 promoter will favor gene transcription mediated by NFκB. BVR also modulates NFκB activity to favor protective gene expression, so the arrow from NFκB is dashed. In addition, as mentioned above, diversion of NFκB to stimulate the protective induction of HO-1 limits its ability to stimulate inflammatory gene expression and allows more Nrf2 to activate transcription of other anti-oxidant genes.

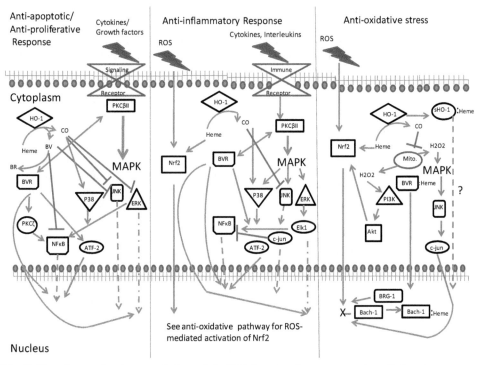

Fig. 2. Signal transduction regulation of the HO-1 protective response to cellular stress signals. The schematic diagram shows the putative signaling pathways responsible for gene induction/repression following different types of cellular stress (apoptotic signals, inflammatory stimuli, and oxidative stress). Arrows ending in the cytoplasm point at downstream kinases or transcription factors activated by the stimuli at the base of the arrow. Arrows ending in the nuclei represent the binding of transcription factors to gene promoters to affect expression and mediate the cytoprotective responses. Double-headed arrows represent kinase reactions that can occur in both directions (see text for details). Dashed arrows indicate attenuated activation, and arrows directed to the same point either have a role in binding together at the promoter or modulating the activity of one another.

7. Conclusions

Hemin is an essential cofactor for heme proteins that carry out a multitude of vital oxidative and oxygen transport-related functions in the cell. Unfortunately, hemin is also reactive and extremely harmful to cells when accumulated in the free form. A highly regulated system has evolved to control the levels of cellular heme. HO-1 and BVR catalyze the steps involved in heme catabolism. Interestingly, the enzymes are also involved in a host of cytoprotective functions mediating anti-oxidant, anti-apoptotic, anti-proliferative, and anti-inflammatory responses that have been proven to be therapeutic in many clinical disease models. HO-1 directly mediates most anti-oxidant effects through the following mechanisms: 1) the removal of heme in coordination with the up-regulation of the iron storage protein, ferritin; 2) the production of a lipophilic, anti-oxidant, biliverdin; 3) the regulation of both cell signaling and gene expression; and 4) the regulation of the cytochrome P450 system. Gene transcription mediated by Nrf2 largely mediates the cellular response to oxidative stress. BVR contributes to the antioxidant response by catalyzing a redox cycle that involves the BVR-mediated conversion of the potent antioxidant, bilirubin. In addition to catalyzing the second step of heme catabolism, BVR also acts as an upstream activator of MAPK and phosphatidylinositol-3-kinase pathway; directly binds to DNA; and participates in the transactivation of AP-1 sites in the HO-1 promoter. The anti-apoptotic effects associated with HO-1 induction are most often caused by BVR-mediated cell signaling and DNA-binding that leads to NFκB activation, but signaling effects related to HO-1-catalyzed CO production work in concert with the effects of BVR to protect against inflammation. Much remains to be learned about the specifics of cytoprotection via BVR-mediated signaling and gene transcription in addition to the roles of biliverdin and bilirubin in altering gene transcription. Similarly, because most in vitro studies of the enzymology of HO-1 have used a shortened mutant that does not bind to membrane or interact with membrane binding partners in the same manner as full length HO-1, almost nothing is known about how interactions between HO-1, BVR, and cytochrome P450 reductase are regulated to influence cell signaling, gene expression, the metabolism by HO-1, and oxidative stress related to P450-mediated, metabolism.

8. References

Abraham NG and Kappas A (2008) Pharmacological and clinical aspects of heme oxygenase. *Pharmacol.Rev.* 60:79-127.

Ahmad Z, Salim M, and Maines MD (2002) Human biliverdin reductase is a leucine zipper-like DNA-binding protein and functions in transcriptional activation of heme oxygenase-1 by oxidative stress. *J.Biol.Chem.* 277:9226-9232.

Alam J and Cook JL (2007) How many transcription factors does it take to turn on the heme oxygenase-1 gene? *Am.J.Respir.Cell Mol.Biol.* 36:166-174.

Alam J, Killeen E, Gong P, Naquin R, Stewart D, Ingelfinger JR, and Nath KA (2003) Heme activates the heme oxygenase-1 gene in renal epithelial cells by stabilizing Nrf2. *Am.J.Physiol.Renal Physiol.* 284:F743-F752.

Angel P and Karin M (1991) The role of Jun, Fos and the AP-1 complex in cell-proliferation and transformation. *Biochim.Biophys.Acta.* 1072:129-157.

Balla G, Vercellotti GM, Muller-Eberhard U, Eaton J, and Jacob HS (1991) Exposure of endothelial cells to free heme potentiates damage mediated by granulocytes and toxic oxygen species. *Lab Invest.* 64:648-655.

Baranano DE, Rao M, Ferris CD, and Snyder SH (2002) Biliverdin reductase: a major physiologic cytoprotectant. *Proc.Natl.Acad.Sci.USA* 99:16093-16098.

Bauer M and Bauer I (2002) Heme oxygenase-1: Redox Regulation and Role in the Hepatic Response to Oxidative Stress. *Antioxid.Redox.Signal.* 4:749-758.

Bellezza I, Mierla AL, and Minelli A (2010) Nrf2 and NF-κB and their concerted modulation in cancer pathogenesis and progression. *Cancers* 2:483-497.

Benbrook DM and Jones NC (1990) Heterodimer formation between CREB and JUN proteins. *Oncogene* 5:295-302.

Bissell DM and Hammaker LE (1976) Cytochrome P-450 Heme and the regulation of hepatic heme oxygenase activity. *Arch.Biochem.Biophys.* 176:91-102.

Bonizzi G and Karin M (2004) The two NF-kappaB activation pathways and their role in innate and adaptive immunity. *Trends Immunol.* 25:280-288.

Brouard S, Otterbein LE, Anrather J, Tobiasch E, Bach FH, Choi AM, and Soares MP (2000) Carbon monoxide generated by heme oxygenase 1 suppresses endothelial cell apoptosis. *J.Exp.Med.* 192:1015-1026.

Bubici, C., Papa, S., Dean, K., and Franzoso, G. Mutual cross-talk between reactive oxygen species and nuclear factor-kappa B: molecular basis and biological significance. Oncogene 25(51), 6731-6748. 2006.

Bulmer AC, Ried K, Blanchfield JT, and Wagner KH (2008) The anti-mutagenic properties of bile pigments. *Mutat.Res.* 658:28-41.

Cardell LO, Ueki IF, Stjärne P, Agusti C, Takeyama K, Lindén A, and Nadel JA (1998) Bronchodilatation in vivo by carbon monoxide, a cyclic GMP related messenger. *Br.J.Pharmacol.* 124:1065-1068.

Chen K, Gunter K, and Maines MD (2000) Neurons overexpressing heme oxygenase-1 resist oxidative stress-mediated cell death. *J.Neurochem.* 75:304-313.

Chen Q and Cederbaum AI (1998) Cytotoxicity and apoptosis produced by cytochrome P450 2E1 in Hep G2 cells. *Mol.Pharmacol.* 53:638-648.

Chiu H, Brittingham JA, and Laskin DL (2002) Differential induction of heme oxygenase-1 in macrophages and hepatocytes during acetaminophen-induced hepatotoxicity in the rat: effects of hemin and biliverdin. *Toxicol.Appl.Pharmacol.* 181:106-115.

Christodoulides N, Durante W, Kroll MH, and Chafer AI (1995) Vascular smooth muscle cell heme oxygenases generate guanylyl cyclase-stimulatory carbon monoxide. *Circulation* 91:2306-2309.

Chun KS, Keum.Y.S., Han SS, Song YS, Kim SH, and Surh YJ (2003) Curcumin inhibits phorbol ester-induced expression of cyclooxygenase-2 in mouse skin through suppression of extracellular signal-regulated kinase activity and NF-kappaB activation. *Carcinogenesis* 24:1515-1524.

Claireaux AE, Cole PG, and Lathe GH (1953) Icterus of the brain in the newborn. *Lancet* 265:1226-1230.

Clark JE, Foresti R, Sarathchandra P, Kaur H, Green CJ, and Motterlini R (2000) Heme oxygenase-1-derived bilirubin ameliorates postischemic myocardial dysfunction. *Am.J.Physiol.Heart Circ.Physiol.* 278:H643-H651.

Converso DP, Taillé C, Carreras MC, Jaitovich A, Poderoso JJ, and Boczkowski J (2006) HO-1 is located in liver mitochondria and modulates mitochondrial heme content and metabolism. *FASEB J.* 20:1236-1238.

Davies KJ, Delsignore ME, and Lin SW (1987) Protein damage and degradation by oxygen radicals. II. Modification of amino acids. *J.Biol.Chem.* 262:9902-9907.

Dennery PA, Spitz DR, Yang G, Tatarov A, Lee CS, Shegog ML, and Poss KD (1998) Oxygen toxicity and iron accumulation in the lungs of mice lacking heme oxygenase-2. *J.Clin.Invest.* 101:1001-1011.

Dérijard B, Raingeaud J, Barrett T, Wu IH, Han J, Ulevitch RJ, and Davis RJ (1995) Independent human MAP-kinase signal transduction pathways defined by MEK and MKK isoforms. *Science* 267:682-685.

Dore S, Takahashi M, Ferris CD, Zakhary R, Hester LD, Guastella D, and Snyder SH (1999) Bilirubin, formed by activation of heme oxygenase-2, protects neurons against oxidative stress injury. *Proc.Natl.Acad.Sci.U.S.A* 96:2445-2450.

Du W, Thanos D, and Maniatis T, (1993) Mechanisms of transcriptional synergism between distinct virus-inducible enhancer elements. *Cell* 74:887-898.

Eisenstein RS, Garcia-Mayol D, Pettingell W, and Munro HN (1991) Regulation of ferritin and heme oxygenase synthesis in rat fibroblasts by different forms of iron. *Proc.Natl.Acad.Sci.USA* 88:688-692.

Emerson MR and LeVine SM (2000) Heme oxygenase-1 and NADPH cytochrome P450 reductase expression in experimental allergic encephalomyelitis: an expanded view of the stress response. *J.Neurochem.* 75:2555-2562.

Fondevila C, Shen XD, Tsuchiyashi S, Yamashita K, Csizmadia E, Lassman C, Busuttil RW, Kupiec-Weglinski JW, and Bach FH (2004) Biliverdin therapy protects rat livers from ischemia and reperfusion injury. *Hepatology* 40:1333-1341.

Galliani G, Monti D, Speranza G, and Manitto P (1985) Biliverdin as an electron transfer catalyst for superoxide ion in aqueous medium. *Experientia* 41:1559-1560.

Gibbs PE and Maines MD (2007) Biliverdin inhibits activation of NF-kappaB: reversal of inhibition by human biliverdin reductase. *Int.J.Cancer* 121:2567-2574.

Gibbs PE, Miralem T, and Maines MD (2010) Characterization of the human biliverdin reductase gene structure and regulatory elements: promoter activity is enhanced by hypoxia and suppressed by TNF-alpha-activated NF-kappaB. *FASEB J.* 24:3239-3254.

Gibson JD, Pumford NR, Samokyszyn VM, and Hinson JA (1996) Mechanism of Acetaminophen-Induced Hepatotoxicity: Covalent Binding versus Oxidative Stress. *Chem.Res.Toxicol.* 9:580-585.

Gong P and Cederbaum AI (2006a) Nrf2 is increased by CYP2E1 in rodent liver and HepG2 cells and protects against oxidative stress caused by CYP2E1. *Hepatology* 43:144-153.

Gong P and Cederbaum AI (2006b) Transcription factor Nrf2 protects HepG2 cells against CYP2E1 plus arachidonic acid-dependent toxicity. *J.Biol.Chem.* 281:14573-14579.

Gong P, Cederbaum AI, and Nieto N (2004) Heme Oxygenase-1 Protects HEPG2 Cells against Cytochrome P450 2E1-dependent Toxicity. *Free Radical Biology and Medicine* 36:307-318.

Gorsky LD, Koop DR, and Coon MJ (1984) On the stoichiometry of the oxidase and monooxygenase reactions catalyzed by liver microsomal cytochrome P-450. Products of oxygen reduction. *J.Biol.Chem.* 259:6812-6817.

Gruenke LD, Konopka K, Cadieu M, and Waskell L (1995) The Stoichiometry of the Cytochrome P-450-catalyzed Metabolism of Methoxyflurane and Benzphetamine in the Presence and Absence of Cytochrome b(5). *J.Biol.Chem.* 270:24707.

Hangai-Hoger N, Tsai AG, Cabrales P, Suematsu M, and Intaglietta M (2007) Microvascular and systemic effects following top load administration of saturated carbon monoxide-saline solution. *Crit.Care Med.* 35:1123-1132.

Hayden MS and Ghosh S (2011) NF-κB in immunobiology. *Cell Res.* 21:223-244.

Herdegen T and Leah JD (1998) Inducible and constitutive transcription factors in the mammalian nervous system: control of gene expression by Jun, Fos and Krox, and CREB/ATF proteins. *Brain Res.Brain Res.Rev.* 28:370-490.

Herr I, van Dam H, and Angel P (1994) Binding of promoter-associated AP-1 is not altered during induction and subsequent repression of the c-jun promoter by TPA and UV irradiation. *Carcinogenesis* 15:1105-1113.

Hibi M, Lin A, Smeal T, Minden A, and Karin M (1993) Identification of an oncoprotein- and UV-responsive protein kinase that binds and potentiates the c-Jun activation domain. *Genes Dev.* 7:2135-2148.

Huber WJ, III and Backes WL (2007) Expression and characterization of full-length human heme oxygenase-1: the presence of intact membrane-binding region leads to increased binding affinity for NADPH cytochrome P450 reductase. *Biochem.* 46:12212-12219.

Huber WJ, III, Scruggs B, and Backes WL (2009) C-Terminal Membrane Spanning Region of Human Heme Oxygenase-1 Mediates a Time Dependent Complex Formation with Cytochrome P450 Reductase. *Biochem.* 48:190-197.

Immenschuh S, Hinke V, Ohlmann A, Gifhorn-Katz S, Katz N, Jungermann K, and Kietzmann T (1998a) Transcriptional activation of the haem oxygenase-1 gene by cGMP via a cAMP response element/activator protein-1 element in primary cultures of rat hepatocytes. *Biochem.J.* 334:141-146.

Immenschuh S, Kietzmann T, Hinke V, Wiederhold M, Katz N, and Muller-Eberhard U (1998b) The rat heme oxygenase-1 gene is transcriptionally induced via the protein kinase A signaling pathway in rat hepatocyte cultures. *Mol Pharmacol* 53:483-491.

Inoue S, Suzuki M, Nagashima Y, Suzuki S, Hashiba T, Tsuburai T, Ikehara K, Matsuse T, and Ishigatsubo Y (2001) Transfer of heme oxygenase 1 cDNA by a replication-deficient adenovirus enhances interleukin 10 production from alveolar macrophages that attenuates lipopolysaccharide-induced acute lung injury in mice. *Hum.Gene Ther.* 12:967-979.

Ishii T, Itoh K, Takahashi S, Sato H, Yanagawa T, Katoh Y, Bannai S, and Yamamoto M (2000) Transcription factor Nrf2 coordinately regulates a group of oxidative stress-inducible genes in macrophages. *J.Biol.Chem.* 275:16023-16029.

Ishii T, Itoh K, and Yamamoto M (2002) Roles of Nrf2 in activation of antioxidant enzyme genes via antioxidant responsive elements. *Methods Enzymol.* 348:190.

Ishikawa M, Kajimura M, Adachi T, Makino N, Goda N, Yamaguchi T, Sekizuka E, and Suematsu M (2005) Carbon monoxide from heme oxygenase-2 Is a tonic regulator against NO-dependent vasodilatation in the adult rat cerebral microcirculation. *Circ.Res.* 97:e104-e114.

Itoh K, Chiba T, Takahashi S, Ishii T, Igarashi K, Katoh Y, Oyake T, Hayashi N, Satoh K, Hatayama I, Yamamoto M, and Nabeshima Y (1997) An Nrf2/small Maf heterodimer mediates the induction of phase II detoxifying enzyme genes through antioxidant response elements. *Biochem.Biophys.Res.Commun.* 236:313-322.

Itoh K, Wakabayashi N, Katoh Y, Ishii T, O'Connor T, and Yamamoto M (2003) Keap1 regulates both cytoplasmic-nuclear shuttling and degradation of Nrf2 in response to electrophiles. *Genes Cells* 8:379-391.

Jackson JH, Schraufstatter IU, Hyslop PA, Vosbeck K, Sauerheber R, Weitzman SA, and Cochrane CG (1987) Role of hydroxyl radical in DNA damage. *Trans.Assoc.Am.Physicians* 100:147-157.

Kapitulnik J and Maines MD (2009) Pleiotropic functions of biliverdin reductase: cellular signaling and generation of cytoprotective and cytotoxic bilirubin. *Cell* 30:129-137.

Kaszubska W, Hooft van Huijsduijnen R, Ghersa P, DeRaemy-Schenk AM, Chen BP, Hai T, DeLamarter JF, and Whelan J (1993) Cyclic AMP-independent ATF family members interact with NF-kappa B and function in the activation of the E-selectin promoter in response to cytokines. *Mol.Cell Biol.* 13:180-190.

Kawamura K, Ishikawa K, Wada Y, Matsumoto H, Kohro T, Itabe H, Kodama T, and Maruyama Y (2005) Bilirubin from heme oxygenase-1 attenuates vascular endothelial activation and dysfunction. *Arterioscler.Thromb.Vasc.Biol.* 25:155-160.

Kawashima A, Oda Y, Yachie A, Koizumi S, and Nakanishi I (2002) Heme oxygenase-1 deficiency: the first autopsy case. *Hum.Pathol.* 33:125-130.

Keum YS, Yu S, Chang PP, Yuan X, Kim JH, Xu C, Han J, Agarwal A, and Kong AN (2006) Mechanism of action of sulforaphane: inhibition of p38 mitogen-activated protein kinase isoforms contributing to the induction of antioxidant response element-mediated heme oxygenase-1 in human hepatoma HepG2 cells. *Cancer Res.* 66:8804-8813.

Keyse SM and Tyrrell RM (1989) Heme oxygenase is the major 32-kDa stress protein induced in human skin fibroblasts by UVA radiation, hydrogen peroxide, and sodium arsenite. *Proc.Natl.Acad.Sci.U.S.A* 86:99-103.

Kikuchi G, Yoshida T, and Noguchi M (2005) Heme oxygenase and heme degradation. *Biochem.Biophys.Res.Commun.* 338:558-567.

Kim HJ, So HS, Lee JH, Park C, Park SY, Kim YH, Youn MJ, Kim SJ, Chung SY, Lee KM, and Park R (2006) Heme oxygenase-1 attenuates the cisplatin-induced apoptosis of auditory cells via down-regulation of reactive oxygen species generation. *Free Radic.Biol.Med.* 40:1810-1819.

Kim HP, Wang X, Galbiati F, Ryter SW, and Choi AM (2004) Caveolae compartmentalization of heme oxygenase-1 in endothelial cells. *FASEB J.* 18:1080-1089.

Kravets A, Hu Z, Miralem T, Torno MD, and Maines MD (2004) Biliverdin reductase, a novel regulator for induction of activating transcription factor-2 and heme oxygenase-1. *J.Biol.Chem.* 279:19916-19923.

Kruger AL, Peterson S, Turkseven S, Kaminski PM, Zhang FF, Quan S, Wolin MS, and Abraham NG (2005) D-4F induces heme oxygenase-1 and extracellular superoxide dismutase, decreases endothelial cell sloughing, and improves vascular reactivity in rat model of diabetes. *Circulation* 111:3126-3134.

Kumar S and Bandyopadhyay U (2005) Free heme toxicity and its detoxification systems in human. *Toxicol.Lett.* 157:175-188.

Elucidating the Role of Biliverdin Reductase in the Expression of Heme Oxygenase-1 as a Cytoprotective
Response to Stress

71

Kutty RK, Daniel RF, Ryan DE, Levin W, and Maines MD (1988) Rat liver cytochrome P-450b, P-420b, and P-450c are degraded to biliverdin by heme oxygenase. *Arch.Biochem.Biophys.* 260:638-644.

Kutty RK and Maines MD (1984) Hepatic heme metabolism: possible role of biliverdin in the regulation of heme oxygenase activity. *Biochem.Biophys.Res.Commun.* 122:40-46.

Kwak JY, Takeshige K, Cheung BS, and Minakami S (1991) Bilirubin inhibits the activation of superoxide-producing NADPH oxidase in a neutrophil cell-free system. *Biochim.Biophys.Acta.* 1076:369-373.

Kwak MK, Wakabayashi N, and Kensler TW (2004) Chemoprevention through the Keap1-Nrf2 signaling pathway by phase 2 enzyme inducers. *Mutat.Res.* 555:133-148.

Lee MY, Jung CH, Lee K, Choi YH, Hong S, and Cheong J (2002) Activating transcription factor-2 mediates transcriptional regulation of gluconeogenic gene PEPCK by retinoic acid. *Diabetes* 5:3400-3407.

Lerner-Marmarosh N, Miralem T, Gibbs PE, and Maines MD (2007) Regulation of TNF-alpha-activated PKC-zeta signaling by the human biliverdin reductase: identification of activating and inhibitory domains of the reductase. *FASEB J.* 21:3949-3962.

Lerner-Marmarosh N, Miralem T, Gibbs PE, and Maines MD (2008) Human biliverdin reductase is an ERK activator; hBVR is an ERK nuclear transporter and is required for MAPK signaling. *Proc.Natl.Acad.Sci.USA* 105:6870-6875.

Lerner-Marmarosh N, Shen J, Torno MD, Kravets A, Hu Z, and Maines MD (2005) Human biliverdin reductase: a member of the insulin receptor substrate family with serine/threonine/tyrosine kinase activity. *Proc.Natl.Acad.Sci.USA* 102:7109-7114.

Lin Q, Weis S, Yang G, Weng YH, Helston R, Rish K, Smith A, Bordner J, Polte T, Gaunitz F, and Dennery PA (2007) Heme oxygenase-1 protein localizes to the nucleus and activates transcription factors important in oxidative stress. *J.Biol.Chem.*

Lin QS, Weis S, Zhuang T, Abate A, and Dennery PA (2008) Catalytic inactive heme oxygenase-1 protein regulates its own expression in oxidative stress. *Free Radic.Biol.Med.* 44:847-855.

Liu Y, Moenne-Loccoz P, Loehr TM, and Ortiz de Montellano PR (1997) Heme oxygenase-1, intermediates in verdoheme formation and the requirement for reduction equivalents. *J.Biol.Chem.* 272:6909-6917.

Liu Y and Ortiz de Montellano PR (2000) Reaction intermediates and single turnover rate constants for the oxidation of heme by human heme oxygenase-1. *J.Biol.Chem.* 275:5297-5307.

Maghzal GJ, Leck MC, Collinson E, Li C, and Stocker R (2009) Limited role for the bilirubin-biliverdin redox amplification cycle in the cellular antioxidant protection by biliverdin reductase. *J.Biol.Chem.* 284:2925-29259.

Maines MD (1988) Heme oxygenase: function, multiplicity, regulatory mechanisms, and clinical applications. *FASEB J.* 2:2557-2568.

Maines MD, Ewing JF, Huang TJ, and Panahian N (2001) Nuclear localization of biliverdin reductase in the rat kidney: response to nephrotoxins that induce heme oxygenase-1. *J.Pharmacol.Exp.Ther.* 296:1091-1097.

Maines MD, Miralem T, Lerner-Marmarosh N, Shen J, and Gibbs PE (2007) Human biliverdin reductase, a previously unknown activator of protein kinase C betaII. *J.Biol.Chem.* 282:810-822.

Maines MD, Trakshel GM, and Kutty RK (1986) Characterization of two constitutive forms of rat liver microsomal heme oxygenase. Only one molecular species of the enzyme is inducible. *J.Biol.Chem.* 261:411-419.

Mancuso C and Barone E (2009) The heme oxygenase/biliverdin reductase pathway in drug research and development. *Curr.Drug Metab.* 10:579-594.

Martin D, Rojo AI, Salinas M, Diaz R, Gallardo G, Alam J, De Galarreta CM, and Cuadrado A (2004) Regulation of heme oxygenase-1 expression through the phosphatidylinositol 3-kinase/Akt pathway and the Nrf2 transcription factor in response to the antioxidant phytochemical carnosol. *J.Biol.Chem.* 279:8919-8929.

McCord JM (1993) Oxygen-derived free radicals. *New Horiz.* 1:70-76.

Miralem T, Hu Z, Torno MD, Lelli KM, and Maines MD (2005) Small interference RNA-mediated gene silencing of human biliverdin reductase, but not that of heme oxygenase-1, attenuates arsenite-mediated induction of the oxygenase and increases apoptosis in 293A kidney cells. *J.Biol.Chem.* 280:17084-17092.

Morse D, Pischke SE, Zhou Z, Davis RJ, Flavell RA, Loop T, Otterbein SL, Otterbein LE, and Choi AM (2003) Suppression of inflammatory cytokine production by carbon monoxide involves the JNK pathway and AP-1. *J.Biol.Chem.* 278:36993-36998.

Motterlini R, Mann BE, Johnson TR, Clark JE, Foresti R, and Green CJ (2003) Bioactivity and pharmacological actions of carbon monoxide-releasing molecules. *Curr.Pharm.Des.* 9:2525-2539.

Murphy K, Haudek SB, Thompson M, and Giroir BP (1998) Molecular biology of septic shock. *New Horiz.* 6:181-193.

Nakahira K, Takahashi T, Shimizu H, Maeshima K, Uehara K, Fujii H, Nakatsuka H, Yokoyama M, Akagi R, and Morita K (2003) Protective role of heme oxygenase-1 induction in carbon tetrachloride-induced hepatotoxicity. *Biochem.Pharmacol.* 66:1091-1105.

Neuzil J and Stocker R (1993) Bilirubin attenuates radical-mediated damage to serum albumin. *FEBS Lett.* 331:281-284.

Noguchi M, Yoshida T, and Kikuchi G (1979) Purification and properties of biliverdin reductases from pig spleen and rat liver. *J.Biochem.* 86:833-848.

Odaka Y, Takahashi T, Yamasaki A, Suzuki T, Fujiwara T, Yamada T, Hirakawa M, Fujita H, Ohmori E, and Akagi R (2000) Prevention of halothane-induced hepatotoxicity by hemin pretreatment: protective role of heme oxygenase-1 induction. *Biochem.Pharmacol.* 59:871-880.

Ossola JO and Tomaro ML (1995) Heme oxygenase induction by cadmium chloride: evidence for oxidative stress involvement. *Toxicology* 104:141-147.

Otterbein L, Sylvester SL, and Choi AM (1995) Hemoglobin provides protection against lethal endotoxemia in rats: the role of heme oxygenase-1. *Am.J.Respir.Cell Mol.Biol.* 13:595-601.

Otterbein LE, Bach FH, Alam J, Soares M, Tao LH, Wysk M, Davis RJ, Flavell RA, and Choi AM (2000) Carbon monoxide has anti-inflammatory effects involving the mitogen-activated protein kinase pathway. *Nat.Med.* 6:422-428.

Pachori AS, Smith A, McDonald P, Zhang L, Dzau VJ, and Melo LG (2007) Heme-oxygenase-1-induced protection against hypoxia/reoxygenation is dependent on biliverdin reductase and its interaction with PI3K/Akt pathway. *J.Mol.Cell Cardiol.* 43:580-592.

Elucidating the Role of Biliverdin Reductase in the Expression of Heme Oxygenase-1 as a Cytoprotective
Response to Stress

73

Paller MS and Jacob HS (1994) Cytochrome P-450 mediates tissue-damaging hydroxyl radical formation during reoxygenation of the kidney. *Proc.Natl.Acad.Sci.USA* 91:7002-7006.

Papa S, Bubici C, Zazzeroni F, Pham CG, Kuntzen C, Dean K, and Franzoso G (2006) The NF-kappaB-mediated control of the JNK cascade in the antagonism of programmed cell death in health and disease. *Cell Death Differ.* 13:712-729.

Parfenova H, Basuroy S, Bhattacharya S, Tcheranova D, Qu Y, Regan RF, and Leffler CW (2006) Glutamate induces oxidative stress and apoptosis in cerebral vascular endothelial cells: contributions of HO-1 and HO-2 to cytoprotection. *Am.J.Physiol.Cell Physiol.* 290:C1399-C1410.

Park SY, Lee SW, Baek SH, Lee SJ, Lee WS, Rhim BY, Hong KW, and Kim CD (2011) Induction of heme oxygenase-1 expression by cilostazol contributes to its anti-inflammatory effects in J774 murine macrophages. *Immunol.Lett.* 136:138-145.

Patel VC, Yellon DM, Singh KJ, Neild GH, and Woolfson RG (1993) Inhibition of nitric oxide limits infarct size in the in situ rabbit heart. *Biochem.Biophys.Res.Commun.* 194:234-238.

Pawson T and Scott JD (2005) Protein phosphorylation in signaling--50 years and counting. *Trends Biochem.Sci.* 30:286-290.

Peng HB, Libby P, and Liao JK (1995) Induction and stabilization of I kappa B alpha by nitric oxide mediates inhibition of NF-kappa B. *J.Biol.Chem.* 270:14214-14219.

Peterson JA, Ebel RE, O'Keeffe DH, Matsubara T, and Estabrook RW (1976) Temperature dependence of cytochrome P-450 reduction. A model for NADPH-cytochrome P-450 reductase:cytochrome P-450 interaction. *J.Biol.Chem.* 251:4010-4016.

Phelan D, Winter GM, Rogers WJ, Lam JC, and Denison MS (1998) Activation of the Ah receptor signal transduction pathway by bilirubin and biliverdin. *Arch.Biochem.Biophys.* 357:155-163.

Piantadosi CA (2008) Carbon monoxide, reactive oxygen signaling, and oxidative stress. *Free Radic.Biol.Med.* 45:562-569.

Piantadosi CA and Zhang J (1996) Mitochondrial generation of reactive oxygen species after brain ischemia in the rat Mitochondrial generation of reactive oxygen species after brain ischemia in the rat. *Stroke* 27:327-31; discussion 332.

Pischke SE, Zhou Z, Song R, Ning W, Alam J, Ryter SW, and Choi AM (2005) Phosphatidylinositol 3-kinase/Akt pathway mediates heme oxygenase-1 regulation by lipopolysaccharide. *Cell Mol.Biol.* 51:461-470.

Ponka P (1997) Tissue-specific regulation of iron metabolism and heme synthesis: distinct control mechanisms in erythroid cells. *Blood* 89:1-25.

Poss KD, Thomas MJ, Ebralidz AK, O'Dell TJ, and Tonegawa S (1995) Hippocampal long-term potentiation is normal in heme oxygenase-2 mutant mice. *Neuron.* 15:867-873.

Poss KD and Tonegawa S (1997a) Heme oxygenase 1 is required for mammalian iron reutilization. *Proc.Natl.Acad.Sci.U.S.A.* 94:10919-10924.

Poss KD and Tonegawa S (1997b) Reduced stress defense in heme oxygenase-1 deficient cells. *Proc.Natl.Acad.Sci.U.S A.* 94:10925-10930.

Pugazhenthi S, Akhov L, Selvaraj G, Wang M, and Alam J (2007) Regulation of heme oxygenase-1 expression by demethoxy curcuminoids through Nrf2 by a PI3-kinase/Akt-mediated pathway in mouse beta-cells. *Am.J.Physiol.Endocrinol.Metab.* 293:E645-E655.

Reed JR, Cawley GF, and Backes WL (2011) Inhibition of cytochrome P450 1A2-mediated metabolism and production of reactive oxygen species by heme oxygenase-1 in rat liver microsomes. *Drug Metab Lett.* 5:6-16.

Reed JR and Hollenberg PF (2003) Comparison of substrate metabolism by cytochromes P450 2B1, 2B4, and 2B6: relationship of heme spin state, catalysis, and the effects of cytochrome b5. *Journal of Inorganic Biochemistry* 93:152-160.

Reed JR, Huber WJ, III, and Backes WL (2010) Human heme oxygenase-1 efficiently catabolizes heme in the absence of biliverdin reductase. *Drug Metab Dispos.* 38:2060-2066.

Robertson P, Jr. and Fridovich I (1982) A reaction of the superoxide radical with tetrapyrroles. *Arch.Biochem.Biophys.* 213:353-357.

Rotenberg MO and Maines MD (1991) Characterization of a cDNA-encoding rabbit brain heme oxygenase-2 and identification of a conserved domain among mammalian heme oxygenase isozymes: possible heme-binding site? *Arch.Biochem.Biophys.* 290:336-344.

Ryan KM, Ernst MK, Rice NR, and Vousden KH (2000) Role of NF-kappaB in p53-mediated programmed cell death. *Nature* 404:892-897.

Ryter SW, Alam J, and Choi MK (2006) Heme oxygenase-1/carbon monoxide: From basic science to therapeutic applications. *Physiol.Rev.* 86:583-650.

Salim M, Brown-Kipphut BA, and Maines MD (2001) Human biliverdin reductase is autophosphorylated, and phosphorylation is required for bilirubin formation. *J.Biol.Chem.* 276:10929-10934.

Schlichting I, Berendzen J, Chu K, Stock AM, Maves SA, Benson DE, Sweet RM, Ringe D, Petsko GA, and Sligar SG (2000) The catalytic pathway of cytochrome p450cam at atomic resolution. *Science* 287:1615-1622.

Sen CK, Traber KE, and Packer L (1996) Inhibition of NF-kappa B activation in human T-cell lines by anetholdithiolthione. *Biochem.Biophys.Res.Commun.* 218:148-153.

Sheftel AD, Kim SF, and Ponka P (2007) Non-heme induction of heme oxygenase-1 does not alter cellular iron metabolism. *J.Biol.Chem.* 282:10480-10486.

Shen G, Jeong WS, Hu R, and Kong AN (2005) Regulation of Nrf2, NF-kappaB, and AP-1 signaling pathways by chemopreventive agents. *Antioxid.Redox.Signal.* 7:1648-1663.

Song R, Kubo M, Morse D, Zhou Z, Zhang X, Dauber JH, Fabisiak J, Alber SM, Watkins SC, Zuckerbraun BS, Otterbein LE, Ning W, Oury TD, Lee PJ, McCurry KR, Choi AM. (2003a) Carbon monoxide induces cytoprotection in rat orthotopic lung transplantation via anti-inflammatory and anti-apoptotic effects. *Am.J.Pathol.* 163:231-242.

Song R, Ning W, Liu F, Ameredes BT, Calhoun WJ, Otterbein LE, and Choi AM (2003b) Regulation of IL-1beta -induced GM-CSF production in human airway smooth muscle cells by carbon monoxide. *Am.J.Physiol.Lung Cell Mol.Physiol.* 284:L50-L56.

Stocker R and Ames BN (1987) Potential role of conjugated bilirubin and copper in the metabolism of lipid peroxides in bile. *Proc.Natl.Acad.Sci.USA* 84:8130-8134.

Stocker R, Glazer AN, and Ames BN (1987) Antioxidant activity of albumin-bound bilirubin. *Proc.Natl.Acad.Sci.USA* 84:5918-5922.

Stocker R and Peterhans E (1989) Synergistic interaction between vitamin E and the bile pigments bilirubin and biliverdin. *Biochim.Biophys.Acta.* 1002:238-244.

Elucidating the Role of Biliverdin Reductase in the Expression of Heme Oxygenase-1 as a Cytoprotective
Response to Stress

75

Sun Jang J, Piao S, Cha YN, and Kim C (2009) Taurine Chloramine Activates Nrf2, Increases HO-1 Expression and Protects Cells from Death Caused by Hydrogen Peroxide. *J.Clin.Biochem.Nutr.* 45:37-43.

Sun J, Hoshino H, Takaku K, Nakajima O, Muto A, Suzuki H, Takahashi S, Shibahara S, Alam J, Taketo MM, Yamamoto M, and Igarashi K (2002) Hemoprotein Bach1 regulates enhancer availability of heme oxygenase-1 gene. *EMBO J.* 21:5216-5224.

Suttner DM and Dennery PA (1999) Reversal of HO-1 related cytoprotection with increased expression is due to reactive iron. *FASEB J.* 13:1800-1809.

Taillé C, Almolki A, Benhamed M, Zedda C, Mégret J, Berger P, Lesèche G, Fadel E, Yamaguchi T, Marthan R, Aubier M, and Boczkowski J (2003) Heme oxygenase inhibits human airway smooth muscle proliferation via a bilirubin-dependent modulation of ERK1/2 phosphorylation. *J.Biol.Chem.* 278:27160-27168.

Tamion F, Richard V, Renet S, and Thuillez C (2006) Protective effects of heme-oxygenase expression against endotoxic shock: inhibition of tumor necrosis factor-alpha and augmentation of interleukin-10. *J.Trauma* 61:1078-1084.

Tan J, Kuang W, Jin Z, Jin F, Yu Q, Kong L, Zeng G, Yuan X, and Duan Y (2009) Inhibition of NFkappaB by activated c-Jun NH2 terminal kinase 1 acts as a switch for C2C12 cell death under excessive stretch. *Apoptosis* 14:764-770.

Tang LM, Wang YP, Wang K, Pu LY, Zhang F, Li XC, Kong LB, Sun BC, Li GQ, and Wang XH (2007) Exogenous biliverdin ameliorates ischemia-reperfusion injury in small-for-size rat liver grafts. *Transplant.Proc.* 39:1338-1344.

Terelius Y and Ingelman-Sundberg M (1988) Cytochrome P-450-dependent oxidase activity and hydroxyl radical production in micellar and membranous types of reconstituted systems. *Biochem.Pharmacol.* 37:1383-1389.

Toda K, Yang LX, and Shizuta Y (1995) Transcriptional regulation of the human aromatase cytochrome P450 gene expression in human placental cells. *J.Steroid Biochem.Mol.Biol.* 53:181-190.

Toda N, Takahashi T, Mizobuchi S, F ujii H, T akahira K, N akahashi S, amashita M, M orita K, H irakawa M, and A kagi R (2002) Tin chloride pretreatment prevents renal injury in rats with ischemic acute renal failure. *Crit.Care Med.* 30:1512-1522.

Tsuji Y, Ayaki H, Whitman SP, Morrow CS, T orti SV, and T orti FM (2000) Coordinate transcriptional and translational regulation of ferritin in response to oxidative stress. *Mol.Cell Biol.* 20:5818-5827.

Tudor C, Lerner-Marmarosh N, Engelborghs Y, Gibbs PE, and Maines MD (2008) Biliverdin reductase is a transporter of haem into the nucleus and is essential for regulation of HO-1 gene expression by haematin. *Biochem.J.* 413:405-416.

Vincent SH (1989) Oxidative effects of heme and porphyrins on proteins and lipids. *Semin.Hematol.* 26:105-113.

Wada T and Penninger JM (2004) Mitogen-activated protein kinases in apoptosis regulation. *Oncogene* 23:2838-2849.

Wagener FADTG, Eggert A, Boerman OC, Oyen WJ, Verhofstad A, Abraham NG, Adema G, van Kooyk Y, de Witte T, and Figdor CG (2001) Heme is a potent inducer of inflammation in mice and is counteracted by heme oxygenase. *Blood* 98:1802-1811.

Wang WW, Smith DL, and Zucker SD (2004) Bilirubin inhibits iNOS expression and NO production in response to endotoxin in rats. *Hepatology* 40:424-433.

Wen T, Wu ZM, Liu Y, Tan YF, Ren F, and Wu H (2007) Upregulation of heme oxygenase-1 with hemin prevents D-galactosamine and lipopolysaccharide-induced acute hepatic injury in rats. *Toxicology* 237:184-193.

White RE and Coon MJ (1980) Oxygen activation by cytochrome P-450. *Annu.Rev Biochem.* 49:315-356.

Williams SE, Wootton P, Mason HS, Bould J, Iles DE, Riccardi D, Peers C, and Kemp PJ (2004) Hemoxygenase-2 is an oxygen sensor for a calcium-sensitive potassium channel. *Science* 306:2093-2097.

Wright MM, Schopfer FJ, Vidyasagar V, Powell P, Chumley P, Iles KE, Freeman BA, and Agarwal A (2006) Fatty acid transduction of nitric oxide signaling: nitrolinoleic acid potently activates endothelial heme oxygenase 1 expression. *Proc.Natl.Acad.Sci.* 103:4299-4304.

Yachie A, Niida Y, Wada T, Igarashi N, Kaneda H, Toma T, Ohta K, Kasahara Y, and Koizumi S (1999) Oxidative stress causes enhanced endothelial cell injury in human heme oxygenase-1 deficiency. *J.Clin.Invest* 103:129-135.

Yang L, Quan S, and Abraham NG (1999) Retrovirus-mediated HO gene transfer into endothelial cells protects against oxidant-induced injury. *Am.J.Physiol.* 277:127-133.

Yao P, Hao L, Nussler N, Lehmann A, Song F, Zhao J, Neuhaus P, Liu L, and Nussler A (2009) The protective role of HO-1 and its generated products (CO, bilirubin, and Fe) in ethanol-induced human hepatocyte damage. *Am.J.Physiol.Gastrointest.Liver Physiol.* 296:G1318-1323.

Yao P, Nussler A, Liu L, Hao L, Song F, Schirmeier A, and Nussler N (2007) Quercetin protects human hepatocytes from ethanol-derived oxidative stress by inducing heme oxygenase-1 via the MAPK/Nrf2 pathways. *J.Hepatol.* 47:253-261.

Yoneya R, Ozasa H, Nagashima Y, Koike Y, Teraoka H, Hagiwara K, and Horikawa S (2000) Hemin pretreatment ameliorates aspects of the nephropathy induced by mercuric chloride in the rat. *Toxicol.Lett.* 116:223-229.

Yoshioka K, Deng T, Cavigelli M, and Karin M (1995) Antitumor promotion by phenolic antioxidants: inhibition of AP-1 activity through induction of Fra expression. *Proc.Natl.Acad.Sci.USA* 92:4972-4976.

Young SC, Storm MV, Speed JS, Kelsen S, Tiller CV, Vera T, Drummond HA, and Stec DE (2009) Inhibition of biliverdin reductase increases ANG II-dependent superoxide levels in cultured renal tubular epithelial cells. *Am.J.Physiol.Integr.Comp.Physiol.* 297:R1546-R1553.

Zangar RC, Davydov DR, and Verma S (2004) Mechanisms that regulate production of reactive oxygen species by cytochrome P450. *Toxicol.Appl.Pharmacol.* 199:316-331.

Zhang J, Ohta T, Maruyama A, Hosoya T, Nishikawa K, Maher JM, Shibahara S, Itoh K, and Yamamoto M (2006) BRG1 interacts with Nrf2 to selectively mediate HO-1 induction in response to oxidative stress. *Mol.Cell Biol.* 26:7942-7952.

3

Unconventional Raw Natural Sustainable Sources for Obtaining Pharmacological Principles Potentially Active on CNS Through Catalytic, Ecologically Clean, Processes

Yanier Nuñez Figueredo[1], Juan E. Tacoronte Morales[2],
Alicia Lagarto Parra[1], Olinka Tiomno Tiomnova[2],
Jorge Tobella Sabater[3] and Jorge Leyva Simeon[2]
*[1]Center for Research and Development of Pharmaceuticals,
CIDEM, Cerro, Ciudad Habana,*
[2]Center for Engineering and Chemical Researches, CIIQ, Cerro, Ciudad Habana
[3]Pharmaceutical Laboratories MEDSOL, La Lisa, Ciudad Habana,
Cuba

1. Introduction

Natural products have been the most successful source of drugs ever (Tulp & Bohlin, 2005). Historically, the most important natural sources have been plants. Research progressed along two mayor lines: ethnopharmacology and toxicology. These strategies have produced many valuable drugs and are likely to continue to produce hit-lead compounds. However, actually exist numerous unconventional natural sources, ecologically sustainable, of potentially medicinal compounds without research.

The development of pharmaceutical and fine chemistry in Cuba and the synthetic or natural product-oriented generation of new pharmacological and molecular entities, in the II decade of XXI century, it´s sustained in several basic conceptual and methodological principles:

- Structure (including isosteric perception) of compounds generates and define properties, which in their order, determinate application and functionality in the related chemical-pharmacological space (SPAF)
- Sustainability – Scalability (scaling-up facilities) –Applicability in real time (SSA-r_t)
- Maximum of atomic efficiency (*click* and *green* chemistry); maximum of analytical efficiency and maximum of environmental efficiency (MAE[3])
- Chemical bioprospecting of the Cuban biodiversity oriented to discovery of new *ecological* molecular fragments-templates with interesting pharmacological properties for their application in therapeutical treatments of several pathologies of CNS including neuroprotection, neuroregeneration after stroke and ischemia.

- Integration of *in silico* screen to natural products or their mixtures with minimal complexity

Taking this into account, in Cuba (2008-2011) it has been attempted, starting from natural products of the forest industry and raw renewable materials ecologically sustainable, such as rosin, colophony and resinic acids isolated from endemic botanic species belonging to gen. *Pinus* (Pinaceae) the development and application of new heterogeneous catalytic procedures, optimization of design and synthesis of new pharmacological agents structurally based on sodium resinate and dehydroabietic acid (DHAA), with a great added value, as therapeutics for medical treatment of pathologies of CNS, including GABA agonist-antagonists, cannabinoid analogues and sedative molecular systems.

Cuban resin acids, an ecological sustainable natural product, derived form Cuban forestry industry, have been shown to have broad and highly active biological properties, potent microbiocidal and fungicidal actions and potential neuroprotective effects on central nervous system (CNS). In this communication, we studied this novel ecologically sustainable source of potentially therapeutic compounds using, as starting raw material, resins from endemic Cuban *Pinus* specie and show their effect on central nervous system in rodents.

2. Materials and methods

2.1 Chemicals and drugs

2.1.1 Oleoresin, colophony and starting resin acids

The Cuban oleoresin, was milked and collected by incision of the bark from mature trees (*Pinus caribbaea* 7-13 years) planted in Viñales Forestry Station, 168 Km West of Havana, serpentine soil) located in the Western zone of the Cuban archipelago. It was submitted to distillation as reported previously (Franich & Gadgil, 1983). The main components, a mixture of colophony (resin acids), turpentine oils and neutral fraction were separated. The acid fraction was submitted to identification of abietane acids (mixture of abietic, dehydroabietic, levopimaric & pimaric acid) and directly used in pharmacological tests.

For the preparation of extracts, approximately 500 mg of colophony were grinding in an agate mortar into 2-mm pieces, extracted with 4 ml methanol, filtered through glass wool, and the extracts stored at −10°C. Extracts were filtered through 0.45-μm Teflon syringe filters prior to HPLC and used in the next steep for obtaining the sodium salt.

The sodium salt (sodium resinate-SR) was prepared as reported in: CU/2006-0144 patent. Crystallized from a mixture of water: ethanol (8: 2 v/v)

2.2 Chromatography conditions

Analytical HPLC-PDA (Kanuer Smart Line-2005): Column: LichroCART 250 x 0.44 cm RP-18, 5μm particle size (Lichropher 100); mobile phase: acetonitrile-water in gradient conditions (40% to 100%) during 45 min, held at 100% for further 2 min; temperature: 25 °C; flow rate: 1mL/min; sample injection 10 μL; detection: 200 nm to 505 nm. Data were analyzed with ChromGate 3.1 (Germany) for LC 3D software.

2.3 Structural elucidation

The structural elucidation was based on FTIR spectroscopy (spectrophotometer FT-IR Jasco, FT/IR-460 Plus, Japan, in a range of 280-7200 cm^{-1} with a sensibility of 0,1 cm^{-1}) and NMR spectrometry (^1H y ^{13}C) at room temperature, using a spectrometer Brucker AC-250 MHz, at 28 ⁰C in DMSO-d_6 ,using as internal reference TMS, given all the signals in ppm (δ).

Diazepam (DZP, Quimefa, Cuba), pentylenetetrazole (PTZ, Sigma, USA, CAS), picrotoxin (PTX, Sigma, USA, CAS), haloperidol (Esteve S.A, España), amphetamine-sulphate (Sigma, USA, CAS), were used in this study. Solvents were analytical grade and were purified by distillation before used. All drugs and their solutions were prepared immediately before use.

2.4 Synthesis of dehydroabietic acid (DHAA)

2.4.1 Catalytic disproportion of colophony using piritic ash as catalyst (0,5 % (m/m) at 230 ⁰C)

500 grams of previously hydrothermally treated colophony is heated during 30 min (130 ⁰C) in a glass pyrex reactor (750 mL) equipped with thermometer and stirrer. 1,0 gram of pyritic ash is added and the reaction temperature increased to 230 ⁰C. The reaction mixture is maintained at this temperature during 3 h under intense stirring (1500 rpm). (The residual concentration of abietic acid is 0,5–0,8 %). 100 grams of disproportionated colophony in 100 mL of alcohol is filtered through SiO_2-Al_2O_3. The solution is heated to 70 ⁰C and then added 18 grams of 2-aminoethanol, and 250 mL of hot water (60-90⁰C). The resulting solution is kept at 70 ⁰C during 10 min., under gentle stirring, then the reaction mixture is extracted with iso-octane, toluene or a mixture of heptane/ciclohexanone 7/3 v/v (3v x 75 mL). The selective crystallization of the quaternary ammonium salt dehydroabietic acid-2-aminoethanol starts at 50 ⁰C. The solution is cooled to 4 ⁰C, collecting crystals which are soluble in cool 50 % ethanol (250 mL) Yield: 51,0 grams with 89,5 % of purity related to dehydroabietic acid (98,5 % overall purity). The obtained salt is dissolved 160 mL of hot ethanol and acidified with aqueous HCl (12 %, pH 4-5) and allowed to stand during 8h at room temperature. The pure dehydroabietic acid is collected, washed, re-crystallized from a mixture of 75 % ethanol/water v/v. and dried 3 h. Yield 39,3 % (overall 98,2 %)

2.5 Animals

2.5.1 Pharmacological studies

Male albino mice (Swiss, 18–22 g) in anticonvulsant activity, elevated plus-maze, amphetamine and thiopental-induced sleep, open field activity and aggressive behaviour test and male rats (Wistar, 150–200 g) in amphetamine-induced behavioural stereotypy test were used.

2.5.1.1 Acute toxicity study

Six female rats (Wistar, 150–200 g) were used for evaluating the acute toxicity of test compounds.

All animals (Laboratory of Biological Control. CIDEM, Havana, Cuba) were housed in groups of five under standard laboratory conditions of temperature, humidity and lighting (12:12-h light/dark). Animals had free access to food and water, except during experiment.

They were deprived of food but not water 6 h before the drug administration and each group consisted of ten animals. All experiments were carried out between 8:00 am and 11:00 am in accordance with the Institutional Animal Ethical Committee approved the study and animal care was in conformity with Canadian Council for Animal Care guidelines

SR was administrated in three doses levels (100, 200 y 400 mg/Kg) in all experiment except the elevated plus-maze behaviour test (50, 100 y 150 mg/Kg). The volume of injection in mouse was 0.4 ml/20 g and in rat was 1 ml/100 g. The SR was dissolved in distilled water and administered orally.

2.5.2 Pharmacological and toxicity evaluation

2.5.2.1 Open field activity

Thirty minutes after the administration of vehicle or test compound a mouse was placed in the centre of a round open field of 30 cm diameter and 25 cm high and the open field activity were measured during 6 minutes recording how many times the animal stay in the centre of cage and the number of rising (Sukma et al., 2002; Tyler, 1982).

2.5.2.2 Aggressive behavior

A group of animal was isolated in individually cage and other group remained grouped during six week. The aggressive behaviors were evaluated through an intruder mouse into the isolated mice's home cage and were recorder the aggressive activity (biting attacks and wrestling) in isolated mice was measure as total fighting time during a 20 min period (Tyler, 1982).

2.5.2.3 Thiopental-induced sleep

Animals were divided into three groups: control (distilled water), diazepam (1 mg/kg)-treated and SR-treated groups. Thiopental sodium (30 mg/kg) was injected intraperitoneally 30 min after administration of vehicle or test compound. An animal was placed on its back on a warmed (35 °C) pad. The number of sleeping animals and the duration of loss of righting reflex were recorded. The duration from loss of righting reflex until a mouse regained its righting reflex was measured (Carlini et al., 1986).

2.5.2.4 Drug-induced convulsion

Mice were divided in groups of ten each. The animals were pre-treated with SR 30 min before the administration of PTZ (85 mg/kg, s.c.) or PTX (10 mg/kg, s.c.). The anticonvulsive effect was assessed by measuring the numbers of convulsing mice and deaths, and the latency of the appearance of the first episode of clonic seizure. The cut off time was set as 30 min. after the convulsant administration (Costa & Greengard, 1975; Fischer & Vander, 1998).

2.5.2.5 Elevated plus-maze behavior

The elevated plus-maze consisted of two closed arms (30_/5_/15 cm) and two open arms (30_/5 cm) emanating from a common central platform (5_/5 cm). The two pairs of identical arms were opposite each other. The entire apparatus was elevated to a height of 54 cm above floor level. Thirty minutes after test compound administration, the mouse was placed at the centre of the maze with its head facing an open arm and allowed to explore the maze for 5 min. Entry into an arm was defined as placement of all four paws into an arm and were recorded: number of entries into each type of arm, the percentage of time spent and the percentage of arm entries in open arms (Sukma et al., 2002).

2.5.2.6 Amphetamine-induced behavioral stereotypy

Amphetamine (1.5 mg/Kg) was injected subcutaneously 30 min after administration of vehicle or test compound in rats and the animals were collocated in individually cage to recorder the behavioral stereotypy each 5 min during 1 h. (Kuczenski et al., 1999).

2.5.2.7 Amphetamine -induced sleep in mice

Mice were divided in four groups of ten each. The animals were pre-treated with SR 30 min before the administration of amphetamine 5 mg/Kg (p sc). An animal was placed on its back on a warmed (35 °C) pad and the number of sleeping animals and the duration of loss of righting reflex were recorded.

2.5.2.8 Acute oral toxicity study

A single dose of SR (2000 mg/kg) or distilled water was administered orally (10 mL/Kg) in equal number female (n=3) animals; and rats were returned to an *ad libitum* diet immediately after dosing. All animals were monitored continuously for 12 h after dosing for signs of toxicosis and daily for changes additional behavioural or clinical signs. The animal weights were recorded weekly. Rats were euthanized on day 14 by ether inhalation, and selected organs removed and examined macroscopically for toxicant-induced changes (OECD, 2001).

2.5.2.9 Statistics

Drug effects were assessed by single factor analysis of variance followed by the Student-/Newman-/Keuls post-hoc test. The level of significance was set at $p < 0.05$.

3. Results and discussion

The Cuban pine oleoresin, was milked and collected by incision of the bark from mature trees *Pinus caribbaea*. After distillation the main components and mixture of colophony (resinic acids), turpentine oils and neutral fraction were separated and hydrothermally treated to minimize the amount of fatty lineal and branched acids. Colophony was analyzed, treated with stecheometrical amount of NaOH, to obtain the desired sodium resinate and submitted directly, after crystallization from a mixture water: ethanol (30:70 v/v), to neuropharmacological evaluations.

The oleoresin collected from *Pinus caribbaea* is hydrothermally treated and purified through redox-acid/base protocols described in (Cuban patents CU 20060144 & CU20060252), generating a practically pure mixture of rosin-colophony as a mixture of resinic acids (RA, FTIR- cm^{-1}: 3426(γO-H), 2931(C_{sp3}-H y C_{sp2}-H), 2869 (v^s CH_2) y 2929 (v^{as} CH_2), 1694(γC=O), 1385-1366(δ_s-CH_3), 1450(δ_{as}-CH_3), 1150-1180 isopropyl system, zone 950-970 olefinic fragments, 830-770 trisubtituted olefins; NMR,δ,ppm: 6 zones observed: *0.5-0,8* methyl groups, *1.0-1.2* methyl groups, *1.3-2.0* methylenic groups, *5.0-6.0* olefinic zone exo- and endocyclic bonds, *6.8-7.3* aromatic protons, *11.9-12.5* COO$\underline{H}$) that was used directly in the evaluation of its neuropharmacological profile. This mixture (50-52 % of abietic acid), without further purification, was used for obtaining dehydroabietic acid (DHAA) by heterogeneous catalytic disproportionation-aromatization treatment of colophony with pyritic ash (Fe_2O_3/FeS/Ba^{2+}/SiO_2, 230°C, stirring, air, 95%) and the selective precipitation of the 2-aminoethanol salt of DHAA (molar ratio 1:1, 50°C, 89 %) in aqueous ethanol solution. The pure DHAA was obtained after acidification (pH 4-5; 98%, TLC: Silicagel G_{60}-254, eluent: n-hexane/ethyl acetate 7:3 v/v, 2 drops of isopropanol; chromophoric agent vainilline/H_2SO_4, mp. 171.5-172.3°C and applied column chromatography; NMR,ppm,δ ^{1}H-^{13}C selected signals: 9,78-O$\underline{H}$/184,32-$\underline{C}$OOH; 7,15 C-11$\underline{H}$/C-11 124,90; 6,95 C-12$\underline{H}$/C-12 124,20; 6,88 C-14$\underline{H}$/C-14 127,0).

The most widely protocol used for resin acid analysis and their derivatives is gas chromatography (GC) of the methyl esters (Zinkel & Engler, 1977) with detection by flame ionization (FID) or mass spectrometry (MS). However, this method has disadvantages for us, including instability of the derivatized samples (Latorre et al., 2003), hazards of methylating reagents (potentially explosive and carcinogenic), and tedious work-up of raw biological material required.

Taking this in consideration, in our laboratory, have been developed a simple analytical methodology for resin acid analysis by high-performance liquid chromatography (HPLC) in gradient conditions. We report a simple protocol for the analysis of abietanes derivatives by reversed-phase HPLC with several advantages including: (1) no sample derivatization is required; (2) extraction and chromatographic conditions are mild, (3) all components of the HPLC mobile (acetonitrile and water) phase are volatile and therefore recovery of compounds from fractionated sample is simplified. These benefits are particularly advantageous in biological studies that require rapid analysis of abietane acid mixtures and screenings for neuroprotective bioactivity.

The results are shown in Fig. 1

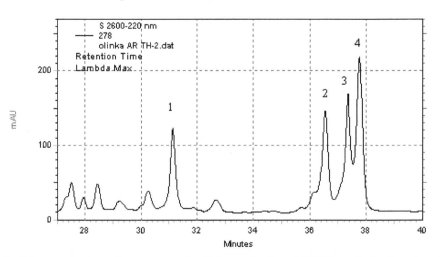

Fig. 1. Abietanes (resin acids present in the Cuban colophony) HPLC analysis of methanol extract obtained from distilled oleoresin. 1= Levopimaric, 2= Palustric, 3= Abietic, 4= Dehydroabietic

The fundamentals (conceptual and methodological) for the analytical technique described here rely on both the optimal combination of wavelengths for detection and the chromatographic resolution of the peaks. Abietanes have distinctive spectra that we used here, together with chromatographic separation, to distinguish and quantify the resin acids by HPLC. The spectra (220-540 nm) of the individual chromatographically separated components (Fig.1), show λ_{max} values of 255 nm (levopimaric), 251 nm (palustric), 266 nm (abietic), and 269, 278 nm (dehydroabietic). The information related is shown in Fig. 2.

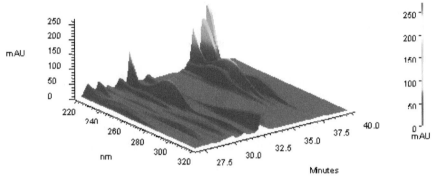

Fig. 2. Spectral chromatogram of analyzed mixture of resin acids present in Cuban colophony

The developed HPLC analysis revealed the main components of the Cuban colophony, a starting raw material for preparing sodium resinate (Fig. 3).

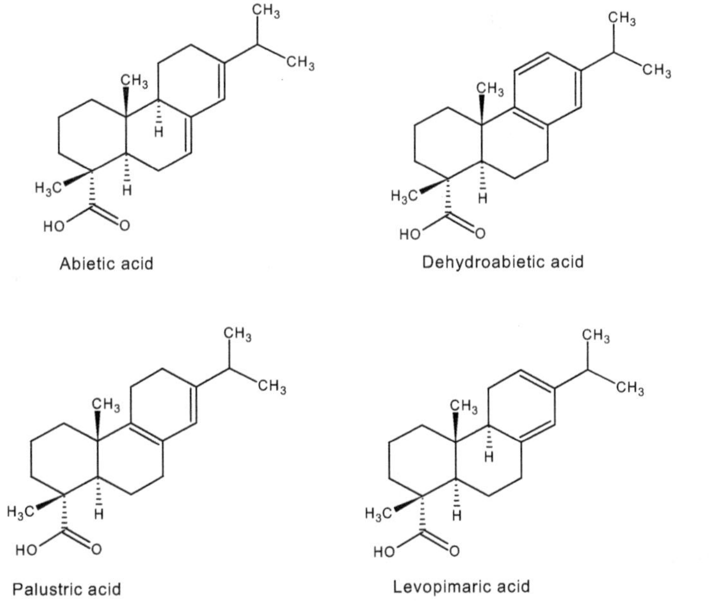

Abietic acid

Dehydroabietic acid

Palustric acid

Levopimaric acid

Fig. 3. Main resin acids present in the Cuban colophony. (abietic acid 40 %; dehydroabietic acid 22 %; palustric acid 18 %; levopimaric acid 18-20 %).

The colophony was administered in 3 dosis levels (100, 200 y 400 mg/Kg) in all experiments, except in the case of bioassay of labyrinth in cross (50, 100 y 150 mg/Kg). The DHAA dosis levels were 50, 100 and 200 mg/Kg. The injection volume of administration in mice was 0.4 ml/20 g and 1mL/100 g in rats. The colophony (sodium salt-SR) was dissolved in distillated water and administered orally.

3.1 Open field activity

SR (100, 200 and 400 mg/kg, po.) reduced locomotor activity and rearing in a dose-dependent manner during the observation period. The observations are given in Table 1. Doses of 400 mg/Kg of SR showed similar behaviour to diazepam (DZP) 1 mg/Kg (standard anxiolytic drugs).

The present study demonstrated that SR prepared from natural and pre-treated (hydro-thermally and by acid-basic reaction) resin extracted from Cuban *Pinus* reduced spontaneous locomotor activity in mice. Usually the rodents show an exploratory behaviour when they are collocated in a novel place. However, if the animals are pre-treated with depressant central nervous system drugs, the locomotor activity is decreased. This result is typical for sedative drugs.

Tested groups	mean±S.E.M
Distilled water	24,5 ± 4,20a
SR 100 mg/Kg.	20,2 ± 3,38 b
SR 200 mg/Kg.	19,6 ± 2,22 b
SR 400 mg/Kg.	12,9 ± 4,48 c
DZP 1 mg/Kg.	10,5 ± 3,39 c

Table 1. Effects of SR (100, 200 and 400 mg/kg, po.) on spontaneous locomotor activity. Groups with unequal letters differ to each other for $p < 0.05$.

3.2 Aggressive behavior

Social isolation induces aggressive behavior in several strains of mice. The isolation-induced aggression is proposed to be useful as an animal model for assessing inhibitory activity on central nervous system. Different neurotransmitters such as serotonin, noradrenaline, dopamine and gamma-aminobutyric acid (GABA) are considered to be involved in mediating aggressive behaviour; there are conflicting results on brain neurotransmitter metabolism (Matsuda et al., 2001; Sakaue et al., 2001). Table 2. shows the effects of SR on aggressive behaviour in isolated mice. Test compound reduces an aggressive behaviour in a dose-dependent manner. A similar result to open field test in between 400 mg/Kg of SR and diazepam 1 mg/Kg doses was obtained. This behaviour was reported by Valzelli in 1973 as a classic pattern for central nervous system depressor (Valzelli, 1973). Our results show an anti-aggressive behaviour in orally SR-treated mice. This result can be mediated by inhibitory effects on brain biogenic amines action or excitatory neurotransmitter release and suggests the inhibitory effect of SR on the central nervous system.

Tested groups	mean±S.E.M
Distilled water	24.90 ± 4.15 a
SR 100 mg/Kg.	17.60 ± 3.38 b
SR 200 mg/Kg.	16.75 ± 2.94 b
SR 400 mg/Kg.	12.90 ± 4.48 c
DZP 1 mg/Kg.	10.50 ± 3.39 c

Table 2. Effects of SR (100, 200 and 400 mg/kg, po.) on aggressive behaviour (biting attacks and wrestling) in isolated mice Groups with unequal letters differ to each other for $p<0.05$.

3.3 Thiopental-induced sleep

SR as well as diazepam, a standard reference drug, increased the number of sleeping animals and prolonged the thiopental-induced sleeping time in mice.

All SR doses increase the number of sleeping animals (Table 3) compared with the control, doses of 200 and 400 mg/Kg caused sleep in all animals.

SR (400 mg/Kg) and diazepam (1 mg/Kg) prolonged thiopental induced sleep in the similar manner (Table 4).

Tested groups	Percentage of sleeping animal
Distilled water	12.50
SR 100 mg/Kg.	56.25
SR 200 mg/Kg.	100
SR 400 mg/Kg.	100
DZP 1 mg/Kg.	100

Table 3. Effect of SR on percentage of sleeping animal.

Tested groups	mean±S.E.M
Distilled water	2,25 ± 6.16 a
SR 100 mg/Kg.	8,25 ± 8.65 b
SR 200 mg/Kg.	33,75 ± 8.83 c
SR 400 mg/Kg.	40,00 ± 0 d
DZP 1 mg/Kg.	40,00 ± 0 d

Table 4. Effect of SR on sleeping time (min). Groups with unequal letters differ to each other for $p<0.05$.

3.4 Drug-induced convulsion

Numerous excitatory drugs such as PTZ and PTX, can induce convulsion *via* GABA receptor antagonism, due to, the anxiolytic-like drugs (ex. diazepam) might be inhibit the drug-induced convulsion via inhibition of GABA-ergic inter-neurons.

To further investigate the inhibitory effect of SR on the central nervous system, drugs that can excite or block excitation in the central nervous system were used. Diazepam (4 mg/kg, po.) was highly effective in delaying the occurrence of clonic convulsion (Table 5 and 6) even in protecting animals against convulsion induced by PTX and PTZ. However the different doses of SR tested were unable to protect animals against convulsion and death, and unable to increase the latency of the clonic convulsion induced by pro-convulsivant drugs. Our findings show an ineffective action of SR to avoid the PTZ and PTX-induced convulsion. These results suggest that the sedative effects of test compound might not be mediated via GABA or glycine systems.

Tested groups	Latency of first convulsion	Latency of first clonic convulsion	Time of death	Percentage of animals with clonic convulsion	Percentage of death
PTX 5 mg/Kg + Distilled water	12.0 ± 1.94a	20.66 ± 4.55a	22.66 ± 5.03a	80	30
PTX 5 mg/Kg + SR 100 mg/Kg.	12.0 ± 6.00a	17.0 ± 4.36a	23.0 ± 8.48a	70	20
PTX 5 mg/Kg + SR 200 mg/Kg.	15.90 ± 8.60a	20.2 ± 4.76a	26.0 ± 1.41a	80	20
PTX 5 mg/Kg + SR 400 mg/Kg.	16.8 ± 6.37a	21.62 ± 5.70a	24.0 ± 2.91a	80	20
PTX 5 mg/Kg + DZP 4 mg/Kg	23.0 ± 3.21b	26.0 ± 3.80b	28.1 ± 2.12b	20	0

Table 5. Effect of SR on clonic convulsion induced by PTX. Groups with unequal letters differ to each other for $p<0.05$.

Tested groups	Latency of first convulsion	Latency of first clonic convulsion	Time of death	Percentage of animals with clonic convulsion	Percentage of death
PTZ 85 mg/Kg + Distilled water	7.30 ± 1.66 a	11.66 ± 3.07 a	14.80 ± 3.83 a	60	50
PTZ 85 mg/Kg + SR 100 mg/Kg	6.00 ± 2.45 a	11.50 ± 1.52 a	13.17 ± 3.97 a	60	60
PTZ 85 mg/Kg + SR 200 mg/Kg	7.27 ± 1.35 a	13.16 ± 2.23 a	13.0 ± 3.16 a	60	40
PTZ 85 mg/Kg + SR 400 mg/Kg	7.90 ± 2.28 a	11.50 ± 3.45 a	13.33 ± 1.86 a	60	40
PTZ 85 mg/Kg + DZP4 mg/Kg	25.0 ± 2.18 b	27.1 ± 3.26 b	29.0 ± 1.18 b	20	0

Table 6. Effect of SR on clonic convulsion induced by PTZ. Groups with unequal letters differ to each other for $p<0.05$.

3.5 Elevated plus-maze behavior

Rodents usually avoid open arms and prefer enclosed arms in an elevated plus-maze. Time spent in open arms and numbers of entries into open arms are indexes of neophobic anxiety in animals. Standard anxiolytic drugs such as diazepam increase open-arm exploration, as reflected by increases in the time spent and the number of entries into the open arms (Pellow, 1985).

Diazepam exhibited the conventional profile of anxiolytics in the elevated plus-maze test; it increased the percentage of open arm entries and time spent in open arms (Table 7). However, SR did not significantly modify the percentage of either time spent or arm entries in open arms at any of the doses tested.

Tested groups	Time spent in open arms	Time spent in close arms	Open arm entries (%)	Open close entries (%)	Number of open arm entries (counts)	Number of closed arm entries (counts)
Distilled water	8.2 ± 8.02 a	198.9 ± 44.70 a	14.81 ± 12.45 a	85.18 ± 12.45 a	1.80± 1.62 a	8.9± 2.33 a
SR 50 mg/Kg	9.12 ± 7.07 a	112.56 ± 30.25 a	16.23 ± 14.36 a	87.26 ± 10.25 a	1.93± 0.98 a	8.03± 2.15 a
SR 100 mg/Kg	9,6 ± 14,35 a	85.4 ± 42,77 a	18,68 ± 23,70 a	81,31 ± 23,70 a	1.50± 2.01 a	7.6± 3.60 a
SR 150 mg/Kg	10.08 ± 8.23 a	93.15 ± 29.15 a	17.59 ± 9.23 a	83.26 ± 15.15 a	1.75± 1.29 a	7.98± 2.23 a
DZP 0.5 mg/Kg	55.23 ± 5.56 b	70.18 ± 7.83 b	65,17 ± 12.18 b	34,83 ± 6.65 b	19.05± 2.15 b	10.18± 1.98 a

Table 7. Effect of SR on the elevated plus-maze test in mice (see Table 6). Groups with unequal letters differ to each other for p<0.05.

3.6 Amphetamine-induced behavioral stereotypy

Psycho stimulants (such as, amphetamine a simpatic-mimetic amine) administration in rats increase dopamine levels in different brain zones, induce stereotyped behaviours, characterized by repetitive sniffing, biting, grooming, and head movements. The dopamine receptor antagonist or sedative drugs can be reducing its behaviour (Ralph et al. 2001). Table 8 shows behavioral stereotypy after subcutaneously administration of amphetamine, 1.5 mg/Kg (p.sc). Rats treated with SR reduced its behaviour in a dose-dependent manner compared with the water-treated group and amphetamine. The observed results reveal that colophony decreases the stimulant effect either for an antagonism of dopaminergic transmission, inhibition of dopamine releasing, blocking of its post-synaptic receptor or by an activation of some inhibitory transmission with the decrease of excitation caused by the dosis of employed amphetamine. The data suggest that the colophony has not a characteristic profile of active antidepressants. It was confirmed by the evaluation of amphetamine (5 mg/Kg)-induced sleeping and its extension in time.

Tested groups	mean±S.E.M
Distilled water	10.45 ± 3.70a
SR 100 mg/Kg. + amphetamine 1,5 mg/Kg.	22,71 ± 4.90b
SR 200 mg/Kg. + amphetamine 1,5 mg/Kg.	23,92 ± 5,75b
SR 400 mg/Kg. + amphetamine 1,5 mg/Kg.	20,70 ± 5,85b
Distilled water + amphetamine 1,5 mg/Kg.	31,64 ± 5,98c
Haloperidol 5 mg/Kg. + amphetamine 1,5 mg/Kg.	12,28 ± 2,56a

Table 8. Effect of SR on behavioural stereotypy induced by amphetamine. Groups with unequal letters differ to each other for $p<0.05$.

3.7 Amphetamine -induced sleep in mice

Mice treated with different doses of SR exhibited similar behaviour against amphetamine - induced sleep in mice compare with water-treated group (Table 9).

Tested groups	Media ± D.S
Distilled water + amphetamine 5 mg/Kg	189.90 ± 9.65
SR 100 mg/Kg. + amphetamine 5 mg/Kg	190.00 ± 11.51
SR 200 mg/Kg. + amphetamine 5 mg/Kg	195.86 ± 5.05
SR 400 mg/Kg. + amphetamine 5 mg/Kg	190.22 ± 7.07

Table 9. Effect of SR on sleep induced by amphetamine in mice.

Although SR showed a sedative effect in evaluated tests (thiopental-induced sleep, open field activity, aggressive behaviours and amphetamine-induced behavioral stereotypy). The interaction of SR with convulsant drugs, confirms that the sedative effect of test compound might not be related via the GABA or glycine systems.

In this context, recently our group found that abietic and dehydroabietic acids might be responsible of the sedative effects of the SR (Unpublished result).

3.8 Acute oral toxicity study

The death of any animal was not observed during the study. The major adverse effects were related with CNS depression (motor impairment and sedation), but these symptoms disappeared within 4 h. With this exception, no outward behavioral abnormalities were noted during the 2-week post-treatment period. The body weight gains were observed in the similar manner in both groups (Figure 4). Macroscopic alterations were not observed in selected organs and tissues removed (stomach, liver, kidney, brain, spleen and lungs). The administration of SR didn't cause significant toxic symptoms for what classifies in 5 category of the GHS or not classified (mortality> 2000 mg/kg).

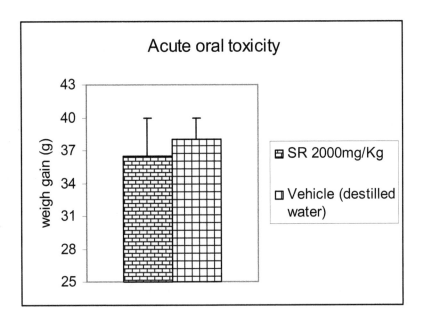

Fig. 4. Effect of SR 2000 mg/Kg on acute oral toxicity test.

Taking into consideration the structural similarity, *grosso modo*,(molecular modeling are underway and are unpublished results yet) between secondary metabolites, DHAA, related derivatives and cannabinoids, the observed pharmacological effects could be attribute to a potential antagonism with glutamate receptors and/or inhibition of noradrenalin-dopamine releasing. The acute toxicity study revealed that no toxic effects were observed, and any symptom (increase of cleaning-up behavior, exploration, decreasing of frequency of movement, etc) disappeared after 4 hrs. In the autopsy were not detected any macroscopic or anatomic effect on organs.

In the case of dehydroabietic acid (DHAA) generated by disproportionation-aromatization of resinic acids the results reveal a dosis depending effect on decreasing of exploratory activity, typical for sedative pharmaceutical compositions. It co-administration (50 mg/Kg) with thiopental, at experimental dosis, increase the number of sleeping animals (65%), a typical depressing action on CNS. The administration of DHAA, at all dosis evaluated, didn't protect animals for PTZ induced convulsions. The experimental data obtained in the Labyrinth in cross model didn't show any relevant results. In the Amphetamine-induced stereotipia model DHAA decreases the stimulant action produced by the subcutaneously administration of 1,5 mg / Kg of amphetamine, in the hypothetically pathways described above. The acute toxicity (DL_{50} > 5000 mg/Kg) study showed that DHAA had not any toxic effects at dosis concentrations used and could be classified in the GSH in the 5 category.

It is noteworthy that synthetic DHAA has a sedative action on CNS and could be employed as starting raw material for designing of new molecular and pharmacological entities potentially useful in the development of formulation for therapy of CNS pathologies where de sedative effect is needed.

Topological studies for determining any QSAR correlation between colophony and derivatives and cannabinoids are underway.

4. Conclusion

The oleoresin, a raw material isolated from Cuban Pinacea (gen. *Pinus, Pinus caribbaea*), constitutes a sustainable resource for developing potentially useful pro-drugs and pharmacologically active substances as resínic acids, sodium resinate (SR) and dehydroabietic acid. The analytical protocol developed (*all in one* wavelengths-retention time) for common abietanes present in Cuban colophony is simple, time-saving, eco-friendly, employing robust reversed-phase HPLC and offer the possibility to determine and quantify the main diterpenic acids (resínico acids) in the natural and modified mixture. The catalytic synthesis of dehydroabietic acid (DHAA) as a principal active pharmaceutical component from colophony for the potential treatment of neuro-psiquiatric dysfunctions and generation of exogenic cannabinoid analogues has been developed under ecological conditions using piritic ash as re-usable catalyst (disproportionation-aromatization) at meso-scale with minimal environmental impact. The neuropharmacological profile (including acute oral toxicity) of SR in rodent behavioural tests was determined; SR reduced spontaneous locomotor activity and aggressive behaviour, increased the number of sleeping animals and prolonged the thiopental-induced sleeping time indicating a the sedative effect of test compound and it might not be related via the GABA or glycine systems. The SR is unable to protect animals against convulsion and death induced by pentylenetetrazole and picrotoxin. The SR (2000 mg/Kg p.o) didn't cause significant toxic symptoms in rats. This finding indicates that the SR can constitute a non conventional source of pharmacological molecular entities with central nervous system depressant activity. The synthetic DHAA has a sedative action on CNS and its acute toxicity (DL_{50} > 5000 mg/Kg) reveals that DHAA had not any toxic effects at dosis concentrations used and could be employed as starting design structural point for developing molecular entities and series leads with potentially remarkable pharmacological properties.

Unconventional Raw Natural Sustainable Sources for Obtaining Pharmacological Principles Potentially
Active on CNS Through Catalytic, Ecologically Clean, Processes

91

5. References

Carlini, E.A., Contar, J.D.P., Silva, A.R., Silveira- Filho, N.G., Frochtengarten, M.L., Bueno, O.F.A. (1986). Pharmacology of lemongrass (Cymbopogon citratus Stapf). I. Effects of teas prepared from the leaves on laboratory animals. *J. Ethnopharmacol.* 17, 37-64.

Costa, E., Greengard, P. (1975). Mechanism of action of benzodiazepines. New York: *Adv Biochem Psychopharmacol*, Raven Press, pp. 14.

CU Patent 20060144, (2006). Tacoronte J.E et al. Disproportionation of Cuban colophony with piritic ash and obtention of dehydroabietic acid.

CU Patent 20060252, (2006). Tacoronte J.E et al. Natural cannabinoid precursors with pharmacological action on CNS.

Franich R A, Gadgil, P. D. (1983). Fungistatic effects of *Pinus radiata* needle epicuticular fatty and resin acids on *Dothistroma pini*. *Physiol. Plant Pathol.* 23:183-195.

Fischer, W., Vander, H. (1998). Effect of clobenpropit, a centrally acting histamine H3-receptors antagonist, on electroshock and pentilenetetrazol-induced seizures in mice. *J-Neural-transm.* 105(6-7), 587-99.

Kuczenski, R., Segal, D.S. (1999). Sensitization of amphetamine-induced stereotyped behaviors during the acute response. *J-Pharmacol-Exp-Ther.* 288(2), 699-709.

Latorre A, Rigol A, Lacorte S, Barcelo D. (2003). Comparison of gas chromatography-mass spectrometry and liquid chromatography-mass spectrometry for the determination of fatty and resin acids in paper mill process waters. *J. Chromatogr.* A 991:205-215.

Matsuda, T., Sakaue, M., Ago, Y., Sakamoto, Y., Koyama, Y., Baba, A. (2001). Functional Alteration of Brain Dopaminergic System in Isolated Aggressive Mice, *Jpn. J. Neuropsychopharmacol.* 21, 71-76.

OECD Guideline For Testing Of Chemical "Acute Oral Toxicity – Acute Toxic Class Method" N° 423 Adopted 20 December 2001.

Pellow, S. (1985). Validation of open: closed arm entries in an elevated plus-maze as a measure of anxiety in the rat. *Journal of Neuroscience* Method 14, 149-167.

Ralph, R.J., Paulus, M.P., Fumagalli, F., Caron, M.G., Geyer, M.A. (2001). Prepulse Inhibition Deficits and Perseverative Motor Patterns in Dopamine Transporter Knock-Out Mice: Differential Effects of D1 and D2 Receptor Antagonists. *Journal of Neuroscience.* 21(1), 305-313.

Sakaue, M., Ago, Y., Murakami, C., Sowa, C., Sakamoto, Y., Koyama, Y., Baba, A., Matsuda, T. (2001). Involvement of benzodiazepine binding sites in an antiaggressive effect by 5-HT1A receptor activation in isolated mice. *European Journal of Pharmacology.* 432, 163-166.

Sukma, M., Chaichantipyuth, C.H., Murakami, Y., Tohda, M., Matsumoto, K., Watanabe, H. (2002). CNS inhibitory effects of barakol, a constituent of Cassia siamia Lamk. *J. Ethnopharmacology.* 83, 87:94.

Tulp M, Bohlin L. (2005) Rediscovery of known natural compounds: Nuisance or goldmine? *Bioorganic & Medicinal Chemistry.* 13 5274–5282

Tyler, C. B.; K. A. (1982) Miczed: effects of phencyclidine on aggressive behavior in mice. *Pharmacol Biochem Behav* 17: 503-10.

Valzelli, L. (1973) The isolation syndrome in mice. *Psychopharmacology 31:305-20.*

4

Antibothropic Action of *Camellia sinensis* Extract Against the Neuromuscular Blockade by *Bothrops jararacussu* Snake Venom and Its Main Toxin, Bothropstoxin-I

Yoko Oshima-Franco et al.[*]
University of Sorocaba/UNISO,
Brazil

1. Introduction

Snake bite envenoming, a serious public health problem in rural areas of tropical and subtropical countries, was included in 2007 as a neglected disease by the World Health Organization (WHO, 2007). Under this geographical perspective Africa, Asia, Oceania and Latin America are the most vulnerable countries to this kind of accident, but also shared by many developing countries (Harrison et al., 2009; Warrel, 2010). An excellent meta-analytic approach about the subject was described by Chippaux (2011), who analysed more than 3,000 references for estimating the burden of snakebites in sub-Saharan Africa. Brazil encloses both requirements, as a developing and a tropical country, and needs to strengthen measures against venomous snake accidents, since, according to Lima et al. (2009), it is the country with the major number of accidents (about 20,000 cases/year), followed by Peru (4,500), Venezuela (2,500-3,000), Colombia (2,675), Ecuador (1,200-1,400) and Argentina (1,150-1.250) (Warrel, 2004).

As mentioned by Nicoleti et al. (2010), venomous snakes in Brazil are represented by *Bothrops, Bothropoides, Bothriopsis, Bothrocophias, Rhinocerophis, Crotalus, Lachesis, Leptomicrurus* and *Micrurus* (see the new taxonomic arrangement proposed by Fenwick et al., 2009). Envenoming by the first five genera produce similar toxic manifestations and treatment assessment are quite the same. They represent 86.9% of accidents, whereas 8.7% were caused by *Crotalus*, 3.6% *Lachesis* and 0.8% by *Leptomicrurus* and *Micrurus* (Ministério da Saúde, 2004).

Bothrops jararacussu snake belongs to the Viperidae family and its venom is able to induce severe signs of local and systemic envenoming, such as necrosis, shock, spontaneous

[*]Luana de Jesus Reis Rosa[1], Gleidy Ana Araujo Silva[1], Jorge Amaral Filho[1], Magali Glauzer Silva[1], Patricia Santos Lopes[2], José Carlos Cogo[3], Adélia Cristina Oliveira Cintra[4] and Maria Alice da Cruz-Höfling[5]
[1]*University of Sorocaba/UNISO, Brazil*
[2]*Federal University of São Paulo/UNIFESP, Brazil*
[3]*University of Vale do Paraiba/UNIVAP, Brazil*
[4]*University of São Paulo/USP, Brazil*
[5]*University of Campinas/UNICAMP/I.B./D.H.E., Brazil*

systemic bleeding and renal failure, incoagulable blood and death (Milani et al., 1997); its venom also blocks *in vitro* the contractile skeletal muscle response (Rodrigues-Simioni et al., 1983). Two myotoxins are responsible for myonecrosis: bothropstoxin-I (Homsi-Brandeburgo et al., 1988), the first myotoxin isolated from the venom that reproduces the effects of the crude venom (Heluany et al., 1992), further characterized as a phospholipase A_2-Lys49 (Cintra et al., 1993); and bothropstoxin-II, a phospholipase A_2 (Gutiérrez et al., 1991), further characterized as an Asp49-PLA$_2$ myotoxin with low catalytic activity (Pereira et al., 1998), although phylogenetically it is more related to Lys49-PLA$_2$s than to other Asp49-PLA$_2$s (dos Santos et al., 2011).

Snake antivenom immunoglobulins (antivenoms) are the only specific treatment for envenoming by snakebites. They are produced by fractionation of plasma usually obtained from large domestic animals hyper-immunized against relevant snake venoms. When injected into an envenomed human patient, antivenom will neutralize any of the effects of the venoms used in its production, and in some instances will also neutralize effects of venoms from closely related species (WHO, 2011a). However, the antibothropic serum effectiveness against the local effects of *Bothrops jararacussu* venom (one of the bothropic venoms used in the serum production) has been debated since the 80's decade (see Correa-Neto et al., 2010). A possible explanation for the lack of effectivenes was given by Battellino et al. (2003) through the use of intravital microscopy after intravenous administration of antibothropic antivenom (BAv), labeled with fluorescein isothiocyanate (FITC). They observed that the antivenom neutralized the systemic effects, but did not efficiently reverse the local effects due to an impaired and/or delayed venom:antivenom interaction at the site of injury. Considering that local effect of venomous snakebites are poorly prevented by specific antivenom, that the access to public health services by people of distant rural regions in tropical and subtropical countries is in general difficult, the use of medicinal plants as a local solution has been a practice of natives of those regions.

Medicinal plants represent a sophisticated biotechnological laboratory that is able to produce a multitude of pharmacologically bioactive substances, with a wide variety of effects (Mahmood et al., 2005). The second beverage (next to water) of major consumption in the world, in its green, black and oolong forms, is the tea from *Camellia sinensis* L. leaves Compounds as polyphenols, polysaccharides, aminoacids, vitamins (Crespy & Williamson, 2004), caffeine and a very small amout of methylxanthines (Yang et al., 1998) can be found in the plant. Catechins, the major component of green tea (fresh leaves are steamed to prevent fermentation, yielding a dry, stable product), and represent the low-molecular-weight polyphenols consisting mainly of flavanol (flavan-3-ol) monomers, such as epicatechin, epicatechin-3-gallate, epigallocatechin and the major, 50-80% of the total catechin, epigallocatechin-3-gallate (Graham, 1992; Khan & Mukhtar, 2007). Catechins account for 6-16% (Zhu & Chen, 1999) up to 30-40% (Phithayanukul et al., 2010) of the dry green tea leaves. The fermentation or semifermentation stage (when the withered leaves are rolled and crushed) during the manufacture of black or oolong tea, respectively, converts catechins to theaflavins (theaflavin, theaflavin-3-gallate, theaflavin-3'-gallate and theaflavin-3,3'-digallate, accounting for 3-6% of solid extract) and thearubigins (accounting for 12-18% of solid extract) (Leung et al., 2001; Khan & Mukhtar, 2007), which are complex polyphenols of poorly-defined chemical structures formed during fermentation of polymerization of theaflavins (Hazarika et al., 1984).

The literature describing the medicinal benefits of tea is extensive, but the report about its consumption to alleviate post game fatigue in players and sportsmen (Krishnamoorthy, 1991) inspired further studies on the mammalian skeletomotor apparatus (Das et al., 1994; 1997). For example, Basu et al. (2005) attributed to theaflavin, but not thearubigin, the facilitatory effect induced at the skeletal myoneural junction. This experimental model has been traditionally used for the pharmacological characterization of snake venoms, and the association between C. sinensis and snake venoms was a natural consequence. Thus, results showing the inhibitory effect of tea polyphenols on local tissue damage induced by snake venoms (Pithayanukul et al., 2010), and the inhibitory effect of Camellia sinensis leaves extracts against the neuromuscular blockade of Crotalus durissus terrificus venom (de Jesus Reis Rosa et al., 2010) were recently published. Here, using the same experimental procedure, the antivenom property of Camellia sinensis leaves extract was assayed against Bothrops jararacussu venom and its main myotoxin, bothropstoxin-I. Commercial theaflavin (from black tea) and epigallocatechin gallate (from green tea), known to be part of the C. sinensis extract, were also tested.

2. Materials and methods

2.1 Hydroalcoholic extract from leaves of *Camellia sinensis*

The leaves of C. sinensis were harvested from plants growing in an orchard at the University of Sorocaba – UNISO (Sorocaba, SP, Brazil). A voucher specimen was deposited in the Instituto Agronômico de Campinas (IAC, number 50.469) herbarium (http://herbario.iac.sp.gov.br) after identification by L.C. Bernacci. Briefly, sixty-four grams of leaves powder were macerated along with 150 mL of 70° GL ethanol, over 3 days. After this period, the resulting suspension was placed into a percolator with 50 mL of 70° GL ethanol, and left for a further 3 days. The macerated drug was percolated and a 20% hydroalcoholic extract was obtained (de Jesus Reis Rosa et al., 2010). The solvent was evaporated until dryness, and the dried extract was then protected from light and humidity at room temperature until the assays.

2.2 Pharmacological study

2.2.1 Animals

Male Swiss white mice (26-32 g) were supplied by the Anilab - Animais de Laboratório (Paulínia, São Paulo, Brazil). The animals were housed at $25 \pm 3°C$ on a 12-h light/dark cycle with access to food and water *ad libitum*. This study was approved (protocol number A077/CEP2007) by the Committee for Ethics in Research from the University of Vale do Paraiba (UNIVAP) and all experiments were performed according to the guidelines of the Brazilian College for Animal Experimentation.

2.2.2 Venom and toxin

The crude venom was obtained from adult Bothrops jararacussu (Bjssu) snakes (Serpentário do Centro de Estudos da Natureza) and certified by Prof. Dr. Jose Carlos Cogo, University of Vale do Paraiba (Univap), São Jose dos Campos, SP, Brazil. Bothropstoxin-I (BthTX-I) was obtained under the conditions described by Homsi-Brandeburgo et al. (1988).

2.2.3 Mouse phrenic-nerve diaphragm muscle (PND) preparation

The PND was obtained from mice anesthetized with halothane and sacrificed by exsanguination. The diaphragm was removed (Bülbring, 1946) and mounted under a tension of 5 g in a 5 mL organ bath containing continuous-aerated Tyrode solution (control) with the following composition: 137 mM NaCl, 2.7 mM KCl, 1.8 mM $CaCl_2$, 0.49 mM $MgCl_2$, 0.42 mM NaH_2PO_4, 11.9 mM $NaHCO_3$, and 11.1 mM glucose. After stabilization with 95% O_2/5% CO_2, the pH was 7.0. The PND myographic recording was performed according to Melo et al. (2009). Briefly, preparations were stimulated indirectly with supramaximal stimuli (4 x threshold, 0.06 Hz, 0.2 ms) delivered from a stimulator (model ESF-15D, Ribeirão Preto, SP, Brazil) to the nerve through bipolar electrodes. Isometric twitch tension was recorded with a force displacement transducer (cat. 7003, Ugo Basile), coupled to a 2-Channel Recorder Gemini physiograph (cat. 7070, Ugo Basile) via a Basic Preamplifier (cat. 7080, Ugo Basile). PND was allowed to stabilize for at least 20 min before addition of the following substances: BthTX-I alone at 20 µg/mL (n=11); Bjssu alone at 40 µg/mL (n=5); 20 µg/mL BthTX-I + 0.05 mg/mL C. sinensis extract (n=5); 40 µg/mL Bjssu + 0.05 mg/mL C. sinensis extract (n=3); 40 µg/mL Bjssu + 0.025 mg/mL epigallocatechin gallate (n=3, Sigma-Aldrich, SP, Brazil); 40 µg/mL Bjssu + 0.05 mg/mL theaflavin (n=3); and the controls nutritive Tyrode solution (n=7) and 0.05 mg/mL C. sinensis extracts (n=7). The plant extract or commercial phytochemicals concentrations were chosen based on the minor changes obtained in comparison with the basal response of PND incubated with Tyrode nutritive solution (control).

2.3 Quantitative histological study

At least three preparations (n=3) resulting from pharmacological assays were analyzed by quantitative morfometry. Preparations used in the controls, nutritive Tyrode solution and C. sinensis hydroalcoholic extract (0.05 mg/mL) were compared to BthTX-I (20 µg/mL), or C. sinensis (0.05 mg/mL) + BthTX-I (20 µg/mL) groups, or Bjssu (40 µg/mL), or C. sinensis (0.05 mg/mL) + Bjssu venom (40 µg/mL) after fixation in Bouin solution and submission to routinely morphological techniques. Cross-sections (5 µm thick) of diaphragm muscle embedded in paraffin were stained with Hematoxylin-Eosin for microscopy examination. Tissue damage was expressed in percentage (number of damaged muscle cells divided by the total number of cells in three non-overlapping, non-adjacent areas of each preparation) according to Cintra-Francischinelli et al. (2008).

2.4 Thin layer chromatography (TLC)

Aliquots of C. sinensis hydroalcoholic extract were spotted onto 0.2 mm thickness silica gel $60F_{254}$ on aluminum plates, 20.10 cm, (Merck, Germany) and developed with ethyl acetate:methanol:water (100:13.5:10, v/v) in a pre-saturated chromatographic chamber along with appropriate phytochemical standards (Simões et al., 2004). These standards (theaflavin and epigallocatechin gallate, Sigma-Aldrich® - USA) were solubilized in methanol (1 mg/mL). The separated spots were visualized (under UV light at 360 nm) with NP/PEG as follows: 5% (v/v) ethanolic NP (diphenylboric acid 2-aminoethyl ester, Sigma Chemical Co., St. Louis, MO, USA) followed by 5% (v/v) ethanolic PEG 4000 (polyethylene glycol 4000, Synth Chemical Co., São Paulo, SP, Brazil). The retention factor (Rf) of each standard was compared with spots exhibited by C. sinensis extracts.

2.5 Statistical analysis

Each pharmacological protocol was repeated at least three times. Results were expressed as the mean ± standard error of the mean (SEM). The Student's t-test or repeated measures ANOVA were used for statistical comparison of the data. The significance level was set at 5%.

3. Results

3.1 Pharmacological assays

3.1.1 BthTX-I neutralization

Figure 1 shows the PND blockade activity of BthTX-I (20 µg/mL, n=11), which was irreversible even after washing (W) of preparations with fresh nutritive Tyrode solution. However, the previous incubation of the toxin with 0.05 mg/mL Camellia sinensis extract totally (100%) prevented the characteristic neurotransmission blockade, showing a better functional outcome of neuromuscular preparation after washing. The 0.05 mg/mL of Camellia sinensis extract was chosen in all protocols since it induced minor changes compared with the basal response of PND.

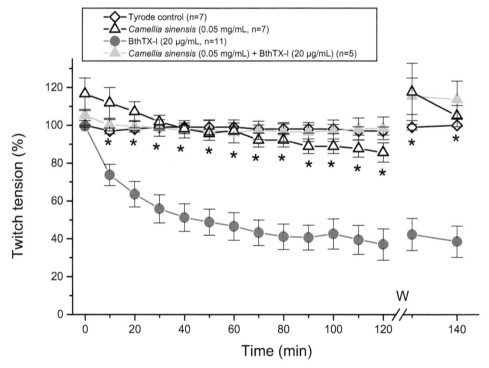

Fig. 1. Isolated mouse phrenic nerve-diaphragm preparations under indirect stimuli. Note the total efficacy of C. sinensis extract in protecting the neuromuscular blockade induced by BthTX-I. Each point represents the mean ± SEM. * = p<0.05 in comparison with the bothropstoxin-I (BthTX-I); W, washing.

3.1.2 Bjssu neutralization

Figure 2 shows the PND blockade activity by Bjssu crude venom. There was no contraction recovery of PND after washing the preparation. *C. sinensis* extract was 78 ± 12 % able to neutralize the venom that, in turn, differently of its myotoxin, contains several constituents.

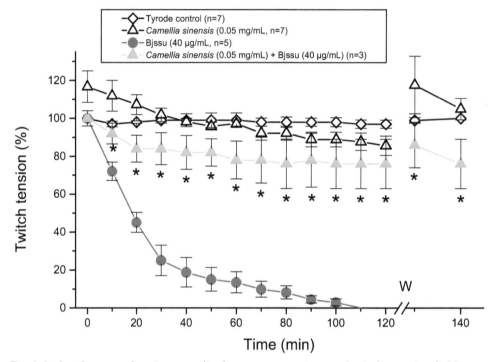

Fig. 2. Isolated mouse phrenic nerve-diaphragm preparations under indirect stimuli. Note the partial efficacy of *C. sinensis* extract in protecting the neuromuscular blockade induced by Bjssu. Each point represents the mean ± SEM. * = $p<0.05$ in comparison with the venom. W, washing. Bjssu, *Bothrops jararacussu* venom.

3.2 Quantitative histological study

Figure 3 shows neuromuscular preparations exposed either to Tyrode (Fig. 3A) or *C. sinensis* extract (Fig. 3B): the muscle fibers were well-preserved, showing changes not significantly different between each other of 15.9 ± 0.8 % or 25.3 ± 1.1 % damaged fibers, respectively. These changes were related mainly to loss of the typical cell cross-sectional polygonal profile. Differently, BthTX-I (Fig. 3C, 66.6 ± 2.3 %) and venom (Fig. 3E, 75.1 ± 1.1 %) alone clearly showed in transversal sections characteristic signals of myonecrosis (m), edematous cells (e), loss of polygonal profile, sarcolemma disruption, delta lesion (arrow), "ghost" cells (g), and nuclei (n) dispersed in the tissue. These changes were already extensively described in the scientific literature. Panel 3D and 3F show cross-sections of PND muscle fibers after *in vitro* neutralization by *C. sinensis* extract of BthTX-I (23.4 ± 1.3 % of lesioned fibers, $p<0.05$) and of Bjssu (27.8 ± 0.9 % of lesioned fibers, $p<0.05$), respectively.

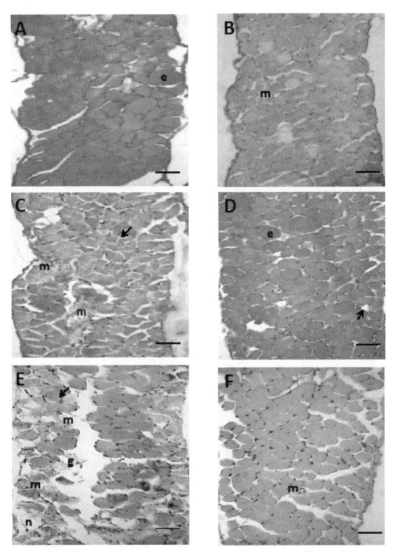

Fig. 3. Cross-sections (5 μm thick) of diaphragm embedded in paraffin and stained with
Hematoxylin-Eosin. (A) Control-sham diaphragm preparation (15.9 ± 0.8 %). (B)
Neuromuscular preparation exposed to 0.05 mg/mL Camellia sinensis extract (25.3 ± 1.1 %).
(C) Muscle incubated with 20 μg/mL BthTX-I (66.6 ± 2.3 %). (E) Muscle incubated with 40
μg/mL Bjssu venom (75.1 ± 1.1 %). The main fibers damage are lettered as follows:
myonecrosis (m), edema (e), delta lesion (arrow), sarcolemmal disruption with nuclei (n)
dispersion, "ghost" cells (g) visualized by spaces optically empty. Note that area with
extensive myonecrosis has a hyaline aspect. Muscles incubated with 0.05 mg/mL Camellia
sinensis extract (D and F) shows fibers maintaining its characteristic polygonal profile in
despite of a number of them being edematous (e). A slow percentage of them · 23.4 ± 1.3 %
for BthTX-I (D); 27.8 ± 0.9 % for Bjssu (F) · · showed myonecrosis (m). Bars = 50 μ m.

3.3 Efficacy of commercial phytochemicals against Bjssu venom

Figure 4 shows the effect of commercial 0.05 mg/mL theaflavin and 0.025 mg/mL epigallocatechin gallate from *C. sinensis* on twitch blockade induced by 40 µg/mL Bjssu venom. This paralysis was completely blocked (n=3, *p<0.05 compared to the venom, but did not show statistical differences with *C. sinensis* extract). In addition, following washing out of treated preparation with fresh physiological salt solution, twitch height was re-established (not shown).

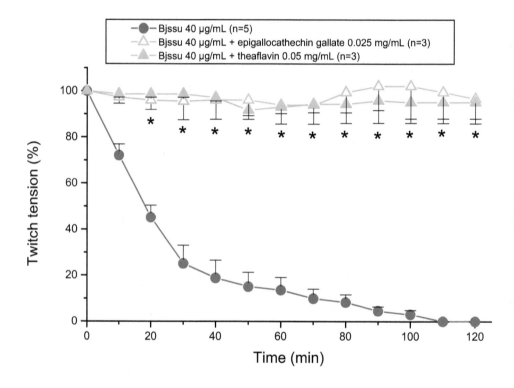

Fig. 4. Isolated mouse phrenic nerve-diaphragm preparations under indirect stimuli. Antibothropic action of commercial phytochemicals from Camellia sinensis. Note total protection against the paralysis of Bjssu (Bothrops jararacussu) venom. Each point represents the mean ± SEM. * = p<0.05 in comparison with the crude venom.

3.4 Thin layer chromatography (TLC)

Figure 5 shows a chromatoplaque of *C. sinensis* leaves extract obtained by TLC exhibiting a complex variety of compounds including theaflavin and epigallocatechin as confirmed by Rf of these commercial phytochemicals. Panel A is the chromatoplaque exposed only to a UV light at 360 nm, whereas Panel B is the same plaque after NP/PEG chromogenic agent pulverization.

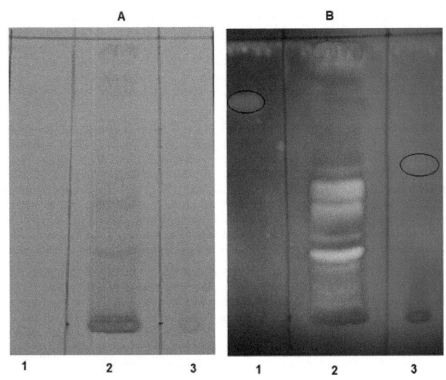

Fig. 5. Thin Layer Chromatography performed by using ethyl acetate:methanol:water
(100:13.5:10) solvent/Developer: NP/PEG. Phytochemical standards: 1 - Epigallocatechin
gallate (Rf=0.80); 2 – Cs, Camellia sinensis leaves extract; 3 – Theaflavin (Rf=0.56). Panel A:
chromatoplaque exposed to UV light at 360 nm. Panel B: is the same plaque after NP/PEG
chromogenic agent pulverization. Cs spots are suggestive of several flavonoids
(yellow/orange fluorescence) and phenolic constituents (blue fluorescence), including
epigallocatechin gallate and theaflavin, respectively. Comparative Rf values between
phytochemicals and extract are highlighted in the circle. Rf, retention factor.

4. Discussion

Although the only specific treatment for envenoming by snakebites is immunoglobulins
(antivenoms), since it can prevent or reverse most of the systemic effects and hence
minimizing mortality and morbidity (WHO, 2011a), any alternative strategy aiming to
interrupt or neutralize the steps of envenoming process can be effective for snakebite local
effects. The clinical features of the bites of venomous snakes reflect the effects of these
venom components that vary between species to species, but can broadly be divided into
categories which include i) cytotoxins, causing local swelling and tissue damage, ii)
haemorrhagins, which disturb the integrity of blood vessels, iii) compounds, which lead to
incoagulable blood, iv) neurotoxins, causing neurotoxicity and iv) myotoxins, which cause
muscle breakdown (WHO, 2011b). *Bothrops jararacussu* venom encloses all of them, except *in
vivo* neurotoxicity (Milani et al., 1997), but it causes an *in vitro* neuromuscular blockade
(Rodrigues-Simioni et al., 1983).

As snake accidents occur by bites and venoms are commonly injected in the subcutaneous muscle tissue, the use of muscle preparations as model for the study of the pharmacological effects of snake venom and toxins is very relevant. Besides, the use of snake venom and toxins as tools to study neuromuscular blockade *in vitro* (Gallacci & Cavalcante, 2010) is very useful given the excitation-contraction coupling process starts with transmission of electrical impulses from nerves towards muscle fibers via release of acetylcholine (ACh) (Hughes et al., 2006).

On the other hand, the plant kingdom represents a rich resource of new molecules able to counteract the venom effects, mainly when the plant is as worldwide as *Camellia sinensis*, an evergreen Asiatic shrub of the Theaceae family. Polyphenols from black or green tea has been shown to be powerful antioxidants with a potent inhibitory effect on low density lipoprotein (LDL) oxidation *in vitro* (Miura et al., 2000), exert anti-carcinogenic (Lambert & Yang, 2003) and anti-inflammatory (Arab & Il'yasova, 2003) effects; act as antibacterial and antiviral agents (Friedman, 2007), and are able to reduce the incidence of coronary heart disease and diabetes (Crozier et al., 2009), among other effects (see Khan & Mukhtar, 2007). Despite its health benefits, there are few studies using *C. sinensis* addressed to snake venom.

Hung et al. (2004) showed an antagonistic effect of 3 mg per mouse of melanin extracted from black tea (MEBT), an unhydrolyzed complex of tea polyphenols (Sava et al., 2001), against *Agkistrodon contortrix laticinctus* (broadbanded copperhead), *Agkistrodon halys blomhoffii* (Japanese mamushi), and *Crotalus atrox* (western diamondback rattlesnake) snake venoms, when administered i.p. immediately after venom administration in the same place of venom injection. Authors demonstrated correlation between antivenom activity of melanin and PLA_2 inhibition as a possible explanation for the protective effect.

Tea polyphenols have been shown to interact with hydrolytic enzymes from *Naja naja kaouthia* Lesson (Elapidae) and *Calloselasma rhodostoma* Kuhl (Viperidae) venoms, inhibiting inflammation and local tissue damage. This effect was attributed to complexation and chelation among the venom proteins and the phenolic contents of the extract. According to the authors, the *Camellia sinensis* extract also inhibited phospholipase A_2, proteases, hyaluronidase and L-amino acid oxidase by *in vitro* neutralization and the hemorrhagic and the dermonecrotic activities of the venoms *in vivo* (Pithayanukul et al., 2010).

Satoh et al. (2002 a,b) reported the protective effect of thearubigin from black tea extract against the neuromuscular blockade caused by botulin neurotoxins and tetanus toxin in synaptosomal membrane preparations. Recently, de Jesus Reis Rosa et al. (2010) reiterate the protective effect of C. sinensis leaves extracts which prevented in vitro the irreversible neuromuscular blockade typical of Crotalus durissus terrificus venom, more specifically caused by crotoxin, the main component of the crude venom (Slotta & Fraenkel-Conrat, 1983). We suggest that the target for C. sinensis protective effect is the motor nerve terminal, since the blockade caused by crotoxin, botulin toxin and tetanus toxin occurs by the inhibition of the neurotransmitter release, differently, from motor nerve terminals (Habermann et al., 1980).

Based on research findings suggesting an effective anti-cancer property attributed mainly to epigallocathechin-3-gallate (Fig. 6A) found primarily in green tea, and theaflavin (Fig. 6B) from black tea, both equally effective antioxidants (Leung et al., 2001), these two compounds were also assayed against *Crotalus durissus terrificus* venom (de Jesus Reis Rosa et al., 2010). Curiously, commercial theaflavin, but not epigallocathechin gallate, maintained partial muscular activity in the presence of 5 µg/mL venom. Coincidently, Basu et al. (2005) showed that only the theaflavin fraction from black tea was able to produce a facilitatory effect at the skeletomotor site, being this facilitation modulated by calcium and nitric oxide signaling.

Concerning the modulation of synaptic nerve-muscle interaction, it was found that ACh and glutamate are co-released from synaptosomes of *Torpedo electric* organ (Vyas & Bradford, 1987), also demonstrated in rat motor nerve terminals (Waerhaug & Ottersen, 1993). Glutamatergic receptors such as N-methyl-D-aspartate (NMDA) have been identified at the postsynaptic membrane in neuromuscular junction of adult rats (Urazaev et al., 1998; Grozdanovic & Gossrau, 1998). Glutamate released from nerve endings probably activates NMDA-receptor mediated Ca^{2+} entry into the sarcoplasm followed by activation of NO (Urazaev et al., 1998). Nonquantal ACh acting through M1-cholinergic receptors (Urazaev et al., 2000; Malomouzh et al., 2007), activates synthesis of NO to serve as a trophic message from motoneurones that keeps the Cl^- transport inactive in the innervated sarcolemma (Urazaev et al., 1999). For a better understanding of the synaptic nerve-muscle modulation, see also the study of Rubem-Mauro et al. (2009) that corroborates the nitric oxide role at the neuromuscular junction.

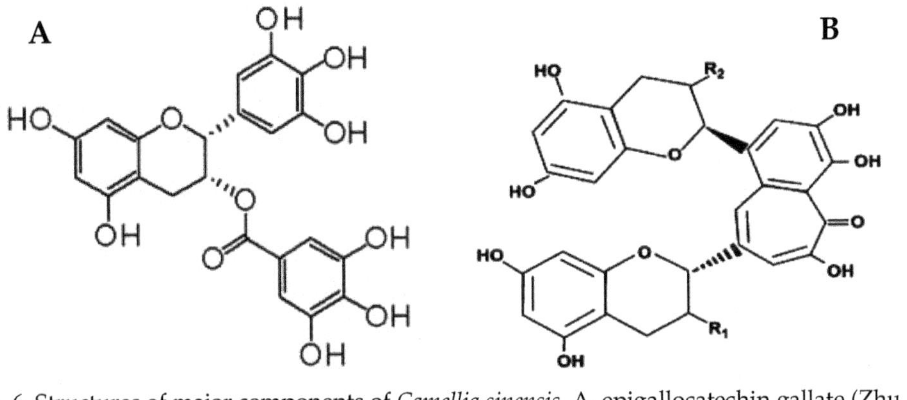

Fig. 6. Structures of major components of *Camellia sinensis*. A, epigallocatechin gallate (Zhu et al., 2008). B, theaflavin (Khan & Mukhtar, 2007).

The well-successful experience between *C. sinensis* leaf extract and presynaptic neurotoxins, and while bothropstoxin-I (BthTX-I) isolated from *Bothrops jararacussu* venom exhibits an earlier presynaptic action (Oshima-Franco et al., 2004) before its well-known myotoxic effect, the same experimental procedure was carried out using *C. sinensis* extract, which protected 100% the neuromuscular blockade (Fig. 1).

Different mechanisms have been proposed for BthTX-I myotoxic effect such as altering the bilayer membrane integrity (Lomonte et al., 2003), binding to the Ca^{2+} -binding region in the pore of Ca^{2+} channels (Oshima-Franco et al., 2004), activating membrane acceptors (Cintra-Francischinelli et al., 2009) or causing a general membrane-destabilizing (Gallacci & Cavalcante, 2009). In order to explain the rationale of this study more details will be given about these mechanisms.

BthTX-I represents a distinct group of PLA$_2$ homologue myotoxins containing Lys49 instead of Asp49 residue, with consequent loss of Ca^{2+}-binding and enzymatic activity, the segment 115-129 of the C-terminal region, which includes a variable combination of positively charged and hydrophobic/aromatic residues, has the ability to alter the bilayer membrane integrity (Lomonte et al., 2003), a possible way by which C. *sinensis* extract could exert its protection against the toxic effect of BthTX-I.

Oshima-Franco et al. (2004) have shown that BthTX-I, at a concentration that does not produce neuromuscular blockade (0.35 mM) caused the appearance of giant miniature endplate potentials, without affecting the resting membrane potential. The authors suggested that the toxin would act through Ca^{2+} channels, since Mn^{2+} antagonized both neurotoxic and myotoxic actions of the myotoxin and are related to Ca^{2+}fluxes. Mn^{2+} is thought to bind to the Ca^{2+} -binding region in the pore of Ca^{2+} channels, thereby preventing the passage of calcium ions (Nachshen, 1984). The influence of the earlier presynaptic action of BthTX-I is relevant from the pharmacological point of view, as shown here using C. *sinensis* leaves extract, although clinically the bothropic envenomation shows no signs of neurotoxicity. However, C. *sinensis* extract also protected against the myotoxic effects of BthTX-I (Fig. 3D), showing a parallelism between neurotoxic and myotoxic effects of the myotoxin.

Cintra-Francischinelli et al. (2009) excluded the possibility that the inactive Lys49 toxins act by binding to a membrane channel, thus increasing its permeability to Ca2+. The authors have shown that the action of myotoxins from snake venoms on muscle cells begins with the activation of membrane acceptors coupled to intracellular Ca^{2+} stores, which is rapidly followed by the toxin dependent alteration of membrane permeability to ions (and other molecules). By this mechanism, C. *sinensis* is able to inactivate the acceptors signalization.

Gallacci & Cavalcante (2010) proposed a hypothetical mechanism for the *in vitro* neuromuscular blockade induced by snake venom Lys49 PLA$_2$ homologues (Fig. 7): the binding of the Lys49 PLA$_2$ homologues to hydrophobic domains in muscle plasma membrane promotes a non-enzymatic alteration of the membrane structure. As a consequence, there is a colapse of the ionic gradient and depolarization of both muscle fiber and nerve terminal, mainly due to re-equilibration of sodium and potassium ions concentration. The persistent cell depolarization could inactivate voltage-dependent sodium channels in the peri-junctional zone. Consequently, the threshold of excitability of the muscle fiber rises out of the reach of the endplate potential; no action potential is triggered and the neuromuscular transmission is blocked. The depolarization of nerve terminal could increase the spontaneous release of acetylcholine, i.e. the frequency of miniature endplate potentials. The action potentials superimposed on the background level of nerve depolarization are reduced since the membrane potential is already shifted nearer to the sodium equilibrium potential. The reduced action potentials promote a decreased calcium influx and consequently a reduction of releasing of evoked acetylcholine. The muscle fiber membrane disruption induced by Lys49 PLA$_2$ homologues also promotes an increase in the concentration of cytosolic calcium that initiates a complex series of degenerative effects on muscle fiber. By this mechanism, C. *sinensis* extract efficiently did avoid the initial trigger.

Antibothropic Action of Camellia sinensis Extract Against the Neuromuscular Blockade by Bothrops jararacussu
Snake Venom and Its Main Toxin, Bothropstoxin-I

105

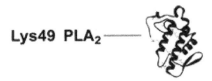

Lys49 PLA₂

Fig. 7. Molecular structure of snake venom Lys49 PLA$_2$ homologue (Gallacci & Cavalcante, 2010).

Basu et al. (2005) showed that the theaflavins-induced facilitation was dependent on the calcium concentration of the physiological solution pointing to an involvement of calcium in the facilitatory action of theaflavins. It is evident that the skeletal muscle can contract in the absence of external calcium, but under physiological conditions, when calcium is present in the medium, it induces the release of stored calcium from the sarcoplasmic reticulum in order to maintain the optimal integrity of the contractile mechanism (Endo, 1985). Considering that C. sinensis extract totally prevent the neuromuscular blockade induced by the myotoxin and calcium seems to be involved in the toxic mechanism of BthTX-I, by different proposed mechanisms as already discussed, the explanation of Basu et al. (2005) that C. sinensis, produces a facilitatory effect, via theaflavin, acting presynaptically as calcium modulating factor is also other possibility.

In spite of the hypothesis discussed here, the actual molecular mechanism involving the C. sinensis extract and the BthTX-I interaction remains to be cleared.

Here, when the efficacy of C. sinensis extract was assayed against the crude venom, 80% of the contractile response was found preserved even after two hours of the venom exposure (Fig. 2), a promising result, since venom has a complex composition, differently from BthTX-I. Histological analyses clearly showed the protective effect of C. sinensis extract against the myotoxic action of venom (Fig. 3E), showing the same positive correlation between neurotoxicity and myotoxicity induced by the venom and the myotoxin.

Whereas only the commercial theaflavin protected against the neuromuscular blockade of Crotalus durissus terrificus (de Jesus Reis Rosa et al., 2010), here, both theaflavin and epigallocatechin gallate, totally protected against the paralysis by Bothrops jararacussu venom (Fig. 4), a result better than that produced by C. sinensis extract, since the amount of these phytochemicals in the extract (as shown in Fig. 5) is lesser than that used in the neutralization assays. However, the C. sinensis extract contains a multitude of other compounds, which real participation against the toxic effects of venom must be assayed, hence using an in vivo model simulating the cronically black or green tea consumption (by humans) followed by subcutaneous injection of the venoms. A comparison between the treatment with commercial antivenom alone and commercial antivenom plus theaflavin or epigallocatechin gallate is also interesting.

It is well-known that C. durissus terrificus and B. jararacussu venoms act differently in inducing clinical symptoms as well as in vitro paralysis at skeletomotor apparatus. Considering that venoms were previously incubated with each commercial phytochemical, and that epigallocatechin gallate, the major catechin in green tea, totally inhibited the toxic compounds of B. jararacussu venom, but did not do so against the rattlesnake venom, it is reasonable to suggest that theaflavin inhibits both presynaptic and postsynaptic venom effects, whereas epigallocatechin gallate inhibits mainly postsynaptic venom effects of these snake venoms, a question that remains to be cleared.

5. Conclusion

Camellia sinensis leaves extract possesses inhibitory effect against the neuromuscular blockade induced by *Bothrops jararacussu* venom and also bothropstoxin-I, by an unclear mechanism of action. Altogether, the data suggest that theaflavin and epigallocatechin gallate have a strong participation on these protective effects.

6. Acknowledgment

This work was supported by a research grant from São Paulo Research Foundation [FAPESP, Proc. 04/09705-8, 07/53883-6, 08/52643-4]. L.J.R.R. is a student of Post-Graduation Course in Pharmaceutical Sciences (Master level) from UNISO. G.A.A.S. had a scholarship (I.C.) from PROBIC/UNISO.

7. References

Arab, L. & Il'yasova, D. (2003). The epidemiology of tea consumption and colorectal cancer incidence. *The Journal of Nutrition* Vol 133, No. 10, (October 2003), pp. 3310S–3318S, ISSN 1541-6100

Basu, S., Chaudhuri, T., Chauhan, S.P.S., Das Gupta, A.K., Chaudhury, L. & Vedasiromoni, J.R. (2005). The theaflavin fraction is responsible for the facilitatory effect of black tea at the skeletal myoneural junction. *Life Sciences*, Vol.76, No.26, (May 2005), pp. 3081–3088, ISSN 1879-0631

Battellino, C., Piazza, R, da Silva, A.M., Cury, Y. & Farsky, S.H. (2003). Assessment of efficacy of bothropic antivenom therapy on microcirculatory effects induced by *Bothrops jararaca* snake venom. *Toxicon*, Vol.41, No.5, (April 2003), pp. 583-593, ISSN 0041-0101

Bülbring, E. (1946). Observation on the isolated phrenic nerve diaphragm preparation of the rat. *British Journal of Pharmacology and Chemotherapy*, Vol.1, (May 1946), pp. 38-61, ISSN 0366-0826

Chippaux, J.P. (2011). Estimate of the burden of snakebites in sub-Saharan Africa: a meta-analytic approach. *Toxicon*, Vol.57, No.4, (March 2011), pp. 586-599. ISSN 0041-0101

Cintra, A.C., Marangoni, S., Oliveira, B. & Giglio, J.R. (1993). Bothropstoxin-I: amino acid sequence and function. *Journal of Protein Chemistry*, Vol.12, No.1, (February 1993), pp. 57-64, ISSN 0277-8033

Cintra-Francischinelli, M., Silva, M.G., Andréo-Filho, N., Gerenutti, M., Cintra, A.C., Giglio, J.R., Leite, G.B., Cruz-Höfling, M.A., Rodrigues-Simioni, L. & Oshima-Franco, Y. (2008). Antibothropic action of *Casearia sylvestris* Sw. (Flacourtiaceae) extracts. *Phytotherapy Research*, Vol.22, No.6, (June 2008), pp. 784-790, ISSN 0951-418X

Cintra-Francischinelli, M., Pizzo, P., Rodrigues-Simioni, L., Ponce-Soto, L.A., Rossetto, O., Lomonte, B., Gutiérrez, J.M., Pozzan, T. & Montecucco, C. (2009). Calcium imaging of muscle cells treated with snake myotoxins reveals toxin synergism and presence of acceptors. *Cellular and Molecular Life Science*, Vol.66, No.10, (March 2009), pp. 1718-1728, ISSN 1420-682X

Correa-Netto, C., Teixeira-Araujo, R., Aguiar A.S., Melgarejo, A.R., De-Simone, S.G., Soares, M.R., Foguel, D. & Zingali, R.B. (2010). Immunome and venome of *Bothrops jararacussu*: a proteomic approach to study the molecular immunology of snake toxins. *Toxicon*, Vol.55, No.7, (June 2010), pp. 1222-1235, ISSN 0041-0101

Crespy, V. & Williamson, G. (2004). A review of the health effects of green tea catechins *in vivo* animal models. *The Journal of Nutrition*, Vol.134, No.12, (December 2004), pp. 3431S-3440S, ISSN 1541-6100

Crozier, A., Jaganath, I.B. & Clifford, M.N. (2009). Dietary phenolics: chemistry, bioavailability and effects on health. *Natural Product Reports*, Vol.26, No.8, (May 2009), pp. 1001-1043, ISSN 0265-0568

Das, M., Vedasiromoni, J.R., Chauhan, S.P.S. & Ganguly, D.K. (1994). Effect of the hot-water extract of black tea (*Camellia sinensis*) on the rat diaphragm. *Planta Medica*, Vol.60, No.5, (October 1994), pp. 470-471, ISSN 0032-0943

Das, M., Vedasiromoni, J.R., Chauhan, S.P.S. & Ganguly, D.K. (1997). Effect of green tea (*Camellia sinensis*) extract on the rat diaphragm. *Journal of Ethnopharmacology*, Vol.57, No.3, (August 1997), pp. 197-201, ISSN 0378-8741

De Jesus Reis Rosa, L., Silva, G.A.A., Amaral Filho, J., Silva, M.G., Cogo, J.C., Groppo, F.C. & Oshima-Franco Y. (2010). The inhibitory effect of *Camellia sinensis* extracts against the neuromuscular blockade of *Crotalus durissus terrificus* venom. *Journal of Venom Research*, Vol.1, No.7, (September 2010), pp. 1-7, ISSN 2444-0324

dos Santos, J.I., Cintra-Francischinelli, M., Borges, R.J., Fernandes, C.A., Pizzo, P., Cintra, A.C., Braz, A.S., Soares, A.M. & Fontes, M.R. (2011). Structural, functional, and bioinformatics studies reveal a new snake venom homologue phospholipase A_2 class. *Proteins*, Vol.79, No.1, (September 2010), pp. 61-78, ISSN 0887-3585

Endo, M. (1985). Calcium release from sarcoplasmic reticulum. In: Bronner, F. (Ed.), *Current Topics in Membrane and Transport*, 25, Academic Press, London, pp. 181-230

Fenwick, A.M., Gutberlet-Jr, R.L., Evans, J. & Parkinson, C.L. (2009). Morphological and molecular evidence for phylogeny and classification of South American pitvipers, genera *Bothrops*, *Bothriopsis*, and *Bothrocophias* (Serpentes: Viperidae). *Zoological Journal of the Linnean Society*, Vol.156, No.3, (March 2009), pp. 617-640, ISSN 0024-4082

Friedman, M. (2007). Overview of antibacterial, antitoxin, antiviral, and antifungal activities of tea flavonoids and teas. *Molecular Nutrition & Food Research*, Vol.51, No.1, (January 2007), pp. 116-134, ISSN 1613-4125

Gallacci, M. & Cavalcante, W.L.G. (2010). Understanding the in vitro neuromuscular activity of snake venom Lys49 phospholipase A2 homologues. *Toxicon*, Vol.55, No.10, (October 2009), pp. 1–11, ISSN 0041-0101

Graham, H. N (1992). Green tea composition, consumption, and polyphenol chemistry. *Preventive Medicine*, Vol.21, No.3, (May 1992), pp. 334-350, ISSN 0091-7435

Grozdanovic, Z. & Gossrau, R. (1998). Co-localization of nitric oxide synthase I (NOS I) and NMDA receptor subunit 1 (NMDAR-1) at the neuromuscular junction in rat and mouse skeletal muscle. *Cell and Tissue Research*. Vol.291, No.1, (January 1998), pp.57-63, ISSN 0302-766X

Gutiérrez, J.M., Núñez, J., Díaz, C., Cintra, A.C., Homsi-Brandeburgo, M.I. & Giglio, J.R. (1991). Skeletal muscle degeneration and regeneration after injection of bothropstoxin-II, a phospholipase A2 isolated from the venom of the snake *Bothrops jararacussu*. *Experimental and Molecular Pathology*, Vol.55, No.3, (December 1991), pp. 217-229, ISSN 0014-4800

Habermann, E., Dreyer, F. & Bigalke, H. (1980). Tetanus toxin blocks the neuromuscular transmission *in vitro* like botulinum A toxin. *Naunyn-Schmiedeberg's Archives of Pharmacology*, Vol.311, No.1, (February 1980), pp. 33-40, ISSN 0028-1298

Harrison, R.A., Hargreaves, A., Wagstaff, S.C., Faragher, B & Lalloo, D.G (2009). Snake envenoming: a disease of poverty. *PLoS Neglected Tropical Diseases*, Vol.3, No.12, (December 2009), pp. e569-e575, ISSN 1935-2735

Hazarika, M., Chakravarty, S. K. & Mahanta, P. K. (1984). Studies on thearubigin pigments in black tea manufacturing systems. *Journal of the Science of Food and Agriculture,* Vol.35, No.11, (November 1984), pp. 1208-1218, ISSN 0022-5142

Heluany, N.F., Homsi-Brandeburgo, M.I., Giglio, J.R., Prado-Franceschi, J. & Rodrigues-Simioni, L. (1992). Effects induced by bothropstoxin, a component from *Bothrops jararacussu* snake venom, on mouse and chick muscle preparations. *Toxicon,* Vol.30, No.10, (October 1992), pp. 1203-1210, ISSN 0041-0101

Homsi-Brandeburgo, M.I., Queiroz, L.S., Santo-Neto, H., Rodrigues-Simioni, L. & Giglio, J.R. (1988). Fractionation of *Bothrops jararacussu* snake venom: partial chemical characterization and biological activity of bothropstoxin. *Toxicon,* Vol.26, No.7, (July 1988), pp. 615-627, ISSN 0041-0101

Hughes, B.W., Kusner, L.L. & Kaminski, H.J. (2006). Molecular architecture of the neuromuscular junction. *Muscle & Nerve,* Vol. 33, No.4, (October 2005), pp. 445–461, ISSN 0148-639X

Hung, Y-C., Sava, V., Hong, M-Y. & Huang, G.S. (2004). Inhibitory effects on phospholipase A_2 and antivenin activity of melanin extracted from *Thea sinensis* Linn. *Life Sciences,* Vol.74, No.16, (March 2004), pp. 2037-2047, ISSN 1879-0631

Khan, N. & Mukhtar, H. (2007). Tea polyphenols for health promotion. *Life Sciences,* Vol.81, No.7, (July 2007), pp. 519-533, ISSN 1879-0631

Krishnamoorthy, K.K. (1991). The nutritional and therapeutic value of tea. In: Yamanishi, T. (Ed.), *Proceedings of the International Symposium on Tea Science,* Japan, pp. 6–11, LC Control Number 92188482

Lambert, J.D. & Yang, C.S. (2003). Mechanisms of cancer prevention by tea constituents. *The Journal of Nutrition,* Vol.133, No.10, (October 2003), pp. 3262S-3267S, ISSN 0022-3166

Leung, L.K., Su, Y., Chen, R., Zhang, Z., Huang, Y. & Chen, Z-Y. (2001). Theaflavins in black tea and catechins in green tea are equally effective antioxidants. *The Journal of Nutrition,* Vol.131, No.9, (September 2001), pp. 2248-2251, ISSN 0022-3166

Lima, A.C.S.F., Campos, C.E.C. & Ribeiro, J.R. (2009). Epidemiological profile of snake poisoning accidents in the State of Amapá. *Revista da Sociedade Brasileira de Medicina Tropical,* Vol.42, No.3, (May-June 2009), pp. 329-335, ISSN 0037-8682

Lomonte, B., Angulo, Y. & Calderón, L. (2003). An overview of lysine-49 phospholipase A2 myotoxins from crotalid snake venoms and their structural determinants of myotoxic action. *Toxicon,* Vol. 42, No. 8, (December 2003), pp. 885–901, ISSN 0041-0101

Mahmood, A., Ahmad, M., Jabeen, A., Zafar, M. & Nadeem, S. (2005). *Pharmacognostic studies of some indigenous medicinal plants of Pakistan,* 26.07.2011, Available from: http://www.siu.edu/~ebl/leaflets/abid.htm

Malomouzh, A.I., Mukhtarov, M.R., Nikolsky, E.E. & Vyskocil, F. (2007). Muscarinic M1 acetylcholine receptors regulate the non-quantal release of acetylcholine in the rat neuromuscular junction via NO-dependent mechanism. *Journal of Neurochemistry,* Vol.102, No.6, (September 2007), pp. 2110-2117, ISSN 0022-3042

Melo, R.F., Farrapo, N.M., Rocha Junior, D.S., Silva, M.G., Cogo, J.C., Dal Belo, C.A., Rodrigues-Simioni, L., Groppo, F.C. & Oshima-Franco, Y. (2009). Antiophidian mechanisms of medicinal plants, In: *Flavonoids: Biosynthesis, Biological Effects and Dietary Sources,* R. B. Keller. (Ed.), 249-262, Nova Science Publishers, ISBN 978-1-60741-622-7, New York, United States of America

Milani Júnior, R., Jorge, M.T., de Campos, F.P., Martins, F.P., Bousso, A., Cardoso, J.L., Ribeiro, L.A., Fan, H.W., França, F.O., Sano-Martins, I.S., Cardoso, D., Ide Fernandez, C., Fernandes, J.C., Aldred, V.L., Sandoval, M.P., Puorto, G., Theakston, R.D. & Warrell, D.A. (1997). Snake bites by the jararacuçu (*Bothrops jararacussu*):

clinicopathological studies of 29 proven cases in São Paulo State, Brazil. *The Quarterly Journal of Medicine*, Vol.90, No.5, (May 1997), pp. 323-334, ISSN 0033-5622

Ministério da Saúde. (2004). Secretaria de Vigilância em Saúde. Sistema de Informação de Agravos de Notificação (SINAN), 07.05.2010, Available from: <http://dtr2004.saude.gov.br/sinanweb/index.php>

Miura, Y., Chiba, T., Miura, S., Tomita, I., Umegaki, K., Ikeda, M. & Tomita, T. (2000). Green tea polyphenols (flavan 3-ols) prevent oxidative modification of low density lipoproteins: an *ex vivo* study in humans. *The Journal of Nutricional Biochemistry*, Vol.11, No.4, (April 2000), pp. 216–222, ISSN 0955-2863

Nachshen, D.A. (1984). Selectivity of the Ca binding site in synaptosome Ca channels: inhibition of Ca influx by multivalent metal cations. *The Journal of General Physiology*, Vol.83, No.6, (June 1984), pp. 941–967, ISSN0022-1295

Nicoleti, A.F., de Medeiros, C.R., Duarte, M.R. & de Siqueira França, F.O. (2010). Comparison of *Bothropoides jararaca* bites with and without envenoming treated at the Vital Brazil Hospital of the Butantan Institute, State of São Paulo, Brazil. *Revista da Sociedade Brasileira de Medicina Tropical*, Vol.43, No.6, (December 2010), pp. 657-661, ISSN 0037-8682

Oshima-Franco, Y., Leite, G.B., Dal Belo, C.A., Hyslop, S., Prado-Franceschi, J., Cintra, A.C.O., Giglio, J.R., Cruz-Höfling, M.A., & Rodrigues-Simioni, L. (2004). The presynaptic pctivity of bothropstoxin-I, a myotoxin from *Bothrops jararacussu* snake venom. *Basic & Clinical Pharmacology & Toxicology*, Vol. 95, No. 4, (October 2004), pp. 175–182, ISSN 1742-7835

Pereira, M.F., Novello, J.C., Cintra, A.C., Giglio, J.R., Landucci, E.T., Oliveira, B. & Marangoni, S. (1998). The amino acid sequence of bothropstoxin-II, an Asp-49 myotoxin from *Bothrops jararacussu* (Jararacuçu) venom with low phospholipase A2 activity. *Journal of Protein Chemistry*, Vol.17, No.4, (May 1998), pp. 381-386, ISSN 0277-8033

Pithayanukul, P., Leanpolchareanchai, J. & Bavovada, R. (2010). Inhibitory effect of tea polyphenols on local tissue damage induced by snake venoms. *Phytotherapy Research*, Vol.24, No.S1, (July 2009), pp. S56–S62, ISSN 0951-418X

Rodrigues-Simioni, L., Borgese, N. & Ceccarelli, B. (1983). The effects of *Bothrops jararacussu* venom and its components on frog nerve-muscle preparation. *Neuroscience*, Vol.10, No.2, (October 1983), pp. 475-489, ISSN 0306-4522

Rubem-Mauro, L., Rocha Jr, D.S., Barcelos, C.C., Costa-Varca, G.H., Andréo-Filho, N., Barberato-Filho, S., Oshima-Franco, Y. & Vila, M.M.D.C. Phenobarbital pharmacological findings on the nerve-muscle basis. *Latin American Journal of Pharmacy*, Vol. 28, No.2, (February 2009), pp. 211-218, ISSN 0326-2383

Satoh, E., Ishii, T., Shimizu, Y., Sawamura, S. & Nishimura, M. (2002a). The mechanism underlying the protective effect of the thearubigin fraction of black tea (*Camellia sinensis*) extract against the neuromuscular blocking action of botulinum neurotoxins. *Pharmacology & Toxicology*, Vol.90, No.4, (April 2002), pp. 199-202, ISSN 0901-9928

Satoh, E., Ishii, T., Shimizu, Y., Sawamura, S. & Nishimura, M. (2002b). A mechanism of the thearubigin fraction of black tea (*Camellia sinensis*) extract protecting against the effect of tetanus toxin. *The Journal of Toxicological Sciences*, Vol.27, No.5, (December 2002), pp. 441-447, ISSN 0388-1350

Sava, V., Yang, S-M., Hong, M-Y., Yan, P-C. & Huang, G.S. (2001). Isolation and characterization of melanic pigments derived from tea and tea polyphenols. *Food Chemistry*, Vol.73, No.2, (March-April 2001), pp. 177–184, ISSN 0308-8146

Simões, C.M.O., Schenkel, E.P., Gosmann, G., Mello, J.C.P., Mentz, L.A. & Petrovick, P.R. (2004). In: *Farmacognosia: da Planta ao Medicamento*, C.M.O. Simões, E.P. Schenkel,

G. Gosmann, J.C.P. Mello, L.A. Mentz, & P.R. Petrovick, (Eds.), UFRGS/UFSC, ISBN 85-7025-682-5, Porto Alegre/Florianópolis, Brazil

Slotta, K.H., Fraenkel-Conrat, H. (1938). Schlangengiffe, III: Mitteilung Reiningung und crystallization des klappershclangengiffes. Berichte der Deutschen Chemischen Gesellschaft, Vol.71, pp.1076-1081, ISSN 0365-9488

Urazaev, A.K., Naumenko, N.V., Nikolsky, E.E. & Vyskocil, F. (1999). The glutamate and carbachol effects on the early post-denervation depolarization in rat diaphragm are directed towards furosemide-sensitive chloride transport. Neuroscience Research, Vol.33, No.2, (February 1999), pp. 81-86, ISSN 0168-0102

Urazaev, A.Kh., Naumenko, N.V., Poletayev, G.I, Nikolsky, E.E., Vyskocil, F. (1998). The effect of glutamate and inhibitors of NMDA receptors on postdenervation decrease of membrane potential in rat diaphragm. Molecular and Chemical Neuropathology, Vol.33, No.3, (April 1998), pp. 163-174, ISSN 1044-7393

Urazaev, A., Naumenko, N., Malomough, A., Nikolsky, E. & Vyskocil, F. (2000). Carbachol and acetylcholine delay the early postdenervation depolarization of muscle fibres through M1-cholinergic receptors. Neuroscience Research,Vol.37, No.4, (August 2000), pp.255-263, ISSN 0168-0102

Vyas, S. & Bradford, H.F. (1987). Co-release of acetylcholine, glutamate and taurine from synaptosomes of Torpedo electric organ. Neuroscience Letters, Vol.82, No.1, (November 1987), pp. 58-64, ISSN 0304-3940.

Waerhaug, O. & Ottersen, O.P. (1993). Demonstration of glutamate-like immunoreactivity at rat neuromuscular junctions by quantitative electron microscopic immunocytochemistry. Anatomy and Embryology, Vol.188, No.5, (November 1993), pp. 501-513, ISSN 0340-2061

Warrel, D.A. (2004). Snakebites in Central and South America: epidemiology, clinical features, and clinical management. In: The venomous reptiles of the Western Hemisphere, J.A. Campbell, W.W. Lamar (Eds.), 709-715, Cornell University Press, ISBN 978-080-1441-41-7, New York, United States of America

Warrell, D.A. (2010). Snake bite. The Lancet, Vol. 375, No. 9708, (January 2010), pp. 77–88, ISSN 0099-5355

WHO – World Health Organization. (2007). Rabies and envenomings: a neglected public health issue, 25.10.2011, Available from: <http://www.who.int/bloodproducts/animal_sera/Rabies.pdf>

WHO – World Health Organization. (2011a). Guidelines for the production control and regulation of snake antivenom immunoglobulins, 27.07.2011, Available from: <http://www.who.int/bloodproducts/snake_antivenoms/SnakeAntivenomGuideline.pdf>.

WHO - World Health Organization. (2011b). Neglected tropical diseases, 24.07.2011, Available from:\ <http://www.who.int/neglected_diseases/diseases/snakebites/en/>.

Yang, C.S., Chen, L., Lee, M.J., Balentine, D., Kuo, M.C. & Schantz, S.P. (1998). Blood and urine levels of tea catechins after ingestion of different amounts of green tea by human volunteers. Cancer Epidemiology, Biomarkers &Prevention, Vol.7, No.4, (April 1998), pp. 351-354, ISSN 1055-9965

Zhu, Q.Y. & Chen, Z.Y. (1999) Isolation and analysis of green tea polyphenols by HPLC. Analytical Laboratory, Vol. 18, pp. 70–72, ISSN 1000-0720

Zhu, S., Li, W., Li, J., Sama, A.E. & Wang H. (2008). Caging a beast in the inflammation arena: use of Chinese Medicinal herbs to inhibit a late mediator of lethal sepsis, HMGB1. International Journal of Clinical and Experimental Medicine, Vol.1, No.1, (January 2008), pp. 64-75, ISSN 1940-5901.

5

The Effects of *Viscum album* (Mistletoe) QuFrF Extract and Vincristine in Human Multiple Myeloma Cell Lines – A Comparative Experimental Study Using Several and Different Parameters

Eva Kovacs
Cancer Immunology Research
Switzerland

1. Introduction

1.1 Multiple myeloma

Multiple myeloma (MM) is a haematological disorder of malignant plasma cells. B lymphocytes start in the bone marrow and move to the lymph nodes.

When they are activated to secrete antibodies, they are known as plasma cells, which are crucial part of the immune system. Due to the fundamental nature of the system affected, multiple myeloma manifests systemic symptoms that make it difficult to diagnose. Multiple myeloma is characterised by slow proliferation of the tumour cells, mainly in the bone marrow, by production of large amounts of immunoglobulins and osteolytic lesions. Multiple myeloma is a generally incurable disease at present, but remissions may be induced with stem cells transplants, steroids, chemotherapy and treatment with vincristine + doxorubicin + dexamethasone or thalidomide + dexamethasone or bortezomib based regimens or lenalidomide. The different therapeutic modalities have different "target location".

1.2 Epidemiology of multiple myeloma

Multiple myeloma mainly affects older adults, but its causes and other risk factors are unknown. Yearly incidence is 3-6/100 000 worldwide, accounts for 1-2 % of all human cancer. Median survival is 50–55 months.

1.3 The role of cytokines in the growth, progression and dissemination of multiple myeloma

Cytokines are soluble proteins, peptides or glycoproteins that are released by cells. Cytokines can affect the cells via an autocrine and/or paracrine regulation mechanisms. In case of an autocrine regulation mechanism the endogenous produced cytokine affects the same type of cell. In case of a paracrine regulation mechanism the target cell is near to the cytokine produced cell. Cytokine binds to a specific receptor and causes a change in function or in development (differentiation) of the target cell. In both cases, i.e. autocrine and paracrine regulation mechanisms the expression of the membrane receptor is altered.

1.3.1 Interleukins are a group of cytokines which are produced by a wide variety of body cells. The majority of interleukins are synthesized by helper CD4+ T lymphocytes, monocytes/macrophages and by endothelial cells. If the produced cytokine is released, then it is measurable in the supernatant, if not then the cytokine is measurable only intracellular.

Interleukin-6 (IL-6) originally defined as a B cell differentiation factor is produced by different cell types and certain tumour cells. Interleukin-6 acts as a pro-inflammatory and an anti-inflammatory cytokine. As a pro-inflammatory cytokine regulates inflammatory reactions either directly or indirectly. As an anti-inflammatory cytokine Interleukin-6 reduces the inflammatory reactions. IL-6 exits in three molecular weights, i.e. 21-30 kDa, 150-200 or 450 kDa. The biological activity of IL-6 depends on binding to its specific receptors. These membrane receptors composed the glycoprotein gp80 Interleukin-6 receptor alpha (IL-6R, also called CD126) and a signal-transducing component gp130 (also called CD 130). The complex IL-6+IL-6R+gp130 initiate a signal transduction cascade through JAKs (Janus kinases) and STATs (Signal Transducer-Activator of Transcription). The membrane receptors are released from the cells as soluble receptor proteins (sIL-6R and sgp130). As agonist, sIL-6R enhances the biological activity of IL-6 and sgp130 is an antagonist against the complex IL-6+sIL-6R.

Interleukin-6 is a major proliferative factor for the malignant plasma cells (multiple myeloma cells). This cytokine produces by the plasma cells and it affects the cells by an autocrine regulation mechanism with an additional paracrine signalling. IL-6 in a concentration of 2pg/ml can induce 50% proliferation in myeloma cells.

The multiple myeloma cells can be classified into three groups depending on exogenous IL-6: (a) both proliferation and survival of the cells are dependent on IL-6, (b) only proliferation of the myeloma cells is affected by IL-6, (c) the cells are dependent on IL-6 only for survival, but not for proliferation. However there are also some cell lines that are independent of IL-6 both for survival and proliferation. The serum values of IL-6 in 35% or in 97% or in 42% of multiple myeloma patients were significantly higher than in healthy persons (Nachbour et al., 1991; DuVillard et al., 1995; Wierzbowska et al., 1999).

Because about 70% of the secreted IL-6 forms a complex with sIL-6R (Gaillard et al., 1987), the amount of the free IL-6 in serum is low. Therefore the serum level of the sIL-6R is an important parameter in the evaluation and in the progression of multiple myeloma (Papadaki et al., 1997; Wierzbowska et al., 1999).

Interleukin-10 (IL-10) is known as a human cytokine synthesis inhibitory factor (CSIF). It produces by Thelper2 cells, monocytes/macrophages, by B lymphocytes and some tumour cells. Interleukin-10 has (1) immunosuppressive effect and (2) immunostimulatory effect. It down-regulates the expression of Thelper1 cytokines, MHC class II antigens and co-stimulatory molecules on macrophages. Interleukin-10 is a pleiotropic cytokine which increases Bcl-2 levels and protects cells from steroid or doxorubicin-induced apoptosis.

How might the presence of IL-10 contribute to a poor prognosis for some cancer? One possibility: Interleukin-10 is a growth factor for tumour cells. Second possibility: Interleukin-10 suppresses the anti-tumour immune responses.

Interleukin-10 enhances the survival and proliferation of B cells. IL-10 is a growth factor for myeloma cells (Kovacs, 2010a), enhances the proliferation of freshly explanted myeloma cells in a short-term bone marrow culture (Lu et al., 1995). Three out of seven human myeloma cell lines produce IL-10. Elevated IL-10 levels were detected in serum from about 50% of patients having multiple myeloma showing a relation to the clinical manifestation (Otsuki et al., 2000; 2002). Interleukin-6 leads to a marked production of Interleukin-10 in several human multiple myeloma cells. Interleukin-10 is an Interleukin-6 related growth factor for these tumour cells (Kovacs, 2010a).

1.4 Cytostatic effect and cytocidal effect

Cytocidal effect: It is known that there are two important pathways against tumours: To inhibit the tumour cell proliferation (**cytostatic effect**) and/or to induce the death of the tumour cells (**cytocidal effect**). **Cytocidal effect**: apoptosis or necrosis.

The apoptosis is a physiological process in the life of healthy cells, whereas necrosis is a pathological process for tumour cells. **Cytotoxicity** is the quality of being toxic to cells. There are a **direct** and an **indirect** (cell-mediated) **cytotoxicity.** In case of direct cytotoxicity the cells are treated with cytotoxic compounds leading to necrosis.

1.5 Viscum album (VA) extract

Viscum album (VA) extract from **European mistletoe** plants has fermented and non-fermented preparations. Active components of VA extracts include mistletoe lectins (I, II, III) and viscotoxin, additionally aminoacids, polysaccharides and lipids. The fermented preparations are used either alone or in combination with chemo/radiotherapy in the treatment of tumour patients.

The Viscum album QuFrF (VAQuFrF) is an aqueous and unfermented extract of mistletoe plants growing in the oak tree. It contains 1 µg lectin and 6 µg viscotoxin in 5 mg/ml or 2 µg lectin and 10 µg viscotoxin in 10 mg/ml. The extract is an experimental drug that is not yet used in the treatment of tumour patients.

1.6 Vincristine

Vincristine is a vinca alkaloid. As a chemotherapeutic agent is used mainly in combination with other chemotherapeutic substances in the therapy of multiple myeloma. Vincristine inhibits the proliferation of these tumour cells and as a CCS blocker (El Alaoui, 1997; Lin et al., 1998; Mastberger et al., 2000) arrests the cell cycle phase G2/M by blocking the mitotic spindle formation (Harmsma et al., 2004).

2. Aim

2.1 Comparison of the effects of Viscum album QuFrF extract with those of Vincristine.

2.2 Mode of action of Viscum album QuFrF extract and Vincristine.

2.3 To assess the effective doses of Viscum album QuFrF extract and to transfer these doses to the in vivo situation.

3. Materials and methods

3.1 Test substances

Viscum album QuFrF (VAQuFrF) extract was obtained from the Hiscia Institute (Arlesheim, Switzerland). According to the manufacturer the aqueous unfermented solution of extract 10 mg/ml contains 2 µg lectin and 10 µg viscotoxin. Vincristine sulfate salt was obtained from Sigma GmbH (Schnelldorf Germany, No 8879). Recombinant human interleukin-6 (rh IL-6) was obtained from R & D Systems (No. 206-IL, United Kingdom) and reconstituted in phosphate-buffered saline with 0.18% bovine serum albumin.

3.2 Cells and culture condition

Human myeloma cell lines (MOLP-8, LP-1, RPMI-8226, OPM-2, U-266, COLO-677, KMS-12-BM, were obtained from DSMZ (Braunschweig, Germany). Five cell lines derived from blood, COLO-677 from lymph node, KMS-12-BM from bone marrow. The cells were cultivated in RPMI 1640 supplemented with 10-20% foetal calf serum, 2mM L-glutamine and 1 % gentamicin in a humidified atmosphere with 5% CO_2 at 37°C. The doubling times of tumour cell lines were between 35 and 96 hours. For the measurement of the parameters the cell cultures were used within 4-6 weeks after thawing.

3.3 Treatment of cells with VAQuFrF extract or vincristine

a. To measure viability, cytokine production, membrane expression of IL-6 receptor, cell cycle phases and apoptosis /necrosis the cells were cultured at a density of $0.5-0.7 \times 10^6$ cells/ml, except for COLO-677 (0.2×10^6 cells/ml). After 24 hours the cells were incubated with VAQuFrF extract or Vincristine (doses: 0, l0, 50 or 100 µg/10^6 cells/ml). The parameters were measured after 24, 48 and 72 hours.

b. To measure proliferation the cells were cultured at a density of $0.5-0.7 \times 10^5$ cells/100 µl, except for COLO-677 (0.2×10^5 cells/100 µl). After 24 hours the cells were incubated with VAQuFrF extract or Vincristine (doses: 0, 1, 5, 10 µg/10^5 cells/100µl). The parameter was measured after 24, 48 and 72 hours.

3.4 Treatment of cells with Interleukin-6

a. To measure viability, cytokine production, membrane expression of IL-6 receptor, cell cycle phases and apoptosis /necrosis the cells were cultured at a density of $0.5-0.7 \times 10^6$ cells/ml, except for COLO-677 (0.2×10^6 cells/ml). After 24 hours the cells were incubated with IL-6 (dose: 5 ng/10^6cells/ml). The parameters were measured after 24, 48 and 72 hours.

b. To measure proliferation the cells were cultured at a density of $0.5-0.7 \times 10^5$ cells/100 µl, except for COLO-677 (0.2×10^5 cells/100 µl). After 24 hours the cells were incubated with IL-6 (dose: 0.5 ng/10^5cells/100µl). The parameter was measured after 24, 48 and 72 hours.

3.5 Measurement of viability

The viabilities of the cultivated tumour cells were determined by 7-aminoactinomycin D (7-AAD), to exclude the non-viable cells in flow cytometric assays. The values are given in %.

3.6 Measurement of cytokine production

The IL-6 production or IL-10 production in the supernatant of the cultured cells was determined by chemiluminescent immunometric assay. The lowest detectable level was 2 pg/ml or 5 pg/ml.

3.7 Measurement of membrane expression of IL-6 receptor

For immunofluorescence staining $3x10^5$ cells/100 µl were incubated with 20 µl phycoerithrin (PE) conjugated monoclonal antibody (CD 126, Immunotech, France) for 30 min at 4 ∘C. Then the cells were washed, sedimented and analysed in the FACSCalibur flow cytometer. For the expression of the membrane IL-6R (CD 126) the signal intensity (geometric mean of the fluorescence intensity x counts) was used as parameter. The signal intensity of the treated samples was compared with that of untreated samples, which were taken as 100%.

3.8 Measurement of the cell cycle phases

The cell cycle phases GO/GI, S, G2/M were assessed using the cycle test plus DNA reagent kit on a flow cytometer (BD, BioSciences, San Jose, USA No 340242). Briefly: $5x105$ cells were incubated at room temperature with trypsin buffer and additionally with trypsin inhibitor+RNAse buffer. The values are expressed in percentage of total viable cell number (100%).

3.9 Measurement of apoptosis and necrosis

Apoptosis was measured using Annexin V-FITC (BD Biosciences Pharmingen, San Diego, USA No 556 570). Necrosis was measured using propidium iodide (PI). Briefly: $1x10^5$ cells were incubated with Annexin V-FITC or PI at room temperature in the dark. Thereafter the samples were analysed in a flow cytometer. Apoptotic cells: Annexin V-FITC positive and PI negative. Necrotic cells: Annexin V-FITC positive and PI positive. The values are given in percent of total cell number.

3.10 Measurement of the proliferation

The proliferation was assessed using cell proliferation reagent WST-1 (Roche, Mannheim, Germany, No 1644 807). The colorimetric assay is based on the reduction of the tetrazolium salt WST-1 by viable cells. The reaction produces the soluble formazan salt. The quantity of the formazan dye is directly correlated to the number of the metabolically active cells. The proliferation rate was measured 1, 2 and 4 h after incubation with the reagents at time points 24, 48 and 72 h. The upper limit of the absorbance was 2.0–2.1. The intra-sample variance of the untreated cells was <10% (3–8%).

3.11 Statistical analysis

Three to four independent measurements were carried out. For the evaluation of the parameters the Mann-Whitney U-test was used. The limit of significance was taken as $P<0.05$.

4. Results

4.1 Production of Interleukin-6 in supernatant of human multiple myeloma cells

Objectives: (a) spontaneous production, (b) production after treatment with VAQuFrF or Vincristine.

Table 1 presents the values of IL-6 in myeloma cell line MOLP-8, LP-1, RPMI-8226, OPM-2, COLO-677. None of the five multiple myeloma cell lines produced Interleukin-6 spontaneously. This means that all the investigated cell lines are IL-6 independent or have **autocrine/paracrine** regulation mechanisms. In case of an **autocrine** regulation mechanism the cytokine is produced endogenously and affects its membrane receptor directly. In case **of paracrine** regulation mechanism the exogenous cytokine also affects the membrane receptor. In two cell lines (RPMI-8226 and OPM-2) exogenous IL-6 led to a high expression of membrane IL-6R and enhanced levels of sIL-6R in the supernatant (Kovacs, 2003; and results are not shown) indicating a paracrine regulation mechanism.

Cell lines	Spontaneous	After treatment with	
		VAQuFrF	Vincristine
MOLP-8	ND	ND	ND
LP-1	ND	ND	ND
RPMI-8226	ND	ND	ND
OPM-2	ND	ND	ND
COLO-677	ND	ND	ND

Maeasurements at 24 and 48 hours after tretment with VAQufrF extractor Vincristine. Dose=50 µg/10^6 cells in both cases.ND = not detectable.

Table 1. Production of Interleukin-6 in human multiple myeloma cell lines.

Treatment with VAQuFrF extract (dose: 50 µg/10^6 cells) and with Vincristine (dose: 50 µg/10^6 cells) also did not lead to IL-6 production in the five multiple myeloma cell lines. These results confirm the findings of previous studies (Kovacs et al., 2006; Kovacs, 2010b).

4.2 Production of interleukin-10 in supernatant of human multiple myeloma cells

Objectives: (a) spontaneous production, (b) production after treatment with IL-6 (dose: 5ng/10^6 cells), (c) production after treatment with VAQuFrF or Vincristine (dose: 50 µg/10^6 cells for both substances), (d) after treatment with IL-6+VAQuFrF or IL-6+Vincristine (doses: 5 ng/10^6 cells +50 µg/10^6 cells in each case). For the combined treatment IL-6 was added 2 hours before the test substances.

Table 2 presents the production of Interleukin-10 in five human multiple myeloma cell lines. Spontaneous IL-10 production was found in 4/5 cell lines: MOLP-8, LP-1, RPMI-8226, COLO-677, however the cell lines MOLP-8 and COLO-677 secreted IL-10 not every time confirming the findings of previous study (Kovacs, 2010a). IL-6 led to a marked increase of

IL-10 production (up to 946 pg/ml) in 5/5 cell lines. VAQuFrF extract and Vincristine reduced the spontaneous IL-10 production in MOLP-8, LP-1 and COLO-677 to non-detectable amounts.

With IL-6+VAQuFrF or IL-6+Vincristine the values were markedly lower after addition of IL-6 but higher than without IL-6 treatment. VAQuFrF and Vincristine reduced the induced IL-10 production to the same degree in cell lines RPMI-8226 and LP-1. In the cell lines OPM-2, MOLP-8, COLO-677 the extract of VAQuFrF inhibited the IL-10 production weaker than Vincristine.

Cell lines	No treatment	After treatment with			IL-6 + VAQuFF	IL-6 + Vincristine
		IL-6	VAQuFrF	Vincristine		
MOLP-8	ND-18	453-862	ND	ND	35-73	8-40
LP-1	10-22	34-95	ND	ND	25-53	31-44
RPMI-8226	32-124	510-946	36-14	15-27	290-334	370-404
OPM-2	ND	8-33	ND	ND	6-14	ND
COLO-677	ND-30	26-105	ND-11	ND	10-32	ND

Maesurements at 24 and 48 hors after tretment. IL-6:5ng/10^6 cells.VAQuFrF and Vincristine: 50 μg/10^6 cells. Range of 4 independent measurements. ND=not detectable

Table 2. Production of Interleukin-10 (pg/ml)in human multiple myeloma cell lines.

No treatment	After treatment with		
	IL-6	VAQuFrF	Vincristine
55-60	49-62	11-17	16-20
82-83	80-85	58-71	30-48
70-72	69-75	30-47	29-53
47-56	49-57	46-55	13-21
67-68	70-81	41-59	21-32

The values are presented in percentage. Range of four independent measurements.

Table 2.A. Viability of human multiple myeloma cells (cell lines see Table 2).

The IL-10 production was measured at 24 and 48 after incubation with IL-6. The results show that in tumour cell lines MOLP-8 and RPMI-8226 the IL-10 production was high during the two days. In the other three cell lines the production decreased slightly at 48 h.

Table 2/A. presents the range of cell viability without treatment and after treatment with the test substances: L-6, VAQuFrF extract and Vincristine. The viability of the untreated MM cells was different: LP-1>RPMI-8226>COLO-677>MOLP-8>OPM-2. The both test substances impaired the viability to different degrees.

IL-6 does not alter the viability, confirming the findings of previous investigations (Kovacs, 2006b, 2010a). It was reported that IL-6 enhances survival of the myeloma cells because it inhibits apoptosis of induction of the anti-Fas (Nordan & Potter, 1986; Hata et al., 1995).

Summarised: The results indicate that the effect of the both test substances on the IL-10 production is due to their apoptotic/necrotic effects. It is possible that VAQuFrF and Vincristine could also impair the membrane expression of IL-10 receptor. To explain this hypothesis further experiments are necessary.

4.3 The effect of Interleukin-6, VAQuFrF and IL-6+VAQuFrF on the membrane expression of Interleukin-6 receptor in human multiple myeloma cells

Objectives: (a) in untreated cells, (b) after treatment with IL-6 (dose: 5 ng/10^6cells), (c) after treatment with VAQuFrF (dose: 50 μg/10^6 cells), (d) after treatment with IL-6+ VAQuFrF(dose: 5 ng/10^6 cells+50 μg/10^6 cells). For the combined treatment IL-6 was added 2 hours before the test substance. For the expression of the membrane IL-6R the signal intensity (geometric mean of the fluorescence intensity x counts) was used as parameter. This parameter was measured at 24 and 48 hours after incubation. The signal intensity of the treated samples, expressed in percentage was compared with that of untreated samples, which were taken as 100%.

Table 3 presents the mean values of the membrane expression of Interleukin -6 receptor in the cell lines LP-1, RPMI-8226 and OPM-2.

Cell lines	No treatment	Treatment with			No treatment	Treatment with		
		IL-6	VAQuFrF	IL-6 + VAQuFrF		IL-6	VAQuFrF	IL-6 + VAQuFrF
LP-1	100	128[a]	28[a]	77[ab]	100	168[a]	34[a]	81[b]
RPMI-8226	100	191[a]	61[a]	81[b]	100	134[a]	42[a]	67[ab]
OPM-2	100	148[a]	94	116[b]	100	104	92	85

Measurements at 24 h after treatment.   Measurements at 48 h after treatment.

The mean values of three independent measurementa are expressed in percentage of untreated samples (100). a=p<0.05 vs.untreated samples, b=p<0.05 vs. with IL-6 treated samples.

Table 3. Membrane expression of Interleukin-6 receptor in human multiple myeloma cell lines.

The surface expressions of IL-6R in untreated cells of all three cell lines were in the similar range (results are not shown). Exogenous IL-6 increased the membrane expression its receptor significantly ($P<0.05$). VAQuFrF reduced the membrane expression markedly in LP-1 and RPMI-8226 ($P<0.05$), it had no effect in OPM-2. With IL-6+VAQuFrF the values were lower than with IL-6 ($P<0.05$), but higher than after treatment with VAQuFrF.

In cell lines MOLP-8, COLO-677 and KMS-12-BM exogenous IL-6 led to down-regulation of its receptor, signalling the possible process of endocytosis (results are not shown). It is interesting that all three cell lines in which IL-6 upregulated its membrane receptor sourced from blood. To investigate of the membrane expression of IL-6 receptor in the cell lines MOLP-8, COLO-677 and KMS-12-BM additional experiments are planned.

4.4 Inhibition of proliferation of multiple myeloma cells (cytostatic effect). Induction of apoptosis and necrosis in multiple myeloma cells (cytocidal effect)

Figure 1 and **Figure 2** present the mean values of the proliferation and those of apoptosis/necrosis in six human multiple myeloma cell lines treated with IL-6 or VAQuFrF or Vincristine. The cell lines MOLP-8, LP-1, RPMI-8226, OPM-2 sourced from blood, COLO-677 which is a derivative of RPMI-8226 from lymph node, KMS-12-BM from bone marrow.

To measure the proliferation the following doses were applied (1) IL-6: 0.5 ng/10^5 cells, (2) VAQuFrF or Vincristine: 1, 5, 10 µg/10^5 cells. To measure apoptosis/ necrosis (1) IL-6: 5 ng/10^6 cells, (2) VAQuFrF or Vincristine; 10, 50, 100 µg/10^6 cells. The parameters were measured at 24, 48 and 72 hours after incubation with the test substances.

Proliferation: The values of the treated samples are expressed as percentages of the untreated samples and are the average of four independent experiments. Significance was assessed versus untreated samples (100%).

Apoptosis/necrosis: The values are expressed as percentage of total cell numbers and are the average of four independent experiments. In the untreated samples the percentage of apoptotic cells lay in the range of 5-38%, that of necrotic cells 10-35% during 72 hours. There were big differences between the tumour cell lines.

4.4.1 MOLP-8

Proliferation: IL-6 increased the proliferation on average up to 130-155%. Comparison of VAQuFrF with Vincristine: 24 and 48 hours after incubation VAQuFrF at the dose of 5 and 10 µg/10^5 cells was more effective than Vincristine. 72 hours after there was no difference between the substances in any dose.

Apoptosis/necrosis: In the untreated tumour cells the values of apoptosis lay either in the range of necrosis or above them. IL-6 treatment did not impair either the apoptosis or necrosis. To measure the effects of the two substances on the apoptosis/necrosis we applied ten times less doses. VAQuFrF increased the apoptosis and necrosis at 5 and 10 µg/10^6 cells ($P<0.05$ and $P<0.01$). Vincristine had the same effect as VAQuFrF.

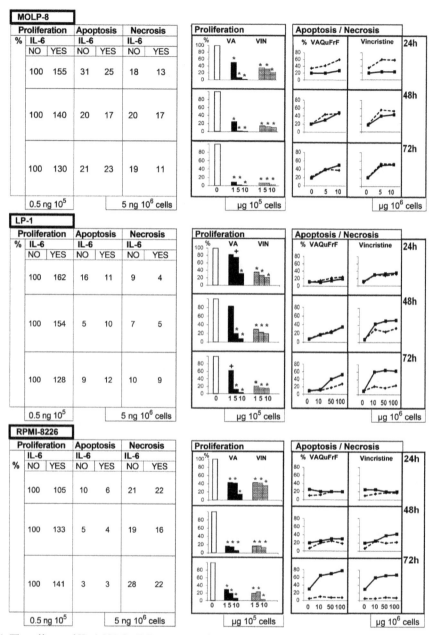

Fig. 1. The effects of IL-6, VAQuFrF extract and Vincristine on the proliferation and on apoptosis/necrosis in human multiple myeloma cell lines MOLP-8, LP-1 and RPMI-8226. The mean values of four independent experiments are expressed as percentage of untreated samples (100%). Proliferation=105 cells. Apoptosis/necrosis=106 cells. •- - -• apoptotic cells, •––• necrotic cells. +P<0.05, *P<0.01 compared with untreated samples (Mann-Whitney U-test).

4.4.2 LP-1

Proliferation: With IL-6 the proliferation rate lay on average between 128-162% during 72 hours. VAQuFrF at the dose of 10 µg/10^5 cells inhibited the proliferation more effectively (P<0.01) than Vincristine.

Apoptosis/necrosis: In the untreated cell the values of apoptosis lay in the range of necrosis. There was no difference between the values of untreated and with IL-6 treated cells. VAQuFrF did not greatly alter the apoptosis during the investigation time. There was a necrotic effect with a dose dependence from 50 up to 100 µg/10^6 cells (P<0.05). Vincristine increased the number of apoptotic cells and that of necrotic cells (P<0.05), however without dose dependence. The number of necrotic cells was higher than that of apoptotic cells at each dose after 48 and 72 hours (P<0.05 and P<0.01).

4.4.3 RPMI-8226

Proliferation: IL-6 increased the proliferation on average up to 105-141%.

The test substances inhibited the proliferation: After 24 and 48 hours VAQuFrF in dose of 10 µg/10^5 cells was more effective than Vincristine (P<0.01). In lower doses (5 µg/10^5 cells and 1 µg/10^5 cells) VAQuFrF had the same effect as Vincristine.

Apoptosis/necrosis: The values of apoptosis in untreated cells lay below the necrosis. There were no differences between the values of cells treated with IL-6 and that those of untreated cells.

VAQuFrF and Vincristine did not alter the apoptosis. At 72 hours after treatment with both substances he numbers of necrotic cells was higher than those of apoptotic cells at each dose (P<0.05 and P<0.01).

4.4.4 OPM-2

Proliferation: IL-6 increased the proliferation on average between 110-130%. Comparison of VAQuFrF with Vincristine: The inhibitory effect of VAQuFrF was weaker than that of Vincristine at each dose and at investigated time point. Additional investigation indicate that higher doses increase the effect of VAQuFrF (results are not presented).

Apoptosis/necrosis: In the untreated cells the values of apoptosis lay in the range of necrosis. IL-6 did not impair either the apoptosis or necrosis of the cells. None of the test substances altered the apoptosis. Vincristine increased markedly the number of necrotic cells between 10 and 100 µg/10^6 cells without dose dependence after 72 hours of treatment. VAQuFrF was ineffective.

4.4.5 COLO-677

Proliferation: With IL-6 the values of proliferation lay on average between 110-115%.

The inhibitory effect of VAQuFrF was weaker than that of Vincristine in doses of 1 and 5 µg/10^5 cells. At the dose of 10 µg/10^5 cells the anti-proliferative effects of VAQuFrF and Vincritine was the same at each investigated time point.

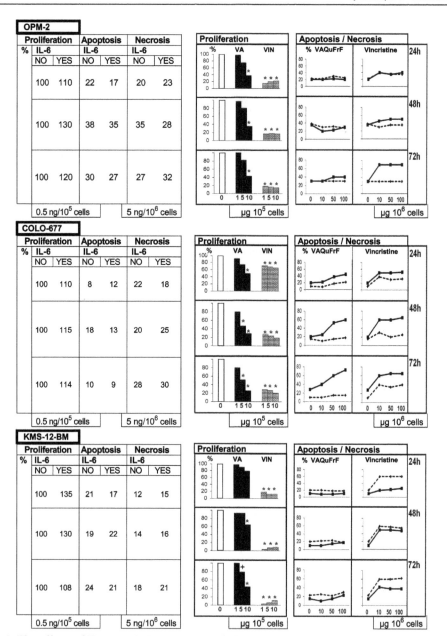

Fig. 2. The effects of IL-6, VAQuFrF extract and Vincristine on the proliferation and on the apoptosis/necrosis in human multiple myeloma cell lines OPM-2, COLO-677 and KMS-12-BM. The mean values of four independent experiments are expressed as percentage of untreated samples (100%). Proliferation=105 cells. Apoptosis/necrosis=106 cells. ●- - -● apoptotic cells, ●--● necrotic cells. +P<0.05, *P<0.01 compared with untreated samples (Mann-Whitney U-test).

Apoptosis/necrosis: In the untreated tumour cells the values of apoptosis lay either in the range of necrosis or below them. There was no alteration after treatment with IL-6. VAQuFrF did not alter the apoptosis. There was a necrotic effect with a dose dependence (from 50 up to 100 µg/10^6 cells) ($P<0.05$). Vincristine increased the number of apoptotic cells ($P<0.05$). The number of necrotic cells was higher than that of apoptotic at each dose and at each time point ($P<0.05$ and $P<0.01$). The apoptotic/necrotic effects of Vincristine were not dose-dependent.

4.4.6 KMS-12-BM

Proliferation: IL-6 increased the proliferation on average between 108 and 135%. VAQuFrF inhibited the proliferation only in dose of 10 µg/10^5 cells after 48 and 72 hours. Vincristine inhibited the proliferation markedly however without dose dependence at each dose and at each investigated time point.

Apoptosis/necrosis: The values of apoptosis in untreated cells lay above the values of necrosis. IL-6 did not alter the apoptosis and necrosis. VAQuFrF did not impair either the apoptosis or the necrosis in this cell line. Vinristine was effective in KMS-12-BM: The number of apoptotic/necrotic cells was significantly higher ($P<0.01$) at each time point, but without dose dependence.

It was reported that that inhibition of cell proliferation is a stronger prognostic indicator than the apoptosis (Stokke et al., 1998). There is a quantitative correlation between the inhibition of proliferation and apoptosis in lymphoma cells (Leoncini, et al., 1993).

Chemotherapeutic agents influence apoptosis through a mitochondrial pathway (Oancea, et al., 2004). Multiple myeloma cells overexpress Bcl-2, a mitochondrial membrane protein which suppresses apoptosis (Chanen-Khan, 2004; Tsujimoto & Shimizu, 2007). VAQuFrF decreases the levels of Bcl-2 in B and T lymphocytes (Duong Van Huyen et al., 2001).

Summarised: In this study the apoptotic/necrotic effect of Vincristine was more marked than its proliferative effect in all cell lines. There was no dose dependence between 10, 50 or 100 µg/10^6 cells/ml in both parameters. It is possible that Vincristine impairs the proliferation and apoptosis/necrosis with dose dependence only in a lower dose range.

VAQuFrF first inhibits the proliferation and then the cells die by apoptosis and/or necrosis in the MM cell lines LP-1, RPMI-8226 and COLO-677, confirming the findings with RPMI-8226 presented in a previous study (Kovacs et al., 2006a). The inhibitory effect of VAQuFrF was markedly weaker than that of Vincristine in cell lines OPM-2 and KMS-12-BM at each dose and at investigated time point.

4.5 The effect of VAQuFrf on the proliferation of cells with high proliferation rate

The effect of VAQuFrF with doses of 5 and 10µg/10^5 cells was investigated in cell line RPMI-8226 with high proliferation rate, which remained unaltered during 2-3 days. VAQuFrF was more effective in cells having high proliferation rates than in those with low proliferation rates (Kovacs et al., 2006a). Recently the same findings were observed in cell lines LP-1 and OPM-2 (results are not shown).

4.6 The effect of combined treatment with Interleukin-6+VAQUFrF on the proliferation in human multiple myeloma cells

The cell lines MOLP-8, LP-1, RPMI-8226 and COLO-677 were treated with Interleukin-6+VAQuFrF for 24, 48 and 72 hours. To measure the proliferation the following doses were used: 0.5 ng/10^5 cells + 1, 5, 10 µg/10^5 cells. For the combined treatment IL-6 was added to the cell cultures 2 hours before VAQuFrF. For comparison the cell lines were treated only with IL-6 or only with VAQuFrF.

Figure 3 presents the range of values expressed in percentage compared with untreated samples (100%). As expected, VAQuFrF inhibited the spontaneous proliferation markedly in all cell lines. The effect was dose-dependent. IL-6 led to enhanced proliferation in each case. We expected that with the combined treatment the values will be lower than after single treatment of IL-6, but higher than after single treatment of VAQuFrF. This situation has been found only in cell lines MOLP-8 and LP-1 for dose 1µg/10^5 cells. It is suggested that the 2 hours pre-treatment with IL-6 is too short.

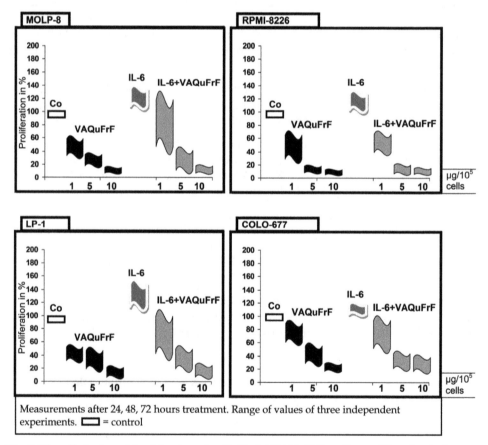

Measurements after 24, 48, 72 hours treatment. Range of values of three independent experiments. ☐ = control

Fig. 3. The effect of combined treatment with IL-6 + VAQuFrF on the proliferation in human multiple myeloma cells. IL-6=0.5 ng/105 cells.

4.7 Investigation of cell cycle phases in human multiple myeloma

Cell division consists of mitosis (M) and interphase, which divides into phases G1, G2, and S. Non dividing cells are in the stable resting phase, called the G0 phase. The blockade in the cell division leads to an arrest in the different cycle phases. This arrest appears as an accumulation of the tumour cells.

The following cell lines: were investigated: MOLP-8, LP-1, RPMI-8226, OPM-2, U-266, COLO-677, KMS-12-BM. The myeloma cells were treated (a) with IL-6 (dose: 5 ng/10^6 cells) (b) with VAQuFrF and with Vincristine (doses: 10, 50, 100 µg/10^6 cells). The investigation was carried out 24, 48 and 72 hours after treatment.

Table 4 presents the range of the values of untreated cells in different cell cycle phases in percentage in the total viable cell number (100%) 24 hours after treatment. **Table 5** presents the mean values resp. the accumulation of treated cells 24 hours after treatment. For the cell lines RPMI-8226, OPM-2 and U-266 the presented values signalize the effects 48 and 72 hours after treatment with VAQuFrF or Vincristine. For a significant increase or decrease, the percentage of the cell number of treated samples was compared with those of untreated samples.

CELL LINES	G0/G1	S	G2/M
MOLP-8	41 - 52	26 - 44	17 - 23
LP-1	50 - 63	27 - 37	8 - 12
RPMI-8226	60 - 78	13 - 28	8 - 15
OPM-2	51 - 62	20 - 38	10 - 19
U-266	48 - 59	17 - 25	9 - 21
COLO-677	36 - 49	42 - 50	10 - 21
KMS-12-BM	45 - 53	39 - 48	3 - 10

Measurements at 24 hour after incubation. Values are expressed in percentage of total viable cell number (100%). Range of four independent experiments.

Table 4. Values of untreated human multiple myeloma cells in different cell cycle phases.

Phases G0/G1: IL-6 did not affect this cell cycle phase. VAQuFrF led to an accumulation of cells in cell line MOLP-8, LP-1 and in KMS-12-BM ($p < 0.05$ and $p < 0.01$). Vincristine had effect in the cell lines MOLP-8 and LP-1 ($p < 0.05$). The both substances were effective at each time point.

Phase S: With IL-6 the number of cells was increased markedly in all cell lines during 72 hours except with OPM-2 and KMS-12-BM. In these cell lines there was no effect at 72 hours. VAQuFrF increased the cell number ($p < 0.01$) in RPMI-8226 and U-266 (p<0.05), Vincristine in RPMI-8226, OPM-2 and U-266 ($p < 0.01$ and $p < 0.05$). Both substances were effective only at 48 and 72 hours after incubation.

CELL LINES	G0/G1			S			G2/M		
	IL-6 5 ng 10^6/cells	VAQuFrF 10 50 100	Vincristine 10 50 100	IL-6 5 ng 10^6/cells	VAQuFrF 10 50 100	Vincristine 10 50 100	IL-6 5 ng 10^6/cells	VAQuFrF 10 50 100	Vincristine 10 50 100
MOLP-8	no effect	↑↑ 46 65	↑↑↑ 51 59 64	↑ 55	no effect	no effect	no effect	no effect	no effect
LP-1	no effect	↑↑ 68 72	↑↑ 78 70	↑ 40	no effect	no effect	no effect	no effect	no effect
RPMI-8226	no effect	no effect	no effect	↑ 37	↑↑ 25 33	↑↑↑ 20 42 45	no effect	no effect	↑↑↑ 49 52 50
OPM-2	no effect	no effect	no effect	↑ 45	no effect	↑↑↑ 30 31 39	no effect	no effect	no effect
U-266	no effect	no effect	no effect	↑ 39	↑↑ 22 31	↑↑↑ 23 23 28	no effect	no effect	no effect
COLO-677	no effect	no effect	no effect	↑ 58	no effect	no effect	no effect	↑↑ 18 22	↑↑↑ 54 62 68
KMS-12-BM	no effect	↑ 54	no effect	↑ 53	no effect	no effect	no effect	no effect	↑↑↑ 44 56 70

Treatment with IL-6(5ng/106 cells) or VAQuFrF or Vincristine(10,50,100 µg/106 cells); The investigation was carried out 24, 48 and 72 hours after treatment. Evaluation of three or four independent experiments ↑=accumulation. The numbers present the mean values in percentage.

Table 5. Accumulation of human multiple myeloma cells in different cell cycle phases.

Phases G2/M: IL-6 treatment led to accumulation of cells in LP-1, RPMI-8226 and OPM-2 after 48 and 72 hours. VAQuFrF was effective in COLO-677 (p < 0.05). Vincristine led to marked increase of the cell numbers in cell lines RPMI-8226, COLO-677 and KMS-12-BM (p < 0.01).

With IL-6 the cell number of each cell line was enhanced in the S phase and in some cell lines in the G2/M phase too. This means that either the DNA synthesis of the cells is increased or the cells are arrested in these cell cycle phases. In this investigation IL-6 led to high proliferation in all cell lines indicating an increased DNA synthesis. This could lead with to arrest in the cycle phase G2/M. In fact we found the accumulation of cells 48 and 72 hours after treatment in some cell lines.

Vincristine blocks the mitotic process by binding to tubulin leading to an arrest of the cycle phase in G2/M (El Alaaoui et al., 1997; Lin et al., 1998). In this study Vincristine led to an accumulation of the cells in cycle phase G2/M in only three out of seven multiple myeloma cell lines. It was effective in S and in G0/G1 phases of five cell lines, indicating that Vincristine also affects these cycle phases. It is interesting that it was effective both in the S and in G2/M cycle phases of the cell line RPMI-8226. VAQuFrF extract had the same effects as Vincristine in five out of seven tumour cell lines; however in a higher dose range. We postulated that different tumour cell lines from the same disorder (multiple myeloma) show a different sensitivity to Vincristine or VAQuFrF.

The inhibition of the G0/G1 phases in different malignancies correlates with anti-proliferative substances (El-Sherbiny et al., 2000; Pellizaro et al., 2008). In fact VAQuFrF blocked the cells in the G0/G1 phases in cell lines MOLP-8 and LP-1 and also inhibited the cell proliferation.

5. Summary and conclusion

In this experimental study we compared **Viscum album (Mistletoe) extract** and **Vincristine** in several human multiple myeloma cell lines using the parameters: (a) the IL-6 production, (b) the IL-10 production, (c) the expression of membrane IL-6 receptor, (d) the proliferation, (e) the apoptosis/necrosis, (f) the cell cycle phases. The following parameters were measured in a "package" i.e. they measured simultaneously: (a) the IL-6 production, (b) the IL-10 production, (c) the proliferation, (d) the apoptosis/necrosis.

The parameters were measured at different times (24, 48 and 72 hours) after incubation with VAQuFrF and Vincristine. Interleukin-6 is a major proliferative factor for the malignant plasma cells (multiple myeloma cells). Therefore this cytokines was measured parallel to the test substances.

Viscum album QuFrF (VAQuFrF) is an experimental drug that is not yet used in the treatment of tumour patients. For this reason it was necessary and important to compare with a well-known clinic-substance. Vincristine is used mainly in combination with other chemotherapeutic substances in the therapy of multiple myeloma.

5.1 Key results

a. Interleukin-6 leads to a markedly increased IL-10 production. Interleukin-6 upregulates markedly the expression of its membrane receptor (IL-6R). IL-6 increases the proliferation and it is effective in the S cell cycle phase. IL-6 does not affect the apoptosis/ necrosis.

b. Neither VAQuFrF nor Vincristine produce IL-6 or lead to an enhanced IL-10 production in any cell line. VAQuFrF and Vincristine inhibits the spontaneous IL-10 production. Both substances **counteract** the increased IL-10 production induced by IL-6. The effects of the two substances are comparable. The results indicate that the effect of the both test substances on the IL-10 production is due to their apoptotic/necrotic effects.

c. VAQuFrF **inhibits** the membrane expression of IL-6 receptor. VAQuFrF **counteracts** the enhanced membrane expression of this receptor induced by IL-6.

d. The **cytocidal effect** of Vincristine is more marked than its **cytostatic** effect in all cell lines.
The effect of VAQuFrF focuses on the inhibition of proliferation (**cytostatic effect**). VAQuFrF first inhibits the proliferation and then the cells die by apoptosis and/or necrosis.

e. VAQuFrF inhibits the proliferation in cells with **high proliferation** rate **more effectively** than in those with **low growth** rate.

f. **Cell cycle phases:** VAQuFrF extract has the same effect as Vincristine in five out of seven tumour cell lines, however in a higher dose range.

The findings indicate that VAQuFrF extract could be a novel drug in the therapy of multiple myeloma.

To assess the effective doses of Viscum album QuFrF extract and to transfer these doses to the in vivo situation.

The Viscum album QuFrF (VAQuFrF) is an aqueous and unfermented extract of mistletoe plants growing in the oak tree. It contains 2 µg lectin and 10 µg viscotoxin in 10 mg/ml. It was tested in dose range of 10, 50, 100 μg/10⁶ cells. 10 μg extract contains 0.002 μg lectin + 0.01 μg viscotoxin, 50 μg extract contains 0.01 μg lectin + 0.05 μg viscotoxin, 100 μg extract contains 0.02 μg lectin + 0.1 μg viscotoxin.

Dosage of Vincristine in the therapy for multiple myeloma: In combination with other chemotherapeutic agents as a part of the VAD regimen 0.4 mg/day intravenously (400 μg/day). In these experimental studies Vincristine was applied in dose range of 10, 50, 100 μg/10⁶ cells. The effects of Vincristine on the proliferation and the apoptosis/necrosis were in each cell line without dose dependence. This means that these doses lay in a saturation range. It is planned to investigate the effects of Vincristine in a lower dose range.

The efficient dose range for VAQuFrF lies between 50 and 100 μg/10⁶ cells (0.01μg lectin + 0.05 μg viscotoxin and 0.02 μg lectin + 0.1 μg viscotoxin). These date concern the cell lines LP-1, RPMI-8226 and COLO-677. For cell lines OPM-2, KMS-12-BM the dose range lies higher. In MOLP-8 cell line VAQuFrF inhibits the proliferation more effectively than Vincristine.

Our findings suggest that the in vivo effective (active) dose for VAQuFrF will be about 10-20 times higher than that of Vincristine.

6. Future research

1. **Viscum album** (VA) QuFrF extract contains two active components: mistletoe lectins (I, II, III) and viscotoxins.
   Question: Which component is responsible for the effects of this extract? Is this the **lectin(s)** or **viscotoxin** or **both**? Further study is planned to clarify this **question.**
   The non-fermented preparation from VAQuFrF extract contains 2 μg lectin and 10 μg viscotoxin in 10 mg/ml **(ratio between lectin and viscotoxin: 0.2).**
   The **ratio between lectin and viscotoxin from the fermented preparations is 0.06** respectively **0.08.** The fermented preparations are used either alone or in combination with chemo /radiotherapy in the treatment of tumour patients. The extract presented in this study is an experimental drug that is not yet used in the treatment of tumour patients.
2. The results presented in this study indicated that VAQuFrF could effect the membrane expression of IL-6 receptor by antagonism. **Question:** Is this substance a competitive- or a non-competitive antagonist? Additional experiments will give answer to this (important) **question.**
3. To investigate more human multiple myeloma cell lines.
   To investigate **tumour cells isolated from bone marrow** of patients with multiple myeloma.
4. To investigate the anti-proliferative and apoptotic/necrotic effects of Vincristine in a lower dose range, respectively the anti-proliferative and apoptotic/necrotic effects of VAQuFrF extract in a higher dose range.

7. Acknowledgements

The measurements of the parameters were carried out in the laboratory of the Society of Cancer Research (Arlesheim, Switzerland). The idea of this study is based on the findings of the author. As principal investigator she wrote the study protocol and co-ordinated the study. The evaluation of the results, the writing and the completion of this manuscript were not supported from the Society of Cancer Research and from any foundation.

8. References

Chanen-Khan, AA. (2004) Bcl-2 antisense therapy in multiple myeloma. *Oncology* Supplement, 21-24.

Duong Van Huyen, JP., Sooryanarayana Delignat, S., Bloch, MF., Kacatchkine, MD., Kaveri, SV. (2001) Variable sensitivity of lymphoblastoid cells to apoptosis induced by Viscum album QuFrF, a therapeutic preparation of mistletoe lectin. *Chemotherapy* 47, 366-376.

DuVillard, L., Guiguet, M., Casasnovas RO., Caillot, D., Monnier-Zeller, V., et al. (1995) Diagnostic serum level of IL-6 in monoclonal gammopathies. *Brit J Haematol* 89, 243-249.

El Alaoui, S., Lawry, J., Griffan, M. (1997) The cell cycle and induction of apoptosis in a hamster fibrosarcoma cell line treated with anti-cancer drugs: its importance to solid tumour chemotherapy. *J Neurol* 31, 195-207.

El-Sherbiny, YM., Cox, MC., Ismail, CA., Shamsuddin, AM., Vucenik, I. (2001) G0/G1 arrest and Sphase inhibition of human cancer cell lines by inositol hexaphosphate (IP6). *Anticancer Research* 21, 2393-2403.

Gaillard, JP., Liautard, J., Klein, P.,Brochier, J. (1997) Major role of the soluble interleukin- 6, interleukin-6 receptor complex for the proliferation of interleukin-6-dependent human myeloma cell lines. *Eur J Immunol* 27, 332-3340.

Harmsma, M., Gromme, M., Ummelen, M., Dignef, W., Tusenius, KJ., et al. (2004) Differential effects of Viscum album extract Iscador[R] Qu on cell cycle progression and apoptosis in cancer cells. *Int J Oncol* 125, 1521-1529.

Hata, H., Matsuzaki, H., Takeya, HM., Yoshida, M., Sonoki, T., et al. (1995) Expression of Fas/Apo-1 (CD95) and apoptosis in tumor cells from patients with plasma cell disorders. *Blood* 86, 1939-1945.

Kovacs, E. (2003). How does interleukin-6 affect the membrane expressions of interleukin-6 receptor and gp130 and the proliferation of the human myeloma cell line OPM-2? *Biomed Pharmacother* 57, 489–94.

Kovacs, E., Link, S., Toffol-Schmidt, U. (2006a). Cytostatic and cytocidal effects of mistletoe (Viscum album L.) Quercus extract Iscador. *Drug Research* 56, 467-473.

Kovacs, E. (2006b) Multiple myeloma and B cell lymphoma. Investigation of IL-6, IL-6 receptor antagonist (IL-6RA) and gp130 antagonist (gp130A) in an in vitro model. *The Scientific World Journal* 6, 888-898.

Kovacs, E. (2010a) Interleukin-6 leads to interleukin-10 production in several human multiple myeloma cell lines. Does interleukin-10 enhance the proliferation of these cells? *Leukemia Research* 34, 912-916.

Kovacs, E. (2010b) Investigation of the proliferation, apoptosis/necrosis and cell cycle phases in several human multiple myeloma cell lines. Comparison of Viscum album QuFrF extract with Vincristine in an in vitro model. *The Scientific World Journal* 10, 311-320.

Leoncini, L., Vecchio, MTD., Megha, T., Barbini, P., Galieni, P., et al. (1993) Correlation between apoptotic and proliferative indices in malignant non-Hodgkin's lymphoma. *Am J Pathol* 142, 755-762.

Lin, Ch-KE., Nguyen, TT., Morgan, TL., Mei, RL., Kaptein, JS., et al. (1998) Apoptosis may be either suppressed or enhanced with strategic combinations of anti-neoplastic drugs or anti-IgM. *Experimental Cell Research* 244, 1-13.

Lu, ZY., Zhang, XG., Rodriguez, C., Wijdenes, J., Gu, ZJ., et al. (1995) Interleukin-10 is a proliferation factor but not a differentiation factor for human myeloma cells. *Blood* 85, 2521–27.

Mastberger, SC., Duivenvoorden, 1., Versteegh, RT., Geldof, AA. (2000) Cell cycle arrest and clonogenic tumour cell kill by divergent chemotherapeutic drugs. *Anticancer Research* 20, 1833-1838.

Nachbaur, DM., Herold, M., Maneschg, A., Huber, H. (1991) Serum levels of interleukin-6 in multiple myeloma and other hematological disorders: correlation with disease activity and other prognostic parameters. *Ann Hematol* 62, 54-58.

Nordan, R., & Potter, M. (1986) A macrophage-derived factor required by plasmocytomas for surivival and proliferation in vitro. *Science* 233, 566-569.

Oancea, M., Mani, A., Hussein, MA., Almasan, A. (2004) Apoptosis of multiple myeloma. *Int JHematol* 8, 224-231.

Otsuki, T., Yamada, O., Yata, K., Sakaguchi, H., Kurebayashi, J., et al. (2000) Expression and production of interleukin 10 in human myeloma cell lines. *Br J Haematol* 111, 835–42.

Otsuki, T., Yata, K., Sakaguchi, H., Uno, M., Fujii, T., et al. (2002) IL-10 in myeloma cells. *Leuk Lymphoma* 43, 969–74.

Papadaki, H., Kyriakou, D., Foudoulakis, A., Markidoum F., Alexandrakis, M. (1997) Serum levels of interleukin-6 receptor in multiple myeloma as indicator of disease activity. *Acta Haematologica* 97, 191-195.

Pellizzaro, C., Speranza, A., Zorzet, S., Crucil, I., Sava, G., et al. (2008) Inhibition of human pancreatic cell line MIA PaCa2 proliferation byHA-But, a hyaluronic butyric ester: a preliminary report. *Pancreas* 36, 15-23.

Shinwari, Z., Manogaran, PS., Alrokayan, SA., Al-Hussein, KA., Aboussekhra, A. (2007) Vincristine and Iomustine induce apoptosis and p21 (WAF1) up-regulation in medulloblastoma and normal human epithelial and fibroblast cells. *Neurooncol* 87, 123-132.

Stokke, T., Holte, H., Smedshammer, L., Smeland, EB., Kaalhus, O., et al. (1998) Proliferation and apoptosis in malignant and normal cells in B-cell non-Hodgkin's lymphomas. *Br J Cancer* 77, 1832-1838.

Tsujimoto, Y. & Shimizu, S. (2007) Role of mitochondrial membrane permeability transition in cell death. *Apoptosis* 12, 835-840.

Wierzbowska, A., Urbanska, H., Robak T. (1999) Circulating IL-6 type cytokines and sIL-.6R in patients with multiple myeloma. *Brit J Haematol* 105, 412-419.

6

Ethanol Toxicity in the Brain: Alteration of Astroglial Cell Function

Metoda Lipnik-Štangelj
University of Ljubljana, Faculty of Medicine,
Department of Pharmacology and Experimental Toxicology
Slovenia

1. Introduction

Ethanol consumption has for a long time been associated with brain damage. Experimental studies and necropsy examinations of chronic alcoholics have shown a variety of structural and functional alterations in the neurons as well as in the glial cells. Such alterations are seen also in children with the alcoholic foetal syndrome. Ethanol is known to be a teratogen. Its abusage can result as dysfunction of the central nerve system (CNS), growth deficiency and facial malformation in the fetus, and behavioural, learning, sensory and motor disabilities (Barret et al., 1996; González & Salido, 2009; Šarc & Lipnik-Štangelj, 2009a). Chronic ethanol consumption in the adult is also intimately associated with brain atrophy. Accumulating evidence indicates that ethanol-induced neurobehavioral dysfunctions may be related to disruptions in the patterns of neuronal and glial developments such as depression of neurogenesis, aberrant migration of neurons and alterations in late gliogenesis and neurogenesis. These changes can further reduce the populations of cortical neurons and glial cells, trigger the biochemical alterations in glial cells and deleterious consequences for neuronal-glial interactions, and eventually lead to damage or apoptosis of these cells (González & Salido, 2009; Šarc & Lipnik-Štangelj, 2009b; Sofroniew & Vinters, 2010).

As the most abundant type of glial cells in the brain, astrocytes provide metabolic and trophic support to neurons, modulate synaptic activities and have a strong capacity to scavenge oxidants and suppress cellular apoptosis. However, when the capacity of cells to eliminate the oxidants is overwhelmed, overproduction of reactive oxygen species (ROS) can cause morphological and functional alterations in the cells, including cellular Ca^{2+} homeostasis and some active molecules tightly associated with neuronal activity (Allansson et al., 2001; Halassa et al., 2007; Sofroniew & Vinters, 2010).

Although astrocytes are more resistant than neurons to the oxidative and neurotoxic stresses and to the chemical and toxic damages in the surrounding environment, any impairment of astrocytes can dramatically affect neuronal functions. The ethanol-induced detrimental alterations of astrocytes would lead to perturbances in neuron–astroglia interactions and developmental defects of the brain (González & Salido, 2009; Šarc & Lipnik-Štangelj, 2009b). Given this important role of astroglial cells in neuronal functioning, they have become a significant object of toxicological evaluation.

2. Astrocytes in the central nerve system

Central nerve system is a complex network, constitutes from several types of cells. Besides neuronal cells, where the information is received, integrated and sent as an output signal, there are several other cell types in the CNS. Oligodendrocytes are specialized for the myelin formation, astrocytes have multiple support functions to neurons, and microglial cells play an important role in defence and inflammation, and act as scavengers when tissue is destroyed. Some other types of cells in the CNS are ependimal cells, which are epithelial cells that line brain ventricles and central canal of spinal and assist in secretion and circulation of cerebral spinal fluid, and endothelial cells which create a blood-brain barrier (González & Salido, 2009).

Glial cells were discovered by the pathologist Rudolf Virchow in 1856. They represent the majority cell population in the CNS. There is a number between 12 and 15 billion neurons in cerebral cortex and about a billion neurons in spinal cord, whereas there are 10 to 50 times more glial cells than neurons in the CNS. When they were discovered, glial cells have been recognised as brain glue. They surround neurons and hold them in place. Later it has been realized that glial cells play a number of other functions in the brain. Astrocytes are the most abundant type of glial cells, and present numerous projections that anchor neurons to their blood supply (Braet et al., 2001; González & Salido, 2009; Grafstein et al., 2000; Haydon, 2001).

2.1 Molecular aspects of astrocyte function

Astrocytes signal each other using Ca^{2+} ions (Verkhratsky et al., 1998). This type of cell-to cell communication has been termed "calcium excitability" that occurs as transient or prolonged elevations in intracellular concentration of Ca^{2+} ions. It can be spontaneous or triggered in response to specific neurotransmitters (Araque et al., 2001; Cornell-Bell et al., 1990). The membrane potential of glia is relatively stable, and although they can express voltage-gated channels (Verkhratsky et al., 1998), they exhibit little or no fluctuation in membrane potential.

Astrocytes respond to a variety of extracellular stimuli by raising intracellular concentration of Ca^{2+} ions that modulates different intracellular processes like differentiation, cytoskeleton reorganisation, and secretion of neuroactive molecules (Araque et al., 1998; Sofroniew & Vinters, 2010; Verkhratsky & Kettenmann, 1996). A rise in intracellular concentration of Ca^{2+} ions, localize to one part of an astrocyte can propagate through-out the entire cell, and Ca^{2+} resposes may be transmitted from one astrocate to others, leading to regenerative Ca^{2+} signal that spread within astrocyte networks (Cornell-Bell et al., 1990; Fam et al., 2000). This cell-to-cell communication could effectively signal to neurons, endothelial or other cell type in the CNS. Obviously, Ca^{2+} signalling in astrocytes is complementary to and interacts with signalling in vascular brain cells (Leybaert et al., 2004) and electrical signalling in neurons (Araque et al., 1999; Parpura et al., 1994). Besides calcium excitability, there are also other mechanisms for transmitting signals between astrocytes, such as releasing of diffusible extracellular messengers. Extracellular release of neurotransmitters like glutamate or adenosine triphosphate (ATP), and consequent activation of specific receptors on neighbouring astrocytes, may also mediate Ca^{2+} wave propagation (Bowser & Khakh, 2007). In addition, astrocytes are able to release other signalling molecules like D-serine and eicosanoids, and more than one of describing mechanisms for neurotransmitter release does operate within astrocytes (Araque et al., 2001; Fellin et al., 2004; Gonzales et al., 2006a; Malarkey & Parpura, 2008; Montana et al. 2006).

Released messengers, in turn, activate Ca²⁺ entry or Ca²⁺ release from intracellular stores by acting on ionotropic and metabotropic receptors, respectively. By this way, ATP and glutamate are the major active neurotransitters involved in the cell-to-cell communication of Ca²⁺ signals in astrocytes and other cell types in the CNS (Bowser & Khakh, 2007; Percea & Araque, 2007). Another putative intercellular signalling molecule for cel-to-cell communication is nitric oxide which is synthesized by enzymatic oxidation of L-arginine by nitric oxide synthase (Willmott et al., 2000). Nitric oxide (NO) activates guanylilcyclase and increases cytoplasmic cyclic guanosine monophosphate (cGMP) signalling cascades (Galione et al, 1993).

Communication between astrocytes thus seems to rely on any communication systems and signalling molecules, which act in parallel or display regional and cellular specialisation. From this point of view, there is a bidirectional signal communication system within the CNS, which might be mainly carried out by extracellular messengers, released from any type of cells. Because of their close apposition to neurons, signalling molecules released by astrocytes can modulate synaptic transmission and neuronal excitability, as well as neuronal plasticity and survival. Even it could be possible that astrocytes could play roles in higher cognitive functions like learning and memory. It is not therefore estrange that an alteration in Ca²⁺ signalling, and hence in the function of astrocytes, could affect synaptic activity and plasticity and bran homeostasis (Gonzalez & Salido, 2009).

2.2 Release of intercellular messengers

Close physical relationship between astrocytes and neurones provides an opportunity for many functional interactions. There is a bidirectional signalling pathway between astrocytes and neurons on one side, and astrocytes and blood vessels on the other, which opens the possibility to an exchange of a huge amount of information in the CNS. There are several mechanisms that have been suggested to underline the release of signalling molecules from astrocytes: reverse operation of glutamate transporters, volume-regulated anion channels, gap-junctional hemichannels, diffusional release through purinergic receptors and Ca²⁺-dependent exocytosis (Araque et al., 2001; Haydon & Carmignoto, 2006; Montana et al., 2006; Parpura et al., 2004). Among the different molecules released, two major signalling messengers, released by astrocytes, are ATP and glutamate (Gonzalez & Salido, 2009).

The mechanisms, by which astrocytes release ATP, appear to be diverse, employing vesicular release, connexion hemi-channels, cystic fibrosis transmembrane regulator, or the P-glycoprotein (Braet et al., 2004). On the other hand, astrocytic glutamate release can be carried out through connexion hemi-channel, excitatory amino acid transporters (EAAT), anion transporter, via P2X₇ receptor channels or exocytosis. Depending on the mechanism employed, ATP and/or glutamate release by astrocytes can be Ca²⁺-dependent or independent (Bowser & Khakh, 2007; Braet et al., 2004).

Besides the mechanisms for ATP and/or glutamate release from astrocytes, exocytosis constitutes the mechanism that has recently received special attention, since it was initially considered to occur only in neurons (Bowser & Khakh, 2007; Fellin et al., 2006; Gonzalez et al., 2006a; Perea & Araque, 2007).

2.3 The role of astroytes in the central nerve system

2.3.1 Astrocytes and development of central nerve system

The developmental generation of astrocytes tends to occur after the initial production of neurons in many CNS regions (Sofroniew & Vinters, 2010). During development of the brain, astrocytes (radial glia) take part in guiding the migration of developing axons and certain neuroblasts (Powel & Geller, 1999). In addition, substantive evidence is accumulating that astrocytes are essential for the formation and function of developing synapses by releasing molecular signals such as thrombospondin (Barres, 2008; Christopherson et al., 2005). Astrocytes appear also to influence developmental synaptic pruning by releasing signals that induce expression of complement C1q in synapses and thereby tag them for elimination by microglia (Barres, 2008).

2.3.2 Blood-brain barrier and regulation of blood flow

Together with brain microvascular endothelial cells astrocytes create the blood-brain barrier that protects the brain from toxic substances in the blood, supplies the brain tissues with nutrients, and filters harmful substances from the brain back to the bloodstream, enabling the proper environment in the CNS. Astrocytes may regulate endothelial cell metabolism, and vasoconstriction and vasodilatation by producing substances with angiogenic properties, such as endothelial growth factor (Proia et al., 2008), ATP (Leybaert et al., 2004), and arachidonic acid, prostagladins and nitric oxide, (Gabryel et al., 2007; Sofroniew & Vinters, 2010), that can increase or decrease CNS blood vessel diameter and blood flow in a coordinated manner. Moreover, astrocytes may be primary mediators of changes in local CNS blood flow in response to changes in neuronal activity (Koehler et al., 2009). Thus, astrocytes play important functions at the level of arterioles where blood flow is controlled, at the level of capillaries where blood-brain barrier is located and at the level of blood immune cells (Leybaert et al., 2004).

2.3.3 Energy, metabolism and homeostasis

Astrocytes play a number of other functions which are crucial for the maintenance of homeostasis and neuronal function. They provide energy supply to neurons and coordinate metabolic reactions. Astrocytes are the principal storage sites of glycogen granules in CNS. The greatest accumulation of astrocytic glycogen occurs in areas of high synaptic density, and its utilisation can sustain neuronal activity during hypoglicemia and during periods of high neuronal activity (Sofroniew & Vinters, 2010).

Astrocytes regulate the external chemical environment by removing excess ions notably potassium, regulate brain cell volume, and participate in recycling neurotransmitters released during synaptic transmission by expressing high levels of transporters for neurotransmitters such as glutamate, GABA, histamine and glycine, that serve to clear the neurotransmitters from the synaptic space. Astrocytes also represent the major site for the detoxification or bioactivation of neurotoxins (Perdan et al., 2009).

2.3.4 Synapse function

There is accumulating evidence that astrocytes play direct roles in synaptic transmission through the regulated release of synaptically active molecules including glutamate, purines

(ATP and adenosine), gamma-aminobutyric acid (GABA), and D-serine. The release of such gliotransmitters occurs in response to changes in neuronal synaptic activity, involves astrocyte excitability as reflected by increases in intracellular concentration of Ca^{2+} ions, and can alter neuronal excitability (Halassa et al., 2007; Perea et al., 2009). Such evidence has given rise to the 'tripartite synapse', which posits that astrocytes play direct and interactive roles with neurons during synaptic activity in a manner that is essential for information processing by neural circuits (Araque et al., 1999; Halassa et al., 2007; Perea et al., 2009).

2.3.5 Immune response

Astrocytes importantly contribute to creation of immune response in the brain. They are an important source of several cytokines and neurotrophic factors in the CNS that have a crucial immunoregulatory role and also promote neuronal survival and neurite growth (Lipnik-Štangelj, 2006). Moreover, cytokines have an impact on neurotoxicity, synaptic transmission and synaptic plasticity in the brain (Allan & Rothwell, 2001). Activation of astrocytes leads to up-regulation of pro-inflammatory cytokines like interleukin-1 beta (IL-1beta), tumour necrosis factor alpha (TNF-alpha), interleukin-6 (IL-6), and inducible nitric oxide synthase (iNOS), and cyclooxygenase 2 (COX2) (Gonzalez & Salido, 2009; Sofroniew & Vinters, 2010).

Research into the actions of IL-1beta in the brain initially focused on its role in host defence responses to systemic disease. IL-1beta can also elicit an array of responses which could inhibit, exacerbate or induce neuronal damage and death (Gonzalez & Salido, 2009).

TNF-alpha has an important function in neurotoxicity, synaptic transmission and synaptic plasticity. It influences homeostatic synaptic scaling by inducing the insertion of AMPA receptors at post-synaptic membranes (Stellwagen & Malenka, 2006). In addition, TNF-alpha may have a pivotal role in augmenting intracerebral immune responses and inflammatory demyelination due to its diverse functional effects on glial cells, such as oligodendrocytes and astrocytes themselves (Šarc et al., 2011).

Unlike TNF-alpha, which is a prototypical pro-inflammatory cytokine, IL-6 affects inflammation and neuronal regeneration via a number of mechanisms. In this sense, besides its immunoregulatory role, IL-6 can also promote neuronal survival and neurite growth. IL-6 can be induced by a variety of molecules including IL-1beta, TNF-alpha, transforming growth factor-beta and prostaglandins, and many other mediators such as beta-amyloid, interferon-g and IL-4 can potentiate these primary inducers, highlighting the complex nature of IL-6 modulation (Šarc et al., 2011; Gonzalez & Salido, 2009).

2.4 Reactive gliosis and glial scar formation

After brain injury, such as a stroke or trauma, astrocytes become reactive, and can undergo to profound proliferation, forming gliosis near or at the site of damage. Astrocyte activity is marked by hypertrophy, resulting in an expression of protein such as glial fibrillary acidic protein (GFAP), adhesion molecules and antigen presenting capabilities, including major histocompatibility antigens. Reactive astrocytes represent an obstacle preventing establishment of normal neural contact and circuitry. On the other hand, reactive astrocytes produce a myriad of neurotoxic substances in various brain pathologies (Mori et al., 2006).

Although reactive astrogliosis is used widely as a pathological hallmark of diseased CNS tissue, definitions of reactive astrogliosis can vary considerably among authors and there are no widely accepted categories of intensity or severity. Recently proposed definition encompasses four key features: (1) reactive astrogliosis is a spectrum of potential molecular, cellular and functional changes in astrocytes that occur in response to all forms and severities of CNS injury and disease including subtle perturbations, (2) the changes undergone by reactive astrocytes vary with severity of the insult along a gradated continuum of progressive alterations in molecular expression, progressive cellular hypertrophy, and in severe cases, proliferation and scar formation, (3) the changes of reactive astrogliosis are regulated in a context-specific manner by inter- and intracellular signalling molecules, (4) the changes undergone during reactive astrogliosis have the potential to alter astrocyte activities both through gain and loss of function that can impact both beneficially and detrimentally on surrounding neural and non-neural cells. Of particular interest as regards function of reactive astrocytes, is recent evidence that reactive astrogliosis and glial scar formation play essential roles in regulating CNS inflammation (Sofroniew, 2009).

In response to different kind of stimulation, reactive astrocytes can make many different kinds of molecules with either pro- or anti-inflammatory potential (John et al., 2003). There is a normal process of reactive astrogliosis and glial scar formation that exerts various beneficial functions including protecting neural cells and function, restricting the spread of inflammation, and promoting tissue repair.

On the contrary, in a manner analogous to inflammation, reactive astrogliosis also has the potential to exert detrimental effects. For example, reactive astrocytes can be stimulated by specific signalling cascades to gain of detrimental effects such as exacerbating inflammation via cytokine production (Brambilla et al., 2009), producing neurotoxic levels of ROS (Hamby et al., 2006), releasing potentially excitotoxic glutamate (Takano et al., 2005), potential contribution to seizure genesis (Tian et al., 2005), compromising blood brain barrier function due to VEGF-production (Argaw et al., 2009), causing cytotoxic edema during trauma and stroke (Zador et al., 2009), and contributing to chronic pain (Milligan et al., 2009).

2.4.1 Molecular mechanisms of reactive gliosis and scar formation

Many different types of intercellular signalling molecules are able to trigger reactive astrogliosis or to regulate specific aspects of reactive astrogliosis, including large polypeptide growth factors and cytokines such as IL-1, IL6, IL-10, TNF-alpha, tumour growth factor beta (TGF-beta), mediators of innate immunity such as lipopolysaccharide and other Toll-like receptor ligands, neurotransmitters such as glutamate and noradrenalin, purines such as ATP, ROS including nitric oxide (NO), hypoxia and glucose deprivation, products associated with neurodegeneration such as beta-amyloid, molecules associated with systemic metabolic toxicity such as NH4, and regulators of cell proliferation such endothelin-1, as reviewed in detail elsewhere (Sofroniew, 2009). Such molecular mediators of reactive astrogliosis can be released by all cell types in CNS tissue, including neurons, microglia, oligodendrocyte lineage cells, pericytes, endothelia, and astrocytes, in response to all forms of CNS insults, ranging from subtle cellular perturbations that release some of the specific factors just listed, to cell stretching as might be encountered during acceleration/deceleration CNS injury and which releases ATP, to intense tissue injury and cell death that release various intracellular molecules that signal intense tissue damage (Sofroniew, 2009).

It is becoming clear that different molecular, morphological, and functional changes in reactive astrocytes are specifically controlled by inter- and intra-cellular signalling mechanisms that reflect the specific contexts of the stimuli and produce specific and gradated responses of reactive astrogliosis. For a long, reactive gliosis and scar formation have been recognized as the main impediment to functional recovery after CNS injury or disease. This absolutely negative viewpoint of reactive astrogliosis is no longer tenable and it is now clear from many different lines of experimental evidence that there is a normal process of reactive astrogliosis that exerts essential beneficial functions and does not do harm. As reviewed in detail elsewhere, many studies using transgenic and experimental animal models provide compelling evidence that reactive astrocytes protect CNS cells and tissue by uptake of potentially excitotoxic glutamate, protection from oxidative stress via glutathione production (Dringen et al., 2000), neuroprotection via adenosine release (Lin et al., 2008), protection from NH4 toxicity (Rao et al., 2005), neuroprotection by degradation of amyloid-beta peptides (Koistinaho et al., 2004), facilitating blood brain barrier repair, reducing vasogenic edema after trauma (Bush et al., 1999), stroke or obstructive hydrocephalus, stabilizing extracellular fluid and ion balance and reducing seizure threshold (Zador et al., 2009), and limiting the spread of inflammatory cells or infectious agents from areas of damage or disease into healthy CNS parenchyma (Bush et al., 1999; Voskuhl et al. 2009).

3. Ethanol in the central nerve system

The deleterious effects of ethanol in CNS could result either from a direct toxic effect of ethanol or from an indirect effect involving its metabolites and/or ROS generation. Ethanol can induce several cellular reactions which result in a modification of cellular redox status that can severely affect the cell's capacity to be protected against the endogenous production of ROS (Gonthier et al., 2004). The consequences derived from the effects of ethanol on cellular structures would end in a morphological and functional impairment of cellular physiology. Among brain cells, astrocytes seem less vulnerable than neurons, but their impairment can dramatically affect neurons because of their protective role towards neurons.

3.1 Ethanol metabolism in the brain

In the CNS, astrocytes represent the major cellular localisation of ethanol metabolism, and have been postulated to protect neurons from ethanol-induced oxidative stress (Watts et al., 2005). The exact enzymatic mechanism responsible for ethanol oxidation in the brain is not clear yet.

Ethanol is normally metabolised in the liver to acetaldehyde by the alcohol dehydrogenase reaction, and acetaldehyde can be further metabolised to acetic acid via aldehyde dehydrogenase reaction. The last step in the pathway is the conversion of acetic acid to acetyl-Co-A. Although theoretically the activity of the latter enzyme is high enough to cope with the rate at which ethanol is oxidized by alcohol dehydrogenase, there is a limit to the rate at which the reaction can continue and can therefore lead to accumulation of acetaldehyde, which is toxic for most tissues, including CNS. Thus, there is always a build up of acetaldehyde which passes out from the liver into the blood, and this acetaldehyde is responsible or some of the unpleasant symptoms of alcohol excess. Once in the bloodstream, the acetaldehyde can also cross the blood-brain barrier and attack the CNS.

In the brain, ethanol can be metabolized by catalase, cytochrome P450 2E1, and alcohol-dehydrogenase, with catalase, playing a pivotal role among the others (Gonzalez et al., 2007).

On the other hand, ethanol also induces up-regulation of antioxidant defences by increasing the enzymatic activities of superoxide-dismutase, catalase, and glutathione-peroxidase (Eysseric et al., 2000; Rathinam et al., 2006). The expression of heat shock proteins like HSP70 (Russo et al., 2001), which have a protective and stabilizing effect on stress-induced injury, is also induced by ethanol. Altogether, this would confer to astrocytes a survival advantage preventing oxidative damage.

3.2 Ethanol influence on astrocyte function

Ethanol has several targets in astrocytes and other cell types, impairing cellular redox status, cell growth and differentiation, interfering with the stimulatory effect of trophic factors or altering the expression of cytoskeletal proteins. In addition, ethanol induces astroglial activation, associated with up-regulation of several pro-inflammatory cytokines, that contribute to neuroinflammation, neurodegeneration and cell apoptosis (Alfonso-Loeches et al., 2010; Šarc & Lipnik-Štangelj, 2009).

3.2.1 The effects of ethanol on developing central nerve system

Ethanol is a known teratogen and has been implicated in the etiology of human fetal alcohol syndrome, which is characterized by distinct craniofacial abnormalities such as microcephaly, agnathia, and ocular aberrations. Prenatal ethanol exposure induces functional abnormalities during brain development affecting neurogenesis and gliogenesis. Thus, ethanol cases a number of changes in several neurochemical systems. Astrocytes are predominant source of postnatal retinoic acid synthesis in the cerebellum, and this acid shows teratogenic effects responsible for the fetal alcohol syndrome.

McCaffery et al. (2004) showed that ethanol could stimulate retinoic acid synthesis leading to abnormal embryonic concentrations of this morphogen and, thus, ethanol could represent a major cause of fetal alcohol syndrome. Additionally, increased sensitivity of glutamate receptors and enhanced trans-membrane transport of glutamate has been observed in the presence of ethanol. This was in relationship to the increase in the expression of the excitatory amino acid transporters EAAT1 and EAAT2. Thus, glutamatergic system is affected by ethanol, which can be viewed as a maladaptive process that disposes the developing brain to fetal alcohol syndrome (Zink et al. 2004).

Furthermore, ethanol affects the synthesis, intracellular transport, distribution, and secretin of N-glicoproteins in different cell types, including astrocytes and neurons (Braza-Boils t al., 2006). Glicoproteins, such as adhesion molecules and growth factors, participate in the regulation of nervous system development. Thus, the alteration in the glycosylation process induced by ethanol could be a key mechanism involved in the teratogenic effects of ethanol exposure on brain development. Further studies by Martinez et al., (2007) showed that long-term ethanol treatment substantially impairs glycosylation and membrane trafficking in primary cultures of rat astrocytes. Ethanol reduced endogenous levels of acive RhoA due to an increase in the activity of small Rho GTP-ases, reduced phosphoinositides levels and induced changes in the dynamics and organization of the actin cytoskeleton.

Ethanol presents as well morphological effects on the developing adolescent brain. There were clear effects immediately and long after drinking cessation of a chronic ethanol administration on two neurotransmitter systems (the serotoninergic and nitrergic), which decreased, and the astrocytic cytoskeleton and neuron, which increased and decreased, respectively (Evrard et al., 2006). The authors concluded that drinking cessation can partially ameliorate the ethanol-induced morphological changes on neurons and astrocytes but cannot fully return it to the basal state.

3.2.2 The effects of ethanol on cholesterol homeostasis

Cholesterol is an essential component of cell membranes and plays an important rule in signal transduction. There are evidences that cholesterol homeostasis may be affected by ethanol, and this may be involved in neurotoxicity (Guizzetti & Costa, 2007). Indeed, the pathogenesis of Alzheimer's disease has been linked to altered cholesterol homeostasis in the brain. Several functions are carried out by cholesterol and are important for brain development, such as glial cell proliferation, synaptogenesis, neuronal survival and neurite outgrowth. In addition, the brain contains high level of cholesterol, mostly synthesized in situ. Furthermore, astrocytes produce large amounts of cholesterol that can be released by these cells and utilized by neurons to form synapses (Gonzalez & Salido, 2009).

3.2.3 The effects of ethanol on synaptic structure

It has been shown that chronic ethanol consumption affects the synaptic structure. The density of dendritic spines was found lower in the nucleus accumbens, and depicted an up-regulation of a subunit of the NMDA receptor. The up-regulated NMDA receptor subunit is a splice variant isoform which is required for membrane-bound trafficking or anchoring into a spine synaptic site. These changes, evoked by ethanol, demonstrated an alteration of micro circuitry for glutamate reception (Zhou et al., 2007).

Adermark and Loviger (2006) showed that ethanol inhibits a Ca^{2+}-insensitive K^+ channel activity, and affects gap junction coupling, demonstrating that astrocytes play a critical role in brain K^+ homeostasis, and that ethanol effects on astrocytic function could influence neuronal activity.

Finally, despite most of the investigations on the effects of ethanol have been performed following its addition to tissue or cell cultures, an interesting study has shown excessive activation of glutamatergic neurotransmission in the cerebral cortex following ethanol withdrawal and its contribution to significant behavioural disturbances and to alcohol craving. These effects were related to the activity of the enzyme glutamine synthetase, which converts released glutamate to glutamine (Miguel-Hidalgo, 2006).

3.2.4 Ethanol and glial oxidative stress

Brain tissue is particularly vulnerable to oxidative damage, possibly due to its high consumption of oxygen and the consequent generation of high quantities of ROS during oxidative phosphorylation. In addition, several regions of the brain are rich in iron, which promotes the production of ROS. On the other hand, the brain counts wit relatively poor levels of antioxidant enzymes and antioxidant compounds. ROS increase intracellular concentration of Ca^{2+} ions, inhibit response of astrocytes to physiological agonists, and stimulate glutamate secretion, which in excess is neurotoxic (Gonzalez et al., 2006a). Although glutamate is the principal excitatory neurotransmitter in the mammalian brain, high levels of this neurotransmitter lead to excitotoxic neuronal death, mediated by Ca^{2+} influx, principally through NMDA-gated channels (Bambrick et al., 2004).

Ca^{2+} signalling is an important medium for neuron-glia interaction, in the sense that neuronal activity can trigger Ca^{2+} signals in glial cells and vice versa. Due to its critical importance for the cellular functions, resting intracellular concentration of Ca^{2+} ions is tightly controlled, and abnormalities in Ca^{2+} regulation lead to impairment of cellular physiology. Ca^{2+}-ROS interplay can be considered as a push-pull relationship. An elevated level of intracellular concentration of Ca^{2+} ions can lead to excessive ROS production, whereas excessive ROS production can lead to cytosolic Ca^{2+} overload (Gonzalez & Salido, 2009). Acute exposure of astrocytes to ethanol increases intracellular concentration of Ca^{2+} ions, probably due to inhibition of plasma membrane Ca^{2+}-ATPase activity (Sepulveda & Mata, 2004). Other changes, evoked by ethanol are cell swelling, and transformation of actin cytoskeleton (Allansson et al., 2001).

Mitochondria represent the major source of intracellular ROS, and Ca^{2+} uptake into the organelle can lead to ROS generation (Gonzalez et al., 2006b; Granados et al., 2004). Ethanol-evoked ROS production takes place in the mitochondria, and accumulated mitochondrial ROS can be released to the cytoplasm leading to damage of different transport mechanisms, ion channel modification, lipid peroxidation, and DNA damage. Furthermore, damage to mitochondrial metabolism may generate additional damaging radial species, thus activating cellular death pathways (Gonzalez et al., 2006a).

Ethanol evokes a dose-dependent increase in glutamate secretion by an exocytosis mechanism, which was dependent on Ca^{2+} mobilisation. The secretory effect of ethanol is reduced in the presence of antioxidants, therefore indicating the participation of ROS in ethanol-evoked glutamate secretion by astrocytes. Glutamate and the attendant increase in intracellular Ca^{2+} play crucial role in triggering excitotoxic cell death in neighbouring cells (Molz et al., 2008). Because astrocytes are the major regulators of glutamate homeostasis, their death can cause and/or aggravate diseases of the CNS.

3.2.5 Ethanol, inflammation and immune response

Ethanol is able to activate glial cells, which is a critical event in the neuroinflammatory processes. Chronic ethanol intake enhances inflammatory mediators like COX-2, and iNOS in rat cerebral cortex and cultured astrocytes. Astrocytes undergo actin cytoskeleton disorganisation, and there is a stimulation of both, interleukin receptor-associated kinase (IRAK)/extracellular signal-regulated kinases (ERK)/nuclear factor-kappaB (NF-kappaB) pathway and the COX-2 expression, which are associated with the inflammatory responses (Guasch et al., 2007).

Ethanol-induced glial activation is also associated with changes in the expression of inflammatory cytokines like IL-1alpha, TNF-alpha, IL-6. Notably, an increased expression of the pro-inflammatory cytokine MCP-1 (monocyte chemoattractant protein 1) and microglial activation as well as astrogliosis have been demonstrated by postmortem analyses in alcoholic brains (Gonzalez & Salido, 2009; He and Crews, 2008).

Besides ethanol, its primary metabolite acetaldehyde is also able to modulate TNF-alpha and IL-6 secretion from cultured astrocytes. Both compounds showed a biphasic, hormetic effect on the IL-6 secretion after the acute as well as after the long-term exposure. It has been shown that long-term exposure to ethanol and acetaldehyde is more toxic than an acute exposure. The maximum stimulation was reached for 50 mM ethanol and 1 mM acetaldehyde after chronic exposure. In contrast, both compounds reduced the TNF-alpha secretion, where the effect was concentration dependent. Acetaldehyde showed to be more potent toxin than ethanol, and the ethanol's toxicity in the brain is at least partially due to its primary metabolite, acetaldehyde (Šarc et al., 2011).

Inflammation is primarily a protective response of the target organism to a noxis. On the other hand, excessive or long-lasting inflammation is often followed by degenerative processes. The stimulatory effect of ethanol and acetaldehyde on IL-6 secretion seems to be involved in both neuroregenerative and survival processes as well as in neurodegeneration. The obtained hormetic dose-response relationship indicates that higher concentrations and long-term exposure could lead in a neurodegenerative direction whereas low concentrations may act as neuroprotective. Unlike TNF-alpha, which is responsible for the induction of multiple pro-inflammatory genes, IL-6 often fails to induce these genes. Moreover, IL-6 can down-regulate the expression of TNF-alpha, which correlate with the data, where the first significant decrease in the TNF-alpha level was found at the highest level of IL-6 after a long-term exposure to ethanol (Šarc et al., 2011).

3.2.6 Ethanol and glial cell death

Apoptosis or programmed cell death is a form of cell death that occurs in multicellular organisms. Apoptosis is a tightly regulated process which engages multiple cell signalling pathways, and involves the altruistic suicide if individual cells in favour of the organism. This process is desirably during organism development and morphological changes, especially at the embryonic stage, as well as during the activation of the immune system. However, defects in apoptosis can result in cancer, autoimmune diseases and neurodegenerative disorders. Studies on Ca^{2+} signalling in apoptosis showed that ethanol potentiates apoptotic cell death induction by thapsigargin, caffeine, and the protonophore, which separately caused similar increases in Ca^{2+} levels, and also induces similar apoptotic death. These effects of ethanol are concentration and time-dependent (Hirata et al., 2006).

The effect of ethanol on the induction of apoptosis in astrocytes, and the formation of ceramide as apoptotic signal was investigated by Schatter et al. (2005). Ethanol induced nuclear fragmentation and DNA laddering, and inhibited phospholipase D-mediated formation of phosphatidic acid, which is a mitogenic lipid messenger. The authors concluded that ethanol induced glial apoptosis during brain development via formation of ceramide. Further studies have shown that astrocytes exposed to ethanol, undergo morphological changes associated with anoikis, a programmed cell death induced by loss of anchorage. Astrocytes depicted peripheral reorganisation of both, focal adhesions and actin-myosin system, cell contraction, membrane blebbing and chromatin condensation (Gonzalez & Salido, 2009).

Recently, it has been shown that ethanol affect intracellular trafficking. In fact, ethanol could interfere with nucleoplasmic transport in astrocytes, in such a way that ethanol induces a delay in both import and export of proteins to the nucleus (Marin et al., 2008).

Neurodegeneration, brain injury, and neuroinflammation are associated not only with increased cell apoptosis but also with the activation of a key proteolytic enzyme in this process, caspase-3. Immunohistochemical findings in mice, fed chronically with ethanol, reveal that inflammatory processes occur concomitantly with caspase-3 activation, suggesting an increase in programmed cell death. Moreover, it seems that the alcohol-induced toll-like receptor 4 (TLR4) response triggers both, inflammatory processes and apoptosis. A recent study suggests that the TLR4 response can also induce oxidative stress and neuronal injury, which agrees with a role of TLR4 in ethanol-induced brain damage and possibly in neurodegeneration (Alfonso-Loeches et al., 2010).

It has been shown that ethanol can activate or inhibit TLR4 by interacting with membrane lipids. Low/moderate ethanol concentrations (10–50 mM, in the range found in the blood of social drinkers and alcoholics) are capable of promoting translocation and clustering of TLR4 and a surface marker protein CD14, and the signalling molecules, like interleukin receptor-associated kinase (IRAK) and extracellular signal-regulated kinases (ERK), into the lipid rafts (Blanco et al., 2008; Fernandez-Lizarbe et al., 2008). Conversely, high ethanol concentrations or lipid raft-disrupting agents (streptolysin-O or saponin) inhibit ethanol-induced activation of the TLR4 signalling pathway (Blanco et al., 2008; Fernandez-Lizarbe et al., 2008). However, the molecular mechanism of ethanol interactions with TLR4 remains unknown.

4. Conclusion

Astrocytes are essential for maintaining a healthy and well-functioning brain. They face the synapses, send end-foot processes that enwrap the brain capillaries, and form an extensive network interconnected by gap junctions. They have the potential to impact on essentially all aspects of neuronal function through regulation of blood flow, provision of energy substrates, or by influencing synaptic function and plasticity. Moreover, astrocytes also protect and aid the brain in the functional recovery from injuries. The activation of glial cells in the CNS is the first defence mechanism against pathological abnormalities that occur in neurodegenerative diseases.

Ethanol has an extensive array of actions on astrocytes, transforming them into activated, potentially injurious cells with negative consequences to neuronal function and survival, and to brain function.

Therefore, it is a pivotal solution to seek molecular mechanisms and molecules that may inhibit or attenuate ethanol-induced neurotoxicity in astrocytes, thus offering an alternative strategy to prevent or treat neurodevelopmental disorders and mental retardation caused by ethanol.

5. Acknowledgment

The work was supported by the grant P3-0067 from the Slovenian Research Agency.

6. References

Adermark, L. & Lovinger, D.M. (2006). Ethanol effects on electrophysiological properties of astrocytes in striatal brain slices. *Neuropharmacology*, Vol.51, No.7-8, (December 2006), pp. 1099-1108.

Alfonso-Loeches, S.; Pascual-Lucas, M.; Blanco, A.M.; Sanchez-Vera, I. & Guerri, C. (2010). Pivotal Role of TLR4 Receptors in Alcohol-Induced Neuroinflammation and Brain Damage. *The Journal of Neuroscience*, Vol. 30, No.24, (June 2010), pp. 8285- 8295.

Allan, S.M. & Rothwell, N.J. (2001). Cytokines and acute neurodegeneration. *Nature Review Neuroscience*, Vol.2, No.10, (October 2001), pp. 734-744.

Allansson, L.; Khatibi, S.; Olsson, T. & Hansson, E. (2001)Acute ethanol exposure induces [Ca2+]i transients, cell swelling and transformation of actin cytoskeleton in astroglial primary cultures. *Journal of Neurochemistry*, Vol.76, No.2, (January 2001), pp. 472-479.

Araque, A.; Parpura, V.; Sanzgiri, R.P. & Haydon, P.G. (1998). Glutamate-dependent astrocyte modulation of synaptic transmission between cultured hippocampal neurons. *European Journal of Neuroscience*, Vol.10, No.6, (June 1998), pp. 2129-2142.

Araque, A.; Parpura, V.; Sanzgiri, R.P. & Haydon, P.G. (1999). Tripartite synapses: glia, the unacknowledged partner. *Trends in Neurosciences*, Vol.22, No.5, (May 1999), pp. 208-215.

Araque, A.; Carmignoto, G. & Haydon, P.G. (2001). Dynamic signaling between astrocytes and neurons. *Annual Review of Physiology*, Vol.63, (2001), pp. 795-813.

Argaw, A.T.; Gurfein, B.T.; Zhang, Y.; Zameer, A. & John, G.R. (2009). VEGF-mediated disruption of endothelial CLN-5 promotes blood-brain barrier breakdown. *Proceedings of the National Academy of Sciences USA*, Vol.106, (2009), pp.1977–1982.

Bambrick, L.; Kristian, T. & Fiskum, G. (2004). Astrocyte mitochondrial mechanisms of ischemic brain injury and neuroprotection. *Neurochemistry Research*, Vol.29, (2004), pp. 601-608.

Barres, B.A. (2008). The mystery and magic of glia: a perspective on their roles in health and disease. *Neuron*, Vol.60, (2008), pp. 430–440.

Barret, L.; Soubeyran, A.; Usson, Y.; Eysseric, H. & Saxod, R. (1996). Characterization of the morphological variations of astrocytes in culture following ethanol exposure. *Neurotoxicology*, Vol.17, No.2, (1996), pp. 497-507.

Blanco, A.M.; Perez-Arago, A.; Fernandez-Lizarbe, S. & Guerri, C. (2008). Ethanol mimics ligand-mediated activation and endocytosis of IL-1RI/TLR4 receptors via lipid rafts caveolae in astroglial cells. *Journal of Neurochemistry*, Vol.106, No.2, (July 2008), pp. 625-639.

Bowser, D.N. & Khakh, B.S. (2007). Vesicular ATP is the predominant cause of intercellular calcium waves in astrocytes. *Journal of General Physiology*, Vol.129, No.6, (June 2007), pp. 485-491.

Braet, K.; Paemeleire, K.; D'Herde, K.; Sanderson, M.J. & Leybaert, L. (2001). Astrocyte-endothelial cell calcium signals conveyed by two signalling pathways. *European Journal of Neuroscience*, Vol.13, No.1, (January 2001), pp 79-91.

Braet, K.; Cabooter, L.; Paemeleire, K. & Leybaert, L. (2004). Calcium signal communication in the central nervous system. *Biology of the Cell*, Vol.94, No.1, (February 2004), pp. 79-91.

Brambilla, R.; Persaud, T.; Hu, X.; Karmally, S.; Shestopalov, V.I.; Dvoriantchikova, G.; Ivanov, D.; Nathanson, L.; Barnum, S.R. & Bethea, J.R. (2009) .Transgenic inhibition of astroglial NF-kappaB improves functional outcome in experimental autoimmune encephalomyelitis by suppressing chronic central nervous system inflammation. *Journal of Immunoloy,* Vol.182, (2009), pp.2628-2640.

Braza-Boïls, A.; Tomás, M.; Marín, M.P.; Megías, L.; Sancho-Tello, M.; Fornas, E. & Renau-Piqueras, J. (2006). Glycosylation is altered by ethanol in rat hippocampal cultured neurons. *Alcohol Alcohol,* Vol.41, No.5, (September-October 2006), pp. 494-504.

Bush, T.G. N.P.; Horner, C.H.; Polito, A.; Ostenfeld, T.; Svendsen, C.N.; Mucke, L.; Johnson, M.H. & Sofroniew. M.V. (1999). Leukocyte infiltration, neuronal degeneration and neurite outgrowth after ablation of scar-forming, reactive astrocytes in adult transgenic mice. *Neuron,* Vol.23, (1999), pp. 297-308.

Christopherson, K.S.; Ullian, E.; Stokes, C.C.; Mullowney, C.E.; Hell, J.W.; Agah, A.; Lawler, J.; Mosher, D.F.; Bornstein, P. & Barres, B.A. (2005). Thrombospondins are astrocyte-secreted proteins that promote CNS synaptogenesis. Cell, Vol.120, (2005), pp. 421-433.

Cornell-Bell, A.H.; Finkbeiner, S.M.; Cooper, M. & Smith S.J. (1990). Glutamate induces calcium waves in cultured astrocytes: long-range glial signaling. *Science,* Vol.26, No.247, (January 1990), pp. 470-473.

Dringen, R.; Gutterer, J.M. & Hirrlinger, J. (2000). Glutathione metabolism in brain metabolic interaction between astrocytes and neurons in the defense against reactive oxygen species. *European Journal of Biochemistry,* Vol.267, No.16, (August 2000), pp. 4912-4916.

Evrard, S.G.; Duhalde-Vega, M.; Tagliaferro, P.; Mirochnic, S.; Caltana, L.R. & Brusco, A. (2006). A low chronic ethanol exposure induces morphological changes in the adolescent rat brain that are not fully recovered even after a long abstinence: an immunohistochemical study. *Experimental Neurology,* Vol. 200, No.2, (August 2006), pp. 438-459.

Eysseric, H.; Gonthier, B.; Soubeyran, A.; Richard, M.J.; Daveloose, D. & Barret, L. (2000). Effects of chronic ethanol exposure on acetaldehyde and free radical production by astrocytes in culture. *Alcohol,* Vol.21, No.2, (June 2000) pp. 117-125.

Fam, S.R.; Gallagher, C.J. & Salter, M.W. (2000). P2Y(1) purinoceptor-mediated Ca(2+) signaling and Ca(2+) wave propagation in dorsal spinal cord astrocytes. *Journal of Neuroscience,* Vol.15, No.20, (April 2000), pp. 2800-2808.

Fellin, T.; Pascual, O.; Gobbo, S.; Pozzan, T.; Haydon, P.G. & Carmignoto, G. (2004). Neuronal synchrony mediated by astrocytic glutamate through activation of extrasynaptic NMDA receptors. *Neuron,* Vol.2, No.43, (September 2004), pp. 729-743.

Fellin, T.; Sul, J.Y.; D'Ascenzo, M.; Takano, H.; Pascual, O. & Haydon, P.G. (2006). Bidirectional astrocyte-neuron communication: the many roles of glutamate and ATP. *Novartis Foundation Symposium,* Vol.276, (2006), pp. 208-217.

Fernandez-Lizarbe, S.; Pascual, M.; Gascon, M.S.; Blanco, A. & Guerri, C. (2008). Lipid rafts regulate ethanol-induced activation of TLR4 signaling in murine macrophages. *Molecular Immunology,* Vol.45, (2008), pp. 2007-2016.

Gabryel, B.; Chalimoniuk, M.; Stolecka, A. & Langfort, J. (2007). Activation of cPLA2 and sPLA2 in astrocytes exposed to simulated ischemia in vitro. *Cell Biology International,* Vol.31, No.9, (September 2007), pp. 958-965.

Galione, A.; White, A.; Willmott, N.; Turner, M.; Potter, B.V. & Watson S.P. (1993). cGMP mobilizes intracellular Ca2+ in sea urchin eggs by stimulating cyclic ADP-ribose synthesis. *Nature*, Vol.365, No.6445, (September 1993), pp. 456-459.

Gonthier, B.; Signorini-Allibe, N.; Soubeyran, A.; Eysseric, H.; Lamarche, F. & Barret, L. (2004). Ethanol can modify the effects of certain free radical-generating systems on astrocytes. *Alcoholism*, Vol.28, (2004), pp. 526-533.

González, A.; Granados, M.P.; Pariente, J.A. & Salido, G.M. (2006). H2O2 mobilizes Ca2+ from agonist- and thapsigargin-sensitive and insensitive intracellular stores and stimulates glutamate secretion in rat hippocampal astrocytes. *Neurochemistry Research*, Vol.31, No.6, (June 2006), pp. 741-750.

González, A.; Núñez, A.M.; Granados, M.P.; Pariente, J.A,. & Salido, G.M. (2006). Ethanol impairs CCK-8-evoked amylase secretion through Ca2+-mediated ROS generation in mouse pancreatic acinar cells. *Alcohol*, Vol.31, No.1, (January 2006), pp. 51-57.

González, A.; Pariente, J.A. & Salido, G.M. (2007). Ethanol stimulates ROS generation by mitochondria through Ca2+ mobilization and increases GFAP content in rat hippocampal astrocytes. *Brain Research*, Vol.31, No.1178, (October 2007), pp. 28-37.

González, A. & Salido G.M. (2009). Ethanol alters the physiology of neuron-glia communication. *Internal review of neurobiology*, Vol.88, (2009), pp. 168-199.

Grafstein, B.; Liu, S.; Cotrina, M.L. & Goldman, S.A. (2000). Nedergaard M. Meningeal cells can communicate with astrocytes by calcium signaling. *Annals of Neurology*, Vol.47, No.1, (January 2000), pp. 18-25.

Granados, M.P.; Salido, G.M.; Pariente, J.A. & González, A. (2004). Generation of ROS in response to CCK-8 stimulation in mouse pancreatic acinar cells. *Mitochondrion*, Vol.3, No.5, (April 2004), pp. 285-296.

Guasch, R.M.; Blanco, A.M.; Pérez-Aragó, A.; Miñambres, R.; Talens-Visconti, R.; Peris, B. & Guerri, C. (2007). RhoE participates in the stimulation of the inflammatory response induced by ethanol in astrocytes. *Experimental Cell Research*, Vol.15, No.313, (October 2007), pp.3779-3788.

Guizzetti, M. & Costa, L.G. (2007). Cholesterol homeostasis in the developing brain: A possible new target for ethanol. *Human and Experimental Toxicology*, Vol.26, (2007), pp. 355-360.

Halassa, M.M.; Fellin, T.; Takano, H.; Dong, J.H. & Haydon, P.G. (2007). Synaptic islands defined by the territory of a single astrocyte. *Journal of Neuroscience*, Vol.27, (2007), pp. 6473–6477.

Hamby, M.E.; Hewett, J.A. & Hewett, S.J. (2006). TGF-beta1 potentiates astrocytic nitric oxide production by expanding the population of astrocytes that express NOS-2. *Glia*, Vol.54, (2006), pp.566–577.

Haydon, P.G. (2001). Glia: listening and talking to the synapse. *Nature Reviews Neuroscience*, Vol.2, (2001), pp. 185-193.

Haydon, P.G. & Carmignoto, G. (2006). Astrocyte control of synaptic transmission and neurovascular coupling. *Physiological Reviews*, Vol.86, (2006), pp. 1009-1031.

He, J. & Crews, F.T. (2008). Increased MCP-1 and microglia in various regions of the human alcoholic brain. *Experimental Neurology*, Vol.210, (2008), pp. 349 –358.

Hirata, H.; Machado, L.S.; Okuno, C.S.; Brasolin, A.; Lopes, G.S. & SmAili, S.S. (2006). Apoptotic effect of ethanol is potentiated by caffeine-iduced calcium release in rat astrocytes. *Neuroscience Letters*, Vol.393, (2006), pp. 136-140.

John, G.R.; Lee, S.C. & Brosnan, C.F. (2003). Cytokines: Powerful regulators of glial cell activation. *Neuroscientist,* Vol.9, (2003), pp. 10–22.

Koistinaho, M.; Lin, S.; Wu, X.; Esterman, M.; Koger, D.; Hanson, J.; Higgs, R.; Liu, F.; Malkani, S.; Bales, K.R. & Paul, S.M. (2004). Apolipoprotein E promotes astrocyte colocalization and degradation of deposited amyloid-beta peptides. *Nature Medicine,* Vol.10, (2004), pp. 719–726.

Leybaert, L.; Cabooter, L. & Braet, K. (2004). Calcium signal communication between glial and vascular brain cells. *Acta Neurologica Belgica,* Vol.104, (2004), pp. 51-56.

Lin, J.H.; Lou, N.; Kang, N.; Takano, T.; Hu, F.; Han, X.; Xu, Q.; Lovatt, D.; Torres, A.; Willecke, K.; Yang, J.; Kang, J. & Nedergaard, M. (2008). A central role of connexin 43 in hypoxic preconditioning. *Journal of Neurosciences,* Vol.28, (2008), pp.681–695.

Lipnik-Štangelj, M. (2006). Multiple role of histamine H1-receptor-PKC-MAPK signalling pathway in histamine stimullated nerve growth factor synthesis and secretion. *Biochemical pharmacology,* Vol.72, No.11, (2006), pp. 1375-1381.

Malarkey, E.B. & Parpura, V. (2008). Mechanisms of glutamate release from atrocytes. *Neurochemistry International,* Vol.52, (2008), pp. 142-154.

Marin, M.P.; Tomas, M.; Esteban-Pretel;, G.; Megias, l.; Lopez-Iglesias, C.; Egea, G. & Renau-Piqueras, J. (2008). Chronic ethanol exposure induces alterations in the nucleocytoplasmic transport in growing astroytes. *Journal of Neurochemistry,* Vol.106, (2008), pp. 1914-1928.

Martinez, S.E.; Lazaro-Dieguez, F.; Selva, J.; Calvo, F.; Piqueras, J.R.; Crespo, P.; Claro, E. & Egea, G. (2007). Lysophosphatidic acid rescues RhoA activation and phosphoinositides levels in astrocytes expoed to ethanol. *Journal of Neurochemistry,* Vol.102, (2007), pp. 1044-1052.

McCaffery, P.; Koul, O.; Smith, D.; Napoli, J.L.; Chen, N. & Ullman, M.D. (2004). Ethanol increases retinoic acid production in cerebellar astrocyes and i cerebellum. *Brain Research. Developmental Brain Research,* Vol.153, (2004), pp. 233-241.

Miguel-Hildago, J.J. (2006). Withdrawal from free-choice ethanol consumption results in increased packing density of glutamine synthetase-immunoreactive astrocytes in the prelimbic cortex of alcohol-preffering rats. *Alcohol Alcoholism,* Vol. 41, (2006), pp. 379-385.

Milligan, E.D. & Watkins, L.R. (2009). Pathological and protective roles of glia in chronic pain. *Nature Reviews Neuroscience,* Vol.10, (2009), pp. 23–36.

Molz, S.; Decker, H.; Dal-Cim, T.; Cremonez, C.; Cordova, F.M.;Leal, R.B. & Tasca, C.I. (2008). Glutamate-induced toxicity in hippocampal slices involves apoptotic features and p38(MAPK) signalling. *Neurochemistry Research,* Vol.33, (2008), pp. 27-36.

Montana, V.; Malarkey, E.B.; Verderio, C.; Matteoli, M. & Parpua, V. (2006).Vesicular transmitter release from astrocytes. *Glia,* Vol.54, (2006), pp. 700-715.

Parpura, V.; Basarsky, T.A.; Liu,F.; Jeftinija, K.; Jeftinija, S. & Haydon P.G. (1994). Glutamate-mediated astrocyte-neuron signaling. *Nature,* Vol.369, (1994), pp. 744-747.

Parpura, V.; Scemes, E. & Spary, D.C. (2004). Mechanisms of glutamate release from astrocytes: Gap junction »hemichanneles«, purinergic receptors and exocytotic release. *Neurochemistry International,*Vol.45, (2004), pp. 259-264.

Percea, G. & Araque, A. (2007). Astrocytes potentiate transmitter release at single hippocampal synapses. *Science,* Vol.317, (2007), pp. 1083-1086.

Perdan, K.; Lipnik-Šangelj, M. & Kržan, M. (2009). The impact of astrocytes in the clearance of neurotransmitters by uptake and inactivation. In: *Advances in planar lipid bilayers and liposomes*, A. Ottova-Leitmannova, H.T. Tien (Eds.), Vol.9, (2009), pp. 211-235, doi: 10.1016/S1554-4516(09)09008-5. Elsevier: Academic Press, Amsterdam.

Perea, G.; Navarrete, M. & Araque, A. (2009). Tripartite synapses: astrocytes process and control synaptic information. Trends in Neurosciences, Vol.32, (2009), pp. t421–t431.

Powell, E.M. & Geller, H.M. (1999). Dissection of astrocyte-mediated cues in neuronal guidance and process extension. *Glia*, Vol.26, (1999), pp. 73–83.

Proia, P.; Schiera, G.; Mineo, M.; Ingrassia, A.M.; Santoro, G.; Savettieri, G. & Di Liegro, I. (2008). Astrocytes shed extracellular vesicles that contain fibroblast growth factor-2 and vascular endothelial growth factor. *International Journal of Molecular Medicine*, Vol.21, (2008), pp. 63-67.

Rao, K.V.; Panickar, K.S.; Jayakumar, A.R. & Norenberg, M.D. (2005). Astrocytes protect neurons from ammonia toxicity. *Neurochemistry Research*, Vol.30, (2005), pp. 1311–1318.

Rathinam, M.L.; Watts, L.T.; Stark, A.A.; Mahimainathan, L.; Stewart, J.; Schenker, S. & Henderson, G.I. (2006). Astrocyte control of fetal cortical neuron glutathione homeostasis: Up-regulation by ethanol. *Journal of Neurochemistry*, Vol.96, (2006), pp. 1289-1300.

Russo, A.; Palumbo, M.; Scifo, C.; Cardil, V.; Barcellona, M.L. & Renis, M. (2001). Ethanol-induced oxidative stress in rat astroytes: Role of HSP70. *Cell Biology and Toxicology*, Vol.17, (2001), pp. 153-168.

Schatter, B.; Jin, S.; Loeffelholz, K. & Klein, J. (2005). Cross-talk between phosphatidic acid and ceramide during ethanol-induced apoptosis in astrocytes. *BMC Pharmacology*, Vol.5, No.3, (2005).

Sepulveda, M.R. & Mata, A.M. (2004). The interaction of ethaol with reconstituted synaptosomal plasma membrane Ca2+-ATPase. *Biochimica et Biophysica Acta*, Vol.1665, (2004), pp. 75-80.

Sofroniew, M.V. & Vinters, H.V. (2010). Astrocytes: biology and pathology. Acta Neuropathol. Vol.119, No.1, (January 2010), pp. 7-35.

Stellwagen, D. & Malenka, R.C. (2006). Synaptic scaling mediated by glial TNF-alpha. *Nature*, Vol.440, (2006), pp. 1054–1059.

Šarc, L. & Lipnik-Štangelj, M. (2009a). Influence of ethanol and its first methabolite acetaldehyde on the central nervous system. *Journal of Slovene Medical Society*, Vol.78, No.2, (2009), pp. 91-96.

Šarc, L. & Lipnik-Štangelj, M. (2009b). Comparison of ethanol and acetaldehyde toxicity in rat astrocytes in primary culture. *Archives of industrial hygiene and toxicology*, Vol.60, No.3, (September 2009), pp. 297-305.

Šarc, L.; Wraber, B. & Lipnik-Štangelj, M. (2011). Ethanol and acetaldehyde disturb TNF-alpha and IL-6 production in cultured astrocytes. *Human and experimental toxicology*, (2011), doi: 10.1177/0960327110388533.

Takano, T.; Kang, J.; Jaiswal, J.K.; Simon, S.M.; Lin, J.H.; Yu, Y.; Li. Y.; Yang, J.; Dienel, G.; Zielke, H.R. & Nedergaard, M. (2005). Receptormediated glutamate release from volume sensitive channels in astrocytes. *Proceedings of the National Academy of Sciences USA*, Vol.102, (2005), pp. 16466–16471.

Tian, G.F.; Azmi, H.; Takano, T.; Xu, Q.; Peng. W.; Lin, J.; Oberheim. N.; Lou, N.; Wang, X.; Zielke, H.R.; Kang, J. & Nedergaard, M. (2005). An astrocytic basis of epilepsy. *Nature Medicine*, Vol.11, (2005), pp. 973–981.

Verkhratsky, A. & Kettenmann, H. (1996). Calcium signalling in glial cells. *Trends in Neurosciences*, Vol.19, (1996), pp. 346-352.

Verkhratsky, A.; Orkland, R.K. & Kettenmann, H. (1998). Glial calcium: Homeostasis and signlling function. *Physiological Rewiev*, Vol.78, (1998), pp. 99-141.

Voskuhl, R.R.; Peterson, R.S.; Song, B.; Ao, Y.; Morales, L.B.; Tiwari-Woodruff, S. & Sofroniew, M.V. (2009). Reactive astrocytes form scar-like perivascular barriers to leukocytes during adaptive immune inflammation of the CNS. *Journal of Neurosciences*, Vol.29, (2009), pp. 11511–11522.

Watts, L.T.; Rathinam, M.L.; Schenker, S. & Henderson, G.I. (2005). Astrocytes protect neurons from ethanol-induced oxidative stress and apoptotic death. *Journal of Neuroscience Research*, Vol.80, (2005), pp. 655-666.

Willmott, N.J.; Wong, K. & Strong, A.J. (2000). A fundamental role for the nitric oxide-G-kinase signalling pathway in mediating intercellular Ca2+ waves in glia. *Journal of Neurosciences*, Vol.20, (2000), pp. 1767-1779.

Zador, Z.; Stiver, S.; Wang, V. & Manley, G.T. (2009). Role of aquaporin-4 in cerebral edema and stroke. *Handbook of Experimental Pharmacology*, Vol.190, (2009), pp.159–170.

Zhou, F.C.; Anthony, B.; Dunn, K.W.; Lindquist, W.B.; Xu, Z.C. & Deng, P. (2007). Chronic alcohol driking alters neuronal dendritic spines in the brain rewardcenter nucleus accumbens. *Brain Research*, Vol.1134, (2007), pp. 148-161.

Zink, M.; Schmitt, A.; Vengeliene, V.; Henn, F.A. & Spanagel, R. (2004). Ethanol induces expression of the glutamate transporters EAAT1 and EAAT2 in organotypic cortical slice cultures. *Alcoholism Clinical and Experimental Research*, Vol.28, (2004), pp. 1752-1757.

Part 2

Future Applications

7

Therapeutic Organometallic Compounds

Beril Anilanmert

Istanbul University, Institute of Forensic Sciences,
Turkiye

1. Introduction

Most drugs used today are purely organic compounds. Especially after the enormous success of the cisplatin (Fig 1) in tumor treatment, interest in metal complexes has grown (Allardyce & Dyson, 2006). Synthetic organometallic compounds are generally considered to be toxic or non-compatible with biological systems. Despite this perception, the medicinal properties of organometallic compounds, in particular organo-transition metal compounds, have been probed for a long time and in the last few years the area has grown considerably.

Transition metals have an important place within medicinal biochemistry (Rafique et al, 2010). Transition metals represent the d block element which includes groups 3 - 12 on the periodic table. They have partially filled d-shells in any of their commonly occuring oxidation state. Metal complex or coordination compound is a structure consisting of a central metal atom, bonded to a surrounding array of ligands (molecules or anions), which donate electron pair to the metal. Research has shown significant progress in utilization of transition metal complexes as drugs to treat several human diseases like carcinomas, lymphomas, infection control, anti-inflammatory, diabetes, and neurological disorders. Transition metals exhibit different oxidation states and can interact with a number of negatively charged molecules. This activity of transition metals has started the development of metal-based drugs with promising pharmacological application and may offer unique therapeutic opportunities.

2. Therapeutic applications of some old and new organometallic complexes and discoveries and ongoing studies

Various metal complexes have been tested in anticancer therapy (Meng et al, 2009). The development of metal complexes with platinum central atoms such as cisplatin or carboplatin had an enormous impact on current cancer chemotherapy (Fig 1, 2) (Ott & Gust, 2007). In particular, cisplatin has become one of the most widely used drugs and is highly effective in treating several cancers such as ovarian and testicular cancers (Meng et al, 2009).

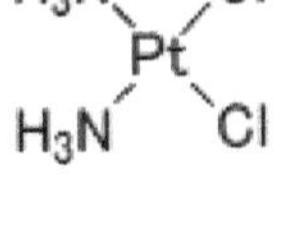

$$H_3N \diagdown \diagup Cl$$
$$Pt$$
$$H_3N \diagup \diagdown Cl$$

Fig. 1. Molecular structure of cisplatin.

Most of the platinum compounds that entered clinical trials follow the same empirical structure-activity relationships (Abu-Surrah & Kettunen, 2006). A necessary prerequisite for an active Pt-drug seems to be *cis*-coordination by bidentate amine ligands or two amines (at least one -NH group on the amine) and two leaving groups with an intermediate binding strength (e.g. Cl^-, SO_4^{2-}, citrate or oxalate) to platinum. The limitations of cisplatin have stimulated research in the field of platinum antitumor chemistry by giving specific goals. These include reduction in toxicity of cisplatin (nausea, ear damage, vomiting, loss of sensation in hands, and kidney toxicity), acquired drug resistance observed in certain tumors, inefficiency of the drug against some of the commonest tumors (e.g. colon and breast).

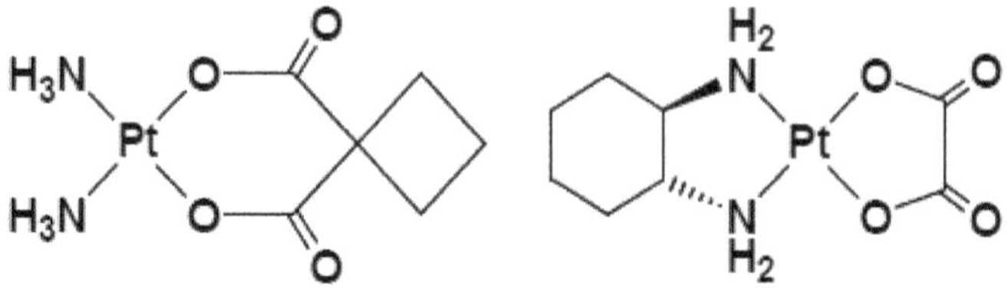

Fig. 2. Structures of carboplatin (left) and oxaliplatin (right) (Hanif, 2010)

Thousands of other platinum complexes have been synthesized and biologically evaluated for their antitumor properties, from which about fourty entered clinical phase I trials but only two carboplatin and oxaliplatin (Fig. 2) have received worldwide approval (Abu-Surrah & Kettunen, 2006). Carboplatin exhibits a tumor inhibiting profile identical to that of cisplatin, however with fewer side effects, whereas oxaliplatin is used in a combination therapy against metastatic colorectal cancer.

Some platinum(II) and palladium(II) complexes with new *trans-l*-dach (1R,2R-cyclohexanediamine) based diamine and diimine donor ligands containing the enantiomerically pure myrtenyl groups as terminal substituents were synthesized in 2008. The anti-proliferative effect of compounds Dichloro[(1R,2R)-(-)-N^1,N^2-bis{(1R)-(-)myrtenyl}-1,2-diamino cyclohexane]-platinum(II).$3H_2O$, Dichloro[1R,2R)-(-)-N^1,N^2-bis{(1R)-(-) myrtenylidene}-1,2-diamino cyclohexane]-platinum(II) and Dichloro [(1R,2R)-(-)-N^1,N^2-bis{(1R)-(-)myrtenyl}-1,2-diaminocyclohexane]-palladium(II).1.5H_2O together with the commercial drugs cisplatin (Cis-Pt) and oxaliplatin (Ox-Pt) were investigated in L1210 Cell line using 3H-thymidine incorporation (Abu-Surrah et. al., 2008). As shown in Figure 3, the platinum compounds Dichloro[(1R,2R)-(-)-N^1,N^2-bis{(1R)-(-)myrtenyl}-1, 2-diaminocyclo hexane]-platinum(II).$3H_2O$ and Dichloro [1R,2R)-(-)-N^1,N^2-bis{(1R)-(-) myrtenylidene}-1,2-diaminocyclohexane]-platinum(II) suppress proliferation more efficiently than the commercial platinum-based drugs with an IC_{50} of 0.6 and 0.7 µL, respectively. Compound Dichloro[(1R,2R)-(-)-N1,N2-bis{(1R)-(-) myrtenyl}-1,2-diaminocyclohexane]- platinum(II).$3H_2O$ is 17-folds more potent than the commercial oxaliplatin and cisplatin. No significant difference could be observed between the complex that contains the diamine nitrogen ligand and the one holding the corresponding diimine ligand. The authors also synthesized the palladium complex; Dichloro[(1R,2R)-(-)-N^1,N^2-bis{(1R)-(-)myrtenyl}-1,2-diaminocyclohexane]-palladium(II).1.5H_2O, which also suppresses proliferation efficiently with an IC_{50} of 4.2 µL. This is about 2-folds more potent than the commercial oxaliplatin and cisplatin.

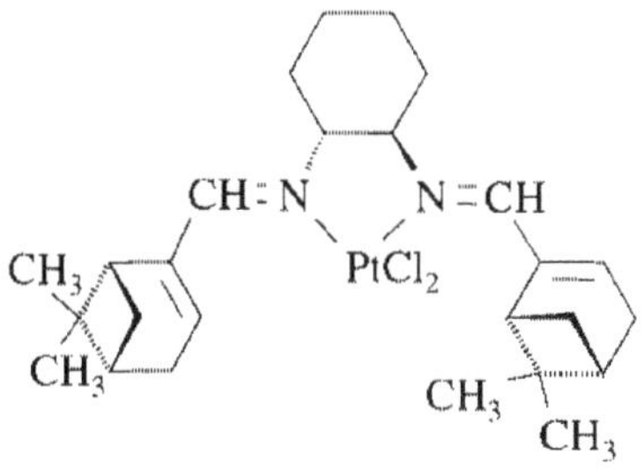

(a) Dichloro[(1R,2R)-(-)-N^1,N^2-bis{(1R)-(-)myrtenyl}-1,2-diamino cyclohexane]-platinum(II).3H$_2$O

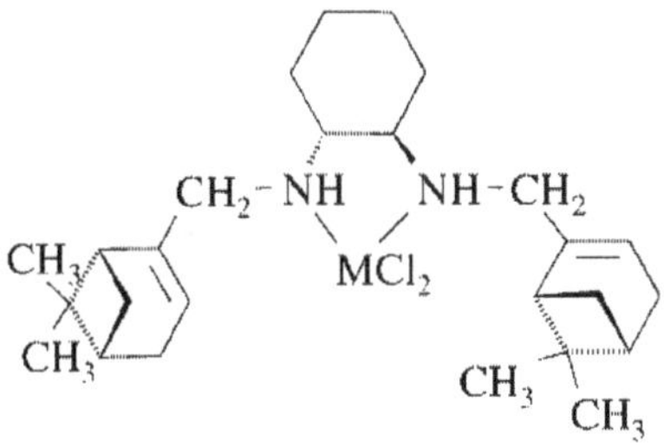

(b) Dichloro[1R,2R)-(-)-N^1,N^2-bis{(1R)-(-) myrtenylidene}-1,2-diamino cyclohexane]-M(II)   M=Pt(II), Pl(II)

Fig. 3. The structure of some platinum(II) and palladium(II) complexes with new *trans-l-* dach based diamine and diimine donor ligands containing the enantiomerically pure myrtenyl groups as terminal substituents (Abu-Surrah & Kettunen, 2006).

In a total look, platinum complexes display, along with other kinds of anticancer drugs, two major drawbacks: (a) severe toxicities (neurotoxicity, nephrotoxicity, etc.) and (b) limited applicability to a narrow range of tumors, as several of them exhibit natural or induced resistance.   These unresolved problems in platinum-based anticancer therapy have stimulated increased research efforts in the search for novel non platinum-containing metal species as cytostatic agents. Non-platinum metals may have different chemical behavior (oxidation state, redox potential, coordination geometry, additional coordination sites, binding preferences to biomolecules according to the HSAB [hard and soft (Lewis) acids and bases] principle etc.), rate of hydrolysis or kinetics of ligand exchange reactions and the ability to replace essential metals (Abu-Surrah & Kettunen, 2006). Therefore, it is likely that non-platinum metal-based compounds may have different mechanisms of action, biodistribution and biological activity.

The antitumor properties of a number of different metal ions and their complexes have been evaluated, but only a few non-platinum metal-based drugs are currently in clinical studies, the most promising ones contain ruthenium and gallium ions (Abu-Surrah & Kettunen, 2006). Preclinical and clinical investigations confirmed that the development of new metal agents with modes of action different from cisplatin is possible (Ott & Gust, 2007). Thus, complexes with iron, cobalt, or gold central atoms have shown promising results in preclinical studies and compounds with titanium, ruthenium, or gallium central atoms (as in Fig 4) have already been evaluated in phase I and phase II trials. Other metal complexes that have shown potential anticancer activity are the complexes of Rh(I), Rh(III), Ir(I), Ir(II), Ir(IV), Os(II) and Os(III). Many platinum and non-platinum metal complexes such as palladium, ruthenium, rhodium, copper, and lanthanum, with aromatic N-containing ligands as pyridine, imidazole and 1,10-phenanthroline, and their derivatives (whose donor properties are somewhat similar to the purine and pyrimidine bases), have shown very promising antitumor properties in vitro and in vivo in cisplatin-resistant model systems or against cisplatin-insensitive cell lines (Zhao & Lin, 2005).

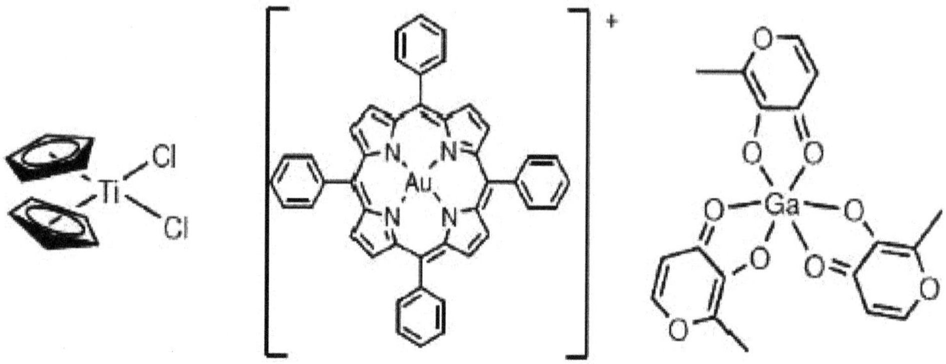

Fig. 4. The chemical structures of titanocene dichloride (a), gold tetraphenylporphyrin (b) and gallium maltolate (c) (Hanif, 2010).

The notable analogy between the coordination chemistry of platinum(II) and palladium(II) compounds has advocated studies of Pd(II) complexes as antitumor drugs (Abu-Surrah & Kettunen, 2006). A key factor that might explain the reason that platinum is most useful, comes from the ligand-exchange kinetics. The hydrolysis of the leaving ligands in palladium complexes is too rapid: 10^5 times faster than their corresponding platinum analogues. They dissociate readily in solution leading to very reactive species that are unable to reach their pharmacological targets. This implies that if an antitumor palladium drug is to be developed, it must somehow be stabilized by a strongly coordinated nitrogen ligand and a suitable leaving group. If this group is reasonably non labile, the drug can maintain its structural integrity *in vivo* long enough. As a way to increase the stability of the palladium(II) complexes, two chelates forming two rings around the central atom were prepared and evaluated. A series of compounds bearing two chelating ligands the N-N and O-O ligand (XO_3: selenite or tellurite) were prepared. The N-N ligand did not influence the activity but the oxygen coordinated leaving group did. Selenite complexes were invariably better cytotoxic agents than tellurite complexes and cisplatin. The complex [(bipy)Pd(SeO_3)] (Fig 5) was found to bind to DNA through a coordinate covalent bond. Another study investigated compounds [((1R,2R)-(-)-1,2-diaminocyclohexane)Pd(3-methylorotate)] which gave a high activity for sarcoma 180 but a low one against P388 leukemia and [(1R,2R)-(-)-1,2-diaminocyclohexane)Pd(5-fluroorot)] which also displayed significant antitumor activity. These strong chelating ligands replacing chloro or nitro ligands induce a reduction in the rate of hydrolysis.

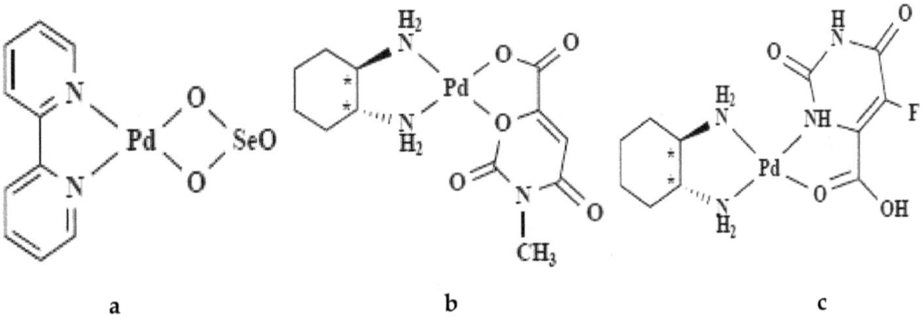

The geometrical structures (a, b, c) are shown at the top of the page.

a   b   c

Fig. 5. The geometrical structure of [bipy)Pd(SeO₃)] (a), [((1R,2R)-(-)-1,2-diaminocyclohexane)Pd(3-methylorotate)] (b), [(1R,2R)-(-)-1,2-diaminocyclohexane)Pd(5-fluroorot) (c)] (Abu-Surrah & Kettunen, 2006)

Both ruthenium and osmium, along with iron, are members of group VIIIB and are placed in the fourth, fifth and sixth row of the periodic table, respectively. They are classified as the 'Platinum group' along with rhodium, palladium, iridium and platinum. All these metals often occur together in the same mineral deposits and have closely related physical and chemical properties. The application of iron in group 8 metal complexes in anticancer drug design is the ferrocenyl derivative of tamoxifen (ferrocifen) (Jauen et al, 2006), and two ruthenium containing drug candidates NAMI-A and KP1019 in clinical trials. In trying to find better alternatives to tamoxifen, Jaouen et al. (Top et al, 2001), have investigated tamoxifen analogs that contain an organometallic moiety. The researchers studied the effects of several hydroxy-substituted ferrocifens on the proliferation of two lines of breast cancer cells, one used for tumors mediated by the ERα receptor, and one used for tumors mediated by ERβ. Three of the ferrocifens (Fig 6) exhibited a strong antiproliferative effect in both cell lines while hydroxytamoxifen, as expected, was effective only against the cells having the ERα receptor. Ferrocifenes exhibit anticancer activity against hormone dependent and hormone independent breast cancers (Rafique et al, 2010). The ferrocene derivatives having hydroxyl group in phenyl ring have high affinity for estrogen receptor. Ferrocene by itself had no effect.

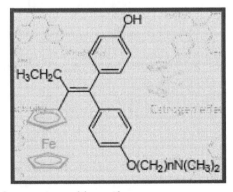

Fig. 6. The main molecular structure of ferrocifenes.

Special attention has been paid to ruthenium compounds because they exhibit cytotoxicity against cancer cells, analogous ligand exchange abilities to platinum complexes, no cross-resistance with cisplatin, and may display reduced toxicity on healthy tissues by using iron transport (Meng et al, 2009). Ruthenium complexes demonstrate similar ligand exchange kinetics to those of platinum(II) antitumor drugs already used in the clinic while displaying only low toxicity (Brabec & Novakova, 2006). This is in part due to the ability of ruthenium complexes to mimic the binding of iron to molecules of biological significance, exploiting the mechanisms that the body has evolved for transport of iron.

Ruthenium complexes tend to accumulate preferentially in neoplastic masses in comparison with normal tissue (Rademaker-Lakhai et al, 2004). They probably use transferrin, for its similarities with iron, to accumulate in the tumor. A transferrin-ruthenium complex can be actively transported into tumor tissues that have high transferrin-receptor densities. Once bound to the transferrin receptor, the complex liberates ruthenium that can be easily internalized in the tumor. Next, ruthenium (III) complexes likely remain in their relatively inactive ruthenium(III) oxidation state until they reach the tumor site. In this environment, with its lower oxygen content and pH than normal tissue, reduction to the more reactive ruthenium(II) oxidation state takes place. This reaction, named "activation by reduction" would provide not only a selective toxicity but also an efficacy toward hypoxic tumors known to be resistant to chemotherapy and/or radiotherapy. Finally, some complexes are more effective against the tumor metastases than against the primary tumor. Due to differing ligand geometry between their complexes, ruthenium compounds bind to DNA affecting its conformation differently than cisplatin and its analogues (Brabec & Novakova, 2006). In addition, non-nuclear targets, such as the mitochondrion and the cell surface, have also been implicated in the antineoplastic activity of some ruthenium complexes. So, ruthenium compounds have a pattern of cytotoxicity and antitumor activity that is different from that of cisplatin tissue (Rademaker-Lakhai et al, 2004). Ruthenium complexes exhibit both nitric oxide release and scavenging functions that can affect vasodilation and synapse firing (Clarke, 2003). Simple ruthenium complexes are unusually effective in suppressing the immune response by inhibiting T cell proliferation. Thus, ruthenium compounds offer the potential over antitumor platinum(II) complexes currently used in the clinic of reduced toxicity, a novel mechanism of action, the prospect of non-cross-resistance and a different spectrum of activity. Although the pharmacological target for antitumor ruthenium compounds has not been completely identified, there is a large body of evidence indicating that the cytotoxicity of many ruthenium complexes correlates with their ability to bind DNA although few exceptions have been reported. One of the first ruthenium compounds described to have anticancer activity was ruthenium red, and further work showed the anticancer potential of ruthenium-containing drugs (Rafique et al, 2010). Since then, several teams have synthesized and characterized new compounds containing ruthenium(II) or ruthenium(III). Ruthenium red and the related Ru360 strongly inhibit calcium ion uptake in the mitochondria (Clarke, 2003).

Ru(II) and Ru(III) complexes have shown very promising properties while the Ru(III) compound NAMI-A (imidazolium *trans*-[tetrachloro(DMSO)(imidazole)ruthenate(III)]) , is the first ruthenium compound that successfully entered phase I clinical trials as an antimetastatic drug candidate (Katsaros & Anagnostopoulou, 2002; Antonarakis & Emadi,

2010). Ruthenium compound KP1019 (indazolium *trans*-[tetrachlorobis(1H-indazole) ruthenate(III)]), as an anticancer drug against colon carcinomas and their metastases has also entered clinical trials so far. It has shown direct antitumor activity against a wide range of primary explants of human tumors by inducing apoptosis (Antonorakis & Emadi, 2010). Both compounds showed relatively little side-effects and better tolerance in clinical phase I trials (Fig. 7). In preclinical studies, NAMI-A has demonstrated inhibitory effects against the formation of cancer metastases in a variety of tumor animal models but appears to lack direct cytotoxic effects (Antonarakis & Emadi, 2010). In case of NAMI-A, DNA is thought to be a less important target, and anti-angiogenic activity based on the NO metabolism has been described (Bharti & Singh, 2009). NAMI-A interaction with the microenvironment involving integrin activation that results in reduced cell invasiveness and migration has been proposed and this may be the reasons for the activity of ruthenium compounds against cisplatin-resistant tumors. Ruthenium compounds ONCO4417 and DW1/2 have been demonstrated to show Pim-1 kinase inhibition in preclinical systems (Sekhon, 2010). A phase I and pharmacokinetic study was also carried out with the new ruthenium complex indazolium trans-[tetrachlorobis(1H-indazole)ruthenate(III)] (KP1019, FFC14A) (Lentz et al, 2009). Seven patients with various types of solid tumours refractory to standard therapy were treated with escalating doses of KP1019 (25-600 mg) twice weekly for 3 weeks. No dose-limiting toxicity occurred. Ruthenium plasma concentration-time profiles after the first dose and under multiple-dose conditions were analysed using a compartmental approach. The pharmacokinetic disposition was characterised by a small volume of distribution, low clearance and long half-life. Only a small fraction of ruthenium was excreted renally.

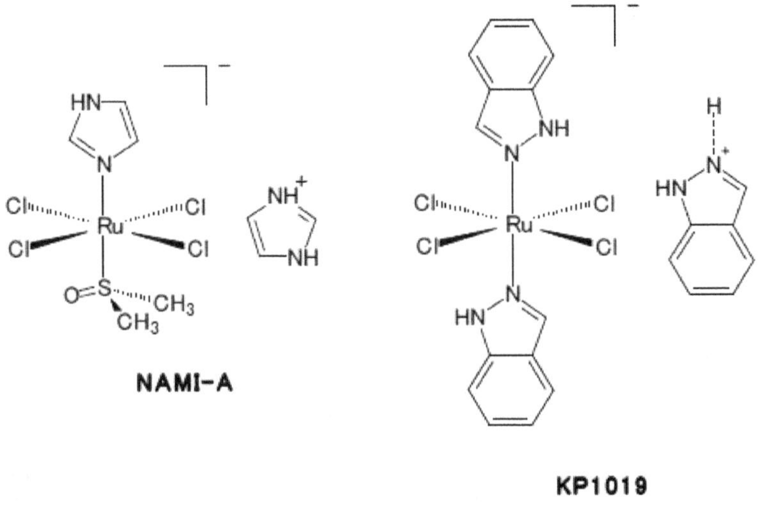

NAMI-A

KP1019

Fig. 7. Structure of ruthenium complexes NAMI-A and KP1019 (Llorca, 2005).

Many biological properties have been attributed to ruthenium complex I (*trans*-[RuCl$_2$(nic)$_4$]) and ruthenium complex II (*trans*-[RuCl$_2$ (i-nic)$_4$]) including nitric oxide synthase inhibition (Valvassori et al, 2006). However, side effects of the ruthenium compounds should also be evaluated. In the investigation of the pharmacological effects of these complexes on anxiety and memory formation on adult male Wistar rats, no effects were observed in the anxiety parameters and habituation to an open-field while memory impairment was observed. The ruthenium complexes impaired memory retention compared with vehicle group in the inhibitory avoidance, as when administrated 30 min prior as immediately after training. The memory impairment induced by ruthenium complexes may be due to their nitric oxide synthase inhibition capacity.

Rhodium belongs to the same group as platinum and ruthenium. However, rhodium compounds, analogues to the corresponding platinum and ruthenium compounds that possess significant antitumor properties, were found to be less effective as anticancer agents mainly due to their toxic effects. Dimeric mu-Acetato dimers of Rh(II) as well as monomeric square planar Rh(I) and octahedral Rh(III) complexes have shown interesting antitumor properties.

In 2009, Meng et al. have studied both in vitro and in vivo the biological properties of RDC11 (Fig 8), which contain a covalent bond between the ruthenium atom and a carbon. RDC11 inhibited the growth of various tumors implanted in mice more efficiently than cisplatin. Importantly, in striking contrast with cisplatin, RDC11 did not cause severe side effects on the liver, kidneys, or the neuronal sensory system. It was shown to interact poorly with DNA and induced only limited DNA damages compared with cisplatin, suggesting alternative transduction pathways. The target genes of the endoplasmic reticulum stress pathway, such as Bip, XBP1, PDI, and CHOP, were activated in RDC11-treated cells. Activation of CHOP led to the expression of several of its target genes, including proapoptotic genes. Acting through an atypical pathway involving CHOP and endoplasmic reticulum stress, RDC11 is thought to provide an interesting alternative for anticancer therapy (Meng et al, 2009).

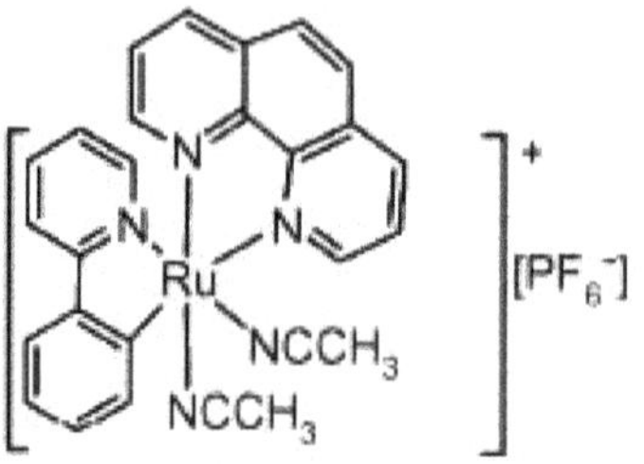

Fig. 8. Molecular structure of RDC11 (Meng et al, 2009).

A class of ruthenium(II)-arene complexes that are weakly cytotoxic in vitro, were also shown to have selective antimetastatic activity in vivo, in the literature (Anga, et. al., 2011). These compounds, [Ru(η6-p-arene)Cl$_2$(1,3,5-triaza-7-phosphaadamantane)] termed RAPTA, interact strongly with proteins, with the ability to discriminate binding to different proteins, but show a relatively low propensity to bind DNA, which is considered to be the main target of many metal-based drugs. The basic RAPTA structure is quite stable in physiological environments, and studies have shown that aquation of the chloride bonds occurs, it may not be an essential step for anticancer drug activity – direct substitution with biomolecular targets is also possible. Based on the concept of bifunctional radiopharmaceuticals (Ogawa et al, 2007), developed a highly stable [186]Remercaptoacetylglycylglycylglycine (MAG3) complex-conjugated bisphosphonate, [[[[(4-hydroxy-4,4-diphosphonobutyl) carbamoylmethyl]carbamoylmethyl]carbamoylmethyl] carbamoylmethane thiolate] oxorhenium (V) ([186]Re-MAG3-HBP), for the treatment of painful bone metastases. [186]Re-MAG3-HBP accumulated at the site where tumor cells were injected in a rat model of bone cancer and significantly inhibited tumor growth and attenuated the allodynia induced by bone cancer without having critical myelosuppressive side effects. The results indicate that [186]Re-MAG3-HBP could be useful as a therapeutic agent for the palliation of metastatic bone pain.

Since DNA has often been proposed as the target of these organometallic antineoplastic agents, there is a particular emphasis on those that can interact with nucleic acids (Clarke et al, 1999). Nevertheless, heavy metals are generally toxic by binding to sulfur and nitrogen sites on proteins and, thus, can interfere with a number of modes of metabolism. Several metals also exhibit action through redox activity. Gallium appears to operate through the displacement of metal ions in iron metabolism or bone. In large part, action of gallium complexes seems to be a consequence of the similarity of gallium(III) to iron(III): Gallium interferes with the cellular transport of iron by binding to transferrin, and also interferes with the action of ribonucleotide reductase, which then results in inhibition of DNA synthesis (Hannon, 2007). The key to activity is making gallium(III) bioavailable, and work is focused on ligands which stabilize gallium against hydrolysis and facilitate membrane permeation. Among the developed gallium comounds, tris(8-quinolinolato)gallium(III) (KP46/FFC11) has entered clinical trials (Fig 9).

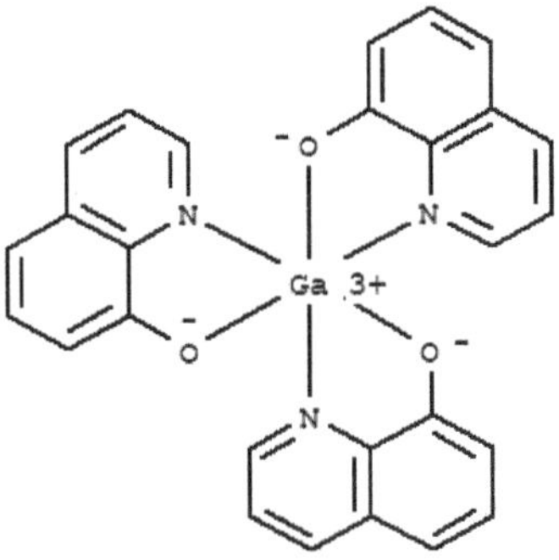

Fig. 9. Molecular structure of Tris(8-quinolinolato)gallium(III)

Gallium-based anticancer chemotherapeutics are appreciably progressing in clinical studies (Timerbaev et al, 2009). The interest of drug developers and clinicians in gallium compounds is due to a proven ability of gallium cations to inhibit tumour growth, and enhanced bioavailability and moderate toxicity provided by the conversion of gallium into chelate complexes. One of the complexes suitable for a more convenient oral administration is tris(8-quinolinolato) gallium(III) (KP46). KP46 is an orally bioavailable gallium complex, which exerts its antitumoral activity via inhibition of ribonucleotide reductase, induction of S phase arrest and apoptosis (Dittrich et al, 2005). In preclinical models KP46 was proved to be a stronger anticancer agent than gallium nitrate and it was effective on a model of tumor-associated hypercalcemia. Nominated from a range of gallium complexes for the clinical stage of development, KP46 has finished phase I trials with the outcome of promising tolerability and evidence of clinical activity in renal cell carcinoma (Timerbaev et al, 2009). The adverse reactions of the complex, observed in a study, where 7 patients were used were neutropenia and anemia, stomatitis and conjunctivitis, dizziness, headache and acne, fatigue and diarrhaea both (Dittrich et al, 2005). In one out of the 4 patients with renal cell carcinoma an unconfirmed partial response has been observed after 8 weeks and in a second patient with renal cell carcinoma the disease was stabilized for 29 weeks. Peak plasma levels were reached 5-7 h after intake and pharmacokinetic analysis revealed a long terminal half-life (28 h). KP46 has been well tolerated with some preliminary evidence of efficacy in renal cell carcinoma.

The low-spin $5d^6$ Ir^{III} organometallic half-sandwich complexes $[(\eta^5\text{-}Cp^x)Ir(XY)Cl]^{0/+}$, Cp^{xph} : tetramethyl(phenyl)cyclopentadienyl, or Cp^{xbiph}: tetramethyl(biphenyl)cyclopentadienyl, XY = 1,10-phenanthroline, 2,2'-bipyridine, ethylenediamine, or picolinate, were investigated at 2011 (Liu et al, 2011). Complexes with N,N-chelating ligands readily form adducts with 9-ethylguanine but not 9-ethyladenine; picolinate complexes bind to both purines. Cytotoxic potency toward A2780 human ovarian cancer cells increases with phenyl substitution on Cp^x: Cp^{xbiph} > Cp^{xph} . The hydrophobicity and intercalative ability of Cp^{xph} and Cp^{xbiph} make a major contribution to the anticancer potency of their Ir^{III} complexes.

Among the metallocene dihalide complexes MX_2Cp_2 (where M=Ti, V, Mo, Nb etc., X= halide and Cp = η5-cyclopentadienide), titanocene (Fig 10), $TiCl_2Cp_2$ or MTK4 is the most successful anticancer agent as shown in phase I/II clinical trials (Bharti & Singh,2009). Titanocene dichloride had been recognized as active anticancer drug against breast and gastrointestinal carcinomas. Previously DNA was supposed to be the target of $[TiCl_2Cp_2]$ in a manner similar to cisplatin due to the similarity in Cl---Cl distances. Later, the aqueous chemistry of $[TiCl_2Cp_2]$ showed that DNA is not the site of action for this drug. The anticancer activity of $TiCl_2Cp_2$ is due to inhibition of collagenase type IV activity, which is involved in regulation of cellular proliferation, protein kinase C and DNA topoisomerase II activities. Titanium may also replace iron in transferrin and facilitate cellular uptake into tumor cells. The titanocene dichloride is believed to be accumulated via the transferrin-dependent pathways. Dose limiting toxicities of titanium compounds include nephrotoxicity and elevation of creatinine and bilirubin levels.

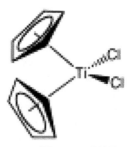

Fig. 10. Molecular structue of titanocene (Hannon, 2007)

Budotitane [cis-diethoxybis(1-phenylbutane-1,3-dionato)titanium (IV)] (Fig 11), was the first non-platinum transition-metal anticancer agent to be tested in clinical trials (Schilling et al, 1995). It is effective against a number of tumors in animals and is well tolerated (Bharti &

Singh, 2009). *In vitro* and *in vivo* experiments with budotitane showed no significant DNA damage. The dose-limiting side effects include cardiac arrhythmia, hepatotoxicity, renal toxicity and a reversible loss of taste (Dabrowiak, 2009; Antonarakis & Emadi, 2010). Ti(IV) compounds are known to inhibit proteases and telomerases. Inhibition of proteases in rapidly growing tumor cells may block the growth of tumor cells. Inhibition of telomerase may control all protein synthesis.

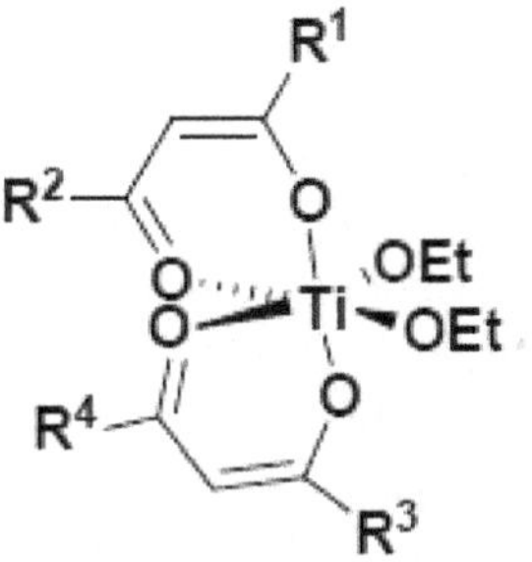

Budotitane (as a mixture of three *cis* **isomers)**

(i) $R^1 = R^3 = Me; R^2 = R^4 = Ph$

(ii) $R^1 = R^3 = Ph; R^2 = R^4 = Me$

(iii) $R^1 = R^4 = Me; R^2 = R^3 = Ph$

Fig. 11. The molecular structure of budotitane (Bharti & Singh, 2009).

Gold compounds are used for treating arthritis and cancer, they have potential for treating AIDS, malaria and Chagas disease (Dabrowiak, 2009). A property of Au^{+3} that greatly complicates its chemistry is that many of its simple complexes can easily be reduced to Au^+ by a variety of ligands, including thiols and thioethers found on cysteine and methionine residues of peptides and proteins. Even the disulfide linkage, R-S-S-R', which is generally considered a poorer ligand than a thiol or a thioether, binds to and reduces Au^{+3} to Au^+. Since there are agents in the biological system that can oxidize Au^+ to Au^{+3}, gold compounds can, in principle, exist in a variety of different coordination states in the biological system. These properties, and the fact that the concentrations of gold compounds normally encountered in therapeutic situations are very low, make it difficult to determine the chemistry of gold in the biological environment. Gold thiolate complexes were found especially effective at slowing the progression of rheumatod arthritis. Sodium aurothiomalate (myochrysine), aurothioglucose (solganol) and aurothiosulfate (sanochrysine) are water-soluble polymeric antiarthritic compounds that are administered to the patient by injection, so-called injectable or parenteral drugs, while auranofin, which is only slightly soluble in water, is given to the patient orally in capsule form. The earlywork on auranofin and its analogs revealed that Au^+ complexes that have phosphine and thioglucose ligands were effective in killing B16 melanoma and P388 leukemia cells in culture. One compound that showed a significantly broader range of activity than auranofin and one of its analogs against a number of different tumor models implanted in mice was the tetrahedral cation [Au(dppe)₂]⁺, bis[1,2-bis(diphenylphosphino) ethane]gold(I).

[Au(dppe)$_2$]$^+$ is active alone, and in combination with cisplatin, against P388 leukemia in mice, and it is also active against various sarcomas in mice. The compound aurocyanide, [Au(CN)$_2$]$^-$, which is a biotransformation product in chrysotherapy, has been found to inhibit proliferation of HIV in a strain of CD$_4$$^+$. A gold complex with two attached thioglucose ligands has been shown to protect MT-4 cells from the HIV virus by binding to a specific cysteine residue on a 120 kDa protein, gp120, which is part of the outer envelope of the virus. The compound [bpza][AuCl$_4$], where bpza is the diprotonated-chloride form of a bis-pyrazole ligand, inhibits both reverse transcriptase and HIV-1 protease. Since these enzymes function differently in the life cycle of the HIV virus, inhibiting both with a single compound is unusual. Reverse transcriptase is responsible for converting viral RNA into double-stranded DNA prior to the integration of the latter into genomic DNA of the T cell, and HIV-1 protease controls the maturation and production of infectious virons (virus particles). Since [bpza][AuCl$_4$] is nontoxic to peripheral blood mononuclear cells in the immune system, the compound is thought to have potential as an anti-HIV agent.

A recent report by Sannella et al. (Sanella et al, 2008) showed that auranofin and other gold compounds inhibit the growth of Plasmodium falciparum, a protozoan parasite carried by Anopheles mosquitoes that causes malaria. The researchers suggested that the mechanism by which the gold compounds inhibit the growth of P. falciparum is related to the ability of the complexes to block the function of the enzyme thioredoxin reductase, TrxR.

Nickel is an essential component in different types of enzymes such as urease, carbon monoxide dehydrogenase, and hydrogenase (Abu-Surrah & Kettunen, 2006). Recently, some results showing also apparent potential of this platinum group element in antitumor studies have been reported. For example the cytotoxicity of the nickel (II) complexes containing 1,2-naphtoquinone-based thiosemicarbazone ligands (NQTS) was tested on MCF7 human breast cancer cell line and compared to free ligand and another naphthoquinone, commercial antitumor drug etoposide. According to the reported data, Ni-NQTS complex has the highest antitumor activity with an IC50 of 2.2 µM. The mechanistic study of action showed inhibition of topoisomerase II. Recent studies showed that the corresponding nickel complexes of semicarbazones (Fig 12) have even greater inhibitory effect on MCF7 cell growth. They display IC50 values in 2-5 µM range and also in general they produce lower side effect than thiosemicarbazones.

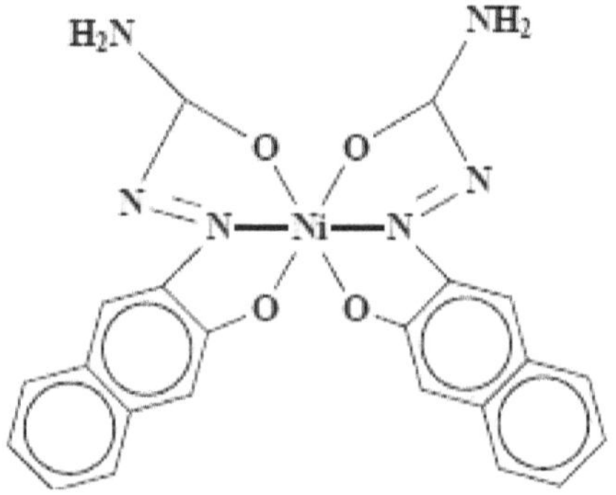

Fig. 12. Structure of a Ni(II)-semicarbazone based antitumor complex (Abu-Surrah & Kettunen, 2006)

In 2010, new methoxy-substituted nickel(II)(salophene) derivatives are synthesized and their anticancer properties were investigated (Lee et al, 2010). It was demonstrated that the most active complex [Ni(II)(3-methoxy-salophene)] (Fig 10) is not necrotic in Burkitt-like lymphoma cells (BJAB) and human B-cell precursor cells (Nalm-6). [Ni(II)(3-methoxy-salophene)] inhibited proliferation and induced apoptosis in a concentration dependent manner, giving evidence for the involvement of CD95 receptor-mediated, extrinsic pathway. Furthermore, [Ni(II)(3-methoxy-salophene)] overcame vincristine drug resistance in BJAB and Nalm-6 cells.

Organometallic compounds like Iron (III)-salophene with selective cytotoxic and antiproliferative properties have also been used in platinum resistant ovarian cancer cells (Rafique et al, 2010).

The low-spin Fe(II) complex sodium nitroprusside (Fig 13) is a clinically used metal-nitrosyl complex (Guo & Sadler, 1999). It is often used to lower blood pressure in humans. Its hypotensive effect is evident within seconds after infusion, and the desired blood pressure is usually obtained within one to two minutes. It is also useful in cases of emergency hypertension, heart attacks, and surgery. Its therapeutic effects depend on release of nitric oxide, which relaxes vascular smooth muscle. Activation in vivo may involve reduction to $[Fe(CN)_5(NO)]^{3-}$, which then releases cyanide to give $[Fe(CN)_4(NO)]^{2-}$ and then nitric oxide.

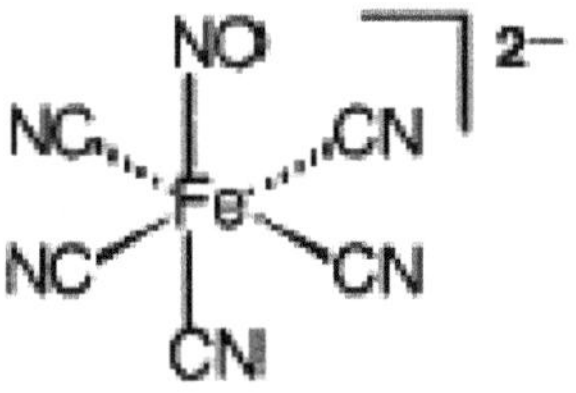

Fig. 13. Fe(II) complex with nitroprusside

The low cytotoxicity of ferrocene, coupled with its lipophilicity ($logP_{octanol/water}$ = 3.28) and its electrochemical behaviour (redox potential of the ferrocene/ferrocenium couple, E^0 =+0.400 V versus SCE (Saturated Calomel Electrode), suggested that this compound could yield interesting results if incorporated into a known drug (Blackie & Chibale, 2008). The ferrocenyl moiety has several characteristics which make it a good addition to known drug molecules. Its lipophilicity, electron density, relative thermal and chemical stability, and interesting redox behaviour are all favourable in this respect. There are several reported successes of increased efficacy of ferrocenyl analogues of known drugs. Brocard and co-workers, combined Chloroquine and ferrocene in the same molecule by inserting a ferrocenyl group into the side chain of Chloroquine, producing a hybrid compound called Ferroquine (Fig 11), which is more potent than Chloroquine. They have shown that incorporation of a ferrocenyl moiety as an integral part of the side chain of chloroquine between the two nitrogens had superior efficacy to other analogues in which the moiety was terminal on the side chain or bonded to the quinoline nitrogen. Some analogues of the compound were produced bearing different alkyl groups on the terminal tertiary nitrogen. They established that the dimethylamino terminal group was superior in efficacy (Fig 14)

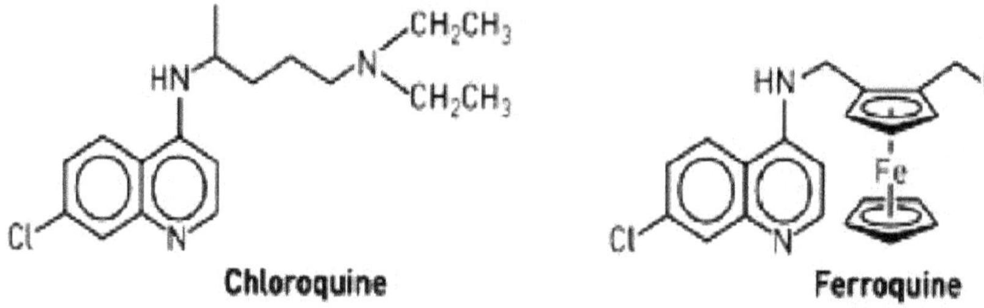

Fig. 14. Molecular structure of Chloroquine and Ferroquine.

The highly established chemistry of ferrocenes that allows an easy and rapid access to a bank of reagents and derivatives has given them a considerable role in the field of analytical chemistry (Rudrangi et al, 2010). Ferrocene-based derivatization of various functional groups and detection techniques is of high interest in particular. The chemistry of ferrocenes is well explored and a wide range of ferrocene derivatives are easily obtained through the established synthetic routes.The ferrocenes allow the use of a large variety of detection techniques like UV/Visible absorption spectroscopy, atomic spectroscopy, atomic absorption spectroscopy (AAS), inductively coupled plasma (ICP) excitation with optical emission spectroscopy (OES) or mass spectrometry (MS), electron impact or electrospray ionization (ESI) MS, and the electrochemical detection (ECD) techniques that include voltammetry or amperometry.

The role of the length of the methylene spacer between the two nitrogens in chloroquine analogues has been shown to have an influence on efficacy in chloroquine resistant strains of *P. falciparum*. Aminoquinolines with short (2-3 carbons) and long (10–12 carbons) methylene side chains are equipotent against chloroquine-sensitive, chloroquineresistant, and multidrug-resistant strains of *P. falciparum*. Whilst aminoquinolines with side chains of intermediate length (4–8 carbons) showed efficacy against chloroquinesensitive strains of *P. falciparum*, they showed a significant decrease in efficacy against chloroquine-resistant strains of *P.Falciparum*. In the chloroquine-sensitive D10 strain, the longer the methylene spacer, the lower the efficacy. It may be that the changes in lipophilicity and *pKa* values and other physicochemical effects of the incorporation of the ferrocenyl moiety into chloroquine are the primary factor in the enhanced efficacy of ferroquine.

As published as a patent application in 2006 (Maurel & Cudennec, 2009), some manganese based organometallic complexes having Mn-SOD like activities, pharmaceutical compositions and dietetic products for use in oxidative stress, including cancer and inflammatory conditions, were also designed. Many human diseases are associated with the overproduction of oxygen free radicals that inflict cell damage (Rafique et al, 2010). Primary reactive oxygen species (ROS) such as superoxide radical, hydrogen peroxide, hydroxyl radicals, and ortho-quinone derivatives of catecholamines exert their cellular effects by modifying DNA, lipids, and proteins to form secondary electrophiles (Zhang & Lippard, 2003). Damage caused by the primary and secondary ROS contributes to the pathogenesis of important human diseases. In particular, one consequence of oxidative metabolism is the generation of superoxide radicals (O_2^-.) which mediate extensive damage to the cellular components of living organisms. The molecular dismutation of O_2^-. to hydrogen peroxide (H_2O_2) and oxygen (O_2) is catalysed by superoxide dismutases (SODs).These enzymes are suggested to form the first line of the cell's defence against oxygen damage. Indeed, mice defective for SOD do not survive and reduction of functional capabilities of this enzyme generates an high increase of oxidative stress in connection with strong mitochondrial disabilities of cells. Fe-containing SODs (FeSOD) are largely confined to prokaryotes and the Cu/Zn enzymes (Cu/ZnSOD) predominantly to eukaryotes. Mn-containing SODs (MnSOD) are universally present. In eukaryotes MnSODs are localised in the mitochondria, while the Cu/ZnSODs reside in the cytosol. SODs from various sources are currently of great interest as potential therapeutic treatments for oxidative damage. SOD has function against certain inflammatory processes (In particular, deficiency in Mn-SOD is supposed to have some significance in the development of rheumatoid arthritis). SOD has also function against inflammatory processes in alcohol-induced liver damage. Additional potential therapeutic effects for SOD include: (i) prevention of oncogenesis, tumour promotion and invasiveness, and UV-induced damage; (ii) protection of cardiac tissue against post-ischemia reperfusion damage; (iii) antiinflamatory effect; (iv) reducing the cytotoxic and cardiotoxic effects of anticancer drugs; (v) endothelial disorders; (vi) degenerative diseases; (vii) coagulation disorders, and; (viii) improving the longevity of living cells. Currently bovine Cu/ZnSOD is being utilised for the treatment of inflamed tendons in horses and for treating osteoarthritis in man. It has been shown that the mitochondrial antioxidant enzyme manganese-containing superoxide dismutase (MnSOD) functions as a tumor suppressor gene and that reconstitution of MnSOD expression in several human cancer cell lines leads to reversion of malignancy.

The use of SOD in therapy is limited by its short plasma half-life (clearance by the kidney) and inability to penetrate cell membranes (i.e., extracellular activity only) (Guo & Sadler, 1999). Low molecular mass mimics of SOD are therefore of much potential pharmaceutical interest. For example, a variety of Mn- and Fe-based porphyrins and macrocyclic complexes exhibit SOD mimic activity.

Among metal complexes (Cu, Fe, Mn) capable of catalyzing dismutation of the superoxide anion, those of manganese are a current focus for developing SOD mimics as drugs because of the low in vivo toxicity of this metal ion (Zhang & Lippard, 2003). Mn(II) and Mn(III) macrocycles appear to be particularly promising (Guo & Sadler, 1999). For example, a manganese (II) complex with bis (cyclohexylpyridine)-substituted macrocyclic ligand has been designed as a functional mimic of SOD which was reported to have a significant of inflammation and reperfusion injury (Aston et al., 2001, Rafique et al, 2010). This complex has remarkably high kinetic and thermodynamic stability with regard to dissociation, is oxidatively stable as well and is excreted intact with no dissociation in vivo This stability profile shows that this is a catalytically active SOD mimic. Manganese complexes have also been used to treat cell and tissue oxidative injuries by acting as superoxide anion scavenger. Nitrogen containing macrocyclic complexes of Manganese (II) have shown anti microbial activity. An octahedral geometry for these complexes has been confirmed by spectroscopic analysis. Many manganese complexes have been screened against a number of pathogenic fungi and bacteria to evaluate their growth and potential. Another example to the therapeutic effects of manganese complexes is Mn(III)5,10,15,20-tetrakis(4-benzoic acid)-porphyrin, which can protect against neurodegeneration and is therefore of potential interest for the treatment of brain diseases such as Parkinson and Alzheimer diseases (Meng et al, 2009). Results from systematic modification of the porphyrin ligand demonstrate that placement of four positively charged ortho-(N-alkyl) pyridyl groups (alkyl: methyl and ethyl) in the meso positions of porphyrin can strongly facilitate the disproportion of O_2^-., owing to favorable electrostatic contributions. SC-52608 (Fig 15) is another complex, able to scavenge superoxide and therefore effectively protect the regionally ischemic and reperfused myocardium from injury. Both complexes reduced oxidative stress injury in vivo and they have high stability and catalytic efficacy (Guo & Sadler, 1999; Zhang & Lippard, 2003). In the search for a lipophilic manganese SOD mimic, a dinuclear manganese(III) complex of biliverdin IX dimethyl ester was discovered to have such activity. In this example O_2^-. dismutation is effected by a Mn(III)/Mn(IV) redox couple. In addition, the manganese complex does not bind to NO and reacts very slowly with H_2O_2, demonstrating specificity towards O_2^-..

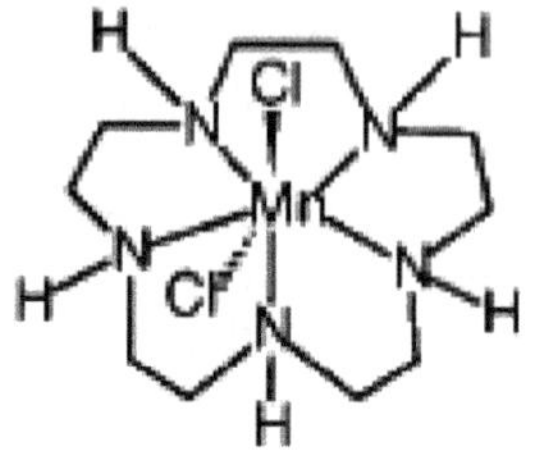

Fig. 15. Molecular structure of SC-52608 (Guo & Sadler, 1999)

The incorporation of manganese into the structure of antioxidants like pyran, pyridine, benzopyran and quinoline i.e., kojic acid, 6-hydroxynicotinic acid, 7-hydroxyflavone, 8-hydroxyquinoline and 8-hydroxyquinoline ethylenediamine, made the complexes possessed the SOD activity and increased radical scavenging activity of antioxidants as expected (Vajgupta et al, 2003). Manganese atom is therefore the essential part for SOD action. 7-hydroxyflavone complex was promising, since it exhibited potent radical scavenging ability and suppressed the MAP-induced hypermotility without reducing the locomotor activity in normal condition, and also improved the impaired learning and memory in transient ischemic mice.

A new approach involves modelling the pharmacological properties of established drugs with organometallic fragments (Ott et al, 2009). The metallocyclic peptide, bacitracin, has an interesting SOD activity. The Mn(II)–bacitracin complex (Piacham et al, 2006) (Fig 16, 17) is potentially useful as an effective agent against oxidative stress (for O_2^-. scavenging). On the other hand, probably this Mn(II)–bacitracin may be involved in the respiratory burst mechanism of white blood cells that could enhance bacterial killing by synergistic process to convert superoxide radical into hydrogen peroxide which is used by enzyme myeloperoxidase to convert normally unreactive halide ions into reactive hypohalous acids that are toxic to bacteria. Also its antibiotic mechanism could be useful for bacterial and oxidative stress treatments.

Bacitracin provides strong affinity to divalent metal ions such as Zn(II), Cu(II), Co(II), and Mn(II) in the formation of 1:1 complex. Structural characterization of metallobacitracin showed that it is composed of a cyclic heptapeptide and a short N-terminal sequence containing a thiazoline ring (Fig 17). The divalent metals interact with the cyclic and the linear peptides to form a strong bending structure that encapsulates the metal inside the coordination sphere. It is interesting to note that the established order of binding affinity of the transition metal ions was found to be inversely correlated with the observed SOD activity reported in this work. The order of metal binding affinity and SOD activity is Cu(II) > Ni(II) > Co(II) ≈Zn(II) >Mn(II) (Brabec & Novakova, 2006) and Mn(II) > Cu(II) > Co(II) > Ni(II), respectively. However, it should be noted that the negative correlation is valid for Mn(II), Co(II), and Ni(II) but not Cu(II).

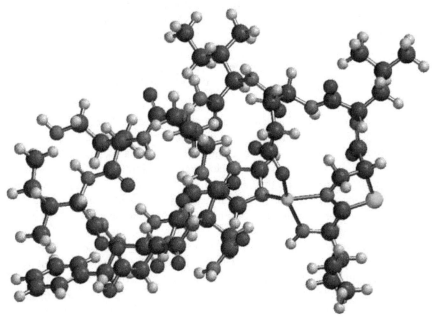

Fig. 16. Molecular modeling of Mn(II)-bacitracin complex (Piacham et al, 2006)

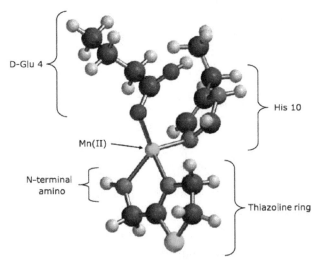

Fig. 17. Mn(II) ligand models derived from metallobacitracin complexes (Piacham et al, 2006)

It is possible that the observed trend, in which Cu(II)–bacitracin did not follow the order of increasing SOD activity with decreasing metal binding affinity, is because Cu(II) takes on a different coordination chemistry from the other divalent metal ions in which Cu(II) forms a tetragonally distorted geometry with two coordinated nitrogens and two coordinated oxygens, particularly, His-10 imidazole nitrogen, thiazoline nitrogen, Glu-4 carboxylate oxygen, and Asp-11 carboxylate oxygen. Proton NMR studies established that Co(II) is coordinated to three nitrogens and one oxygen, namely, His-10 imidazole nitrogen, thiazoline nitrogen, Ile-1 amino nitrogen, and Glu-4 carboxylate oxygen. For the construction of the molecular models of metallobacitracin, it was assumed that Mn(II) and Ni(II) adopt a similar coordination chemistry to that of Co(II) because they all have a vacant d shell.

Cobalt–aspirin complexes are investigated as potential cytostatics (Ott et al, 2009). Aspirin (acetylsalicylic acid) belongs to the family of nonsteroidal antirheumatics (NSAR), which have anti-inflammatory and pain-relieving effects The pharmacological effects of NSARs stem from the inhibition of enzymes in the cyclooxygenase family (COX). Besides the role of NSARs in inflammatory processes, they also seem to be involved in tumor growth. NSARs have thus come into focus as potential cytostatics. It may be possible to improve anti-tumor activity in the case of aspirin by binding it to an organometallic fragment. A hexacarbonyldicobalt–aspirin complex (Fig 18), is shown to inhibit COX activity differently from aspirin. Whereas the effect of aspirin stems from the acetylation of a serine residue in the active center of COX, Co-Aspirin complex does not attack this side chain, but acetylates several other sites instead. This may block access to the active center of the enzyme, resulting in a different activity spectrum for the drug. Experiments with zebra fish embryos showed that in contrast to aspirin, Co-Aspirin inhibits both cell growth and the formation of small blood vessels (angiogenesis). Tumors are dependent on newly formed blood vessels for their nutrients and can be starved out by the inhibition of angiogenesis. In addition, Co-Aspirin modulates other tumor-relevant metabolic pathways. For example, it activates the enzyme caspase, which is involved in processes that lead to apoptosis (programmed cell death).

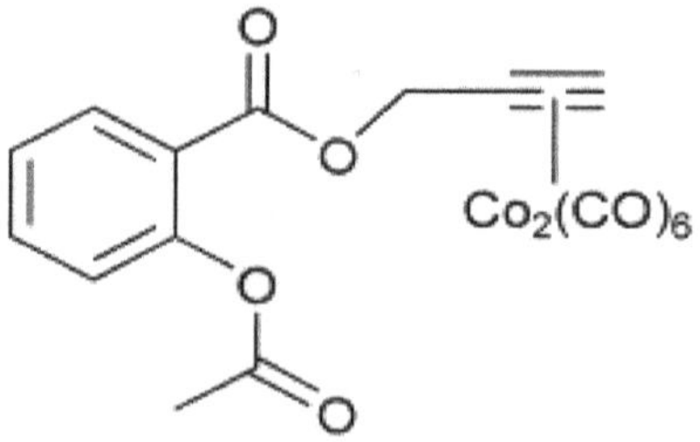

Fig. 18. The structure of hexacarbonyldicobalt–aspirin complex (Ott et al, 2009)

Sadler and coworkers (Meggers, 2007) investigated the binding of metal complexes of 1,4,8,11-tetraazacyclotetradecane (cyclam) macrocycles to the CXCR4 coreceptor and lysozyme as a model protein. In such metallocyclam complexes, the metal is supposed to function by controlling the conformation and configuration of the macrocycle. Additional direct coordinative bonds with the target protein can be formed with the vacant axial coordination sites. One of the most potent members of this family is the xylyl-bicyclam AMD3100 (Fig 19), a CXCR4 receptor inhibitor, which is in clinical trials for the treatment of AIDS. The anti-HIV activity correlates with its binding to the coreceptor protein CXCR4. CXCR4 is a chemokine receptor that transduces signals of its endogenous ligand, CXCL12/stromal cell-derived factor-1 (SDF-1) (Tamamura et al, 2006). CXCR4 is classified into 7TMGPCR and plays a physiological critical role by the action of CXCL12 in the migration of progenitors during embryologic development of the cardiovascular, hemopoietic, central nervous systems, etc. In addition, CXCR4 was previously identified as a coreceptor that is used by X4-HIV-1 in its entry into T cells and has recently been proven to be involved in several problematic diseases, including HIV infection, metastasis of several types of cancer, leukemia cell progression, rheumatoid arthritis. Thus, CXCR4 is thought to be a great therapeutic target to overcome these diseases, and several inhibitors directed against CXCR4 have been developed to date. Research performed on AMD3100 analogs have revealed that if it is complexed with certain metals it will increase the bonding affinity to CXCR4 by causing the cyclam rings to take on a folded cis configuration (Snell, 2005). When Zn(II)–xylyl-bicyclam binds with acetate, it undergoes a configuration change and becomes cis folded. The cyclam ring can function as a tetradentate coordination ring for transition metals, and it has been shown that chelation of such metal ions by the macrocyclic rings of AMD3100 alters its binding affinity to the CXCR4 receptor (Gerlach et al, 2003). Thus, the Zn^{2+} complex of AMD3100 binds with a 10-fold higher affinity to the receptor as compared to AMD3100 alone and has an up to 6-fold increased potency as an anti-HIV agent. Zn^{2+} is located in the center of the cyclam ring, coordinating the four nitrogens in a planar fashion. Since Zn^{2+} does not coordinate in a square planar conformation, it either obtains a square pyramidal or an octahedral geometry with one or two vacant coordination sites. Zn^{2+} has the option to make strong interactions with both histidine and cysteine residues, as well as acidic residues such as aspartates. The CXCR4 receptor does not contain any free extracellular cysteines; however, the main interaction points for AMD3100 are two aspartates, and furthermore, several histidine residues are located in TM-III, TM-V, and TM-VII (TM: transmembrane domain) pointing toward the main ligand binding crevice (Figure 20). Thus, metal ion coordination could either improve the binding mode of AMD3100 to one or more of the two aspartates, Asp171 and Asp262, or it could pick up interaction with one or more of the His residues that potentially could serve as partners in the coordination of Zn^{2+} bound by the bicyclam.

The level of anti-HIV activity expressed by these metal complexes were Zn>Ni>Cu>Co>Pd in decreasing order. The affinity of AMD3100, a symmetrical nonpeptide antagonist composed of two 1,4,8,11-tetraazacyclotetradecane (cyclam) rings connected through a 1,4-dimethylene(phenylene) linker to the CXCR4 chemokine receptor was increased 7, 36, and 50-fold, respectively, by incorporation of Cu^{2+}, Zn^{2+}, or Ni^{2+} into the cyclam rings of the compound. The rank order of the transition metal ions correlated with the calculated binding energy between free acetate and the metal ions coordinated in a cyclam ring. Construction of AMD3100 substituted with only a single Cu^{2+} or Ni^{2+} ion demonstrated that the increase in binding affinity of the metal ion substituted bicyclam is achieved through an enhanced interaction of just one of the ring systems.

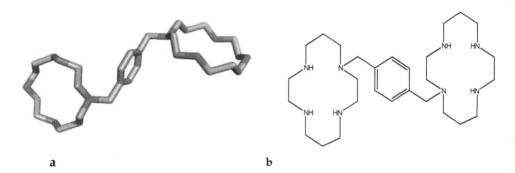

a   b

Fig. 19. The 3D (a) and 2D (b) structure of AMD3100 (New Indications for AMD-3100, In: Drug Discovery Opinion, 2008; (Snell, 2005)]

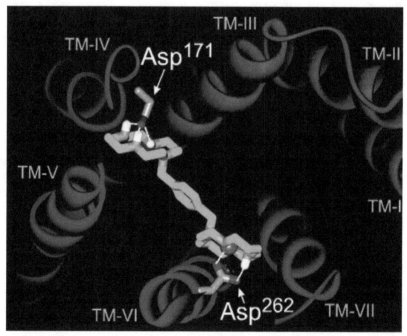

Fig. 20. Molecular model of the main ligand-binding pocket of the CXCR4 receptor with AMD3100(Zn) manually docked into favorable interactions with Asp171 in TM-IV and Asp262 in TM-VI. The receptor model is built over the rhodopsin model of Palcewski et al (Palczewski et al, 2000). The conformation of AMD3100 is based on structural requirements of high antiviral effects of AMD3100 and the crystallographic X-ray structure of 6,6′-spirobis- (1,4,8,11-tetraazacyclotetradecane)-dinickel(II)tetraperchlorate, obtained from the Cambridge Structural Database (Gerlach et al, 2003).

Several low molecular weight nonpeptide compounds having the dipicolylamine-zinc(II) complex structure were also identified as potent and selective antagonists of the chemokine receptor CXCR4 (Tamamura et al, 2006). These compounds showed strong inhibitory activity against CXCL12 binding to CXCR4, and one of them (which has two sets of the [bis(pyridin-2-ylmethyl) amino]methylene unit with zinc(II) complexation at the para-position of benzene) exhibited significant anti-HIV activity.

The use of organometallic complexes are also investigated in the treatment of leishmania. The drugs for treating cutaneous lesions, or, in the case of visceral leishmaniasis (kala-azar), caused by the species L. donovani or L. infantum have traditionally been pentavalent antimonials, aromatic diamidines and fungicides such as amphotericine B (Mesa-Valle et al, 1996). However, these are extremely toxic and cause a great number of side effects. Many recent efforts have been made to synthesize and evaluate alternative compounds for treating these parasites. In the last few years, certain metal complexes have proven anti-tumoral against such protozoan parasites as Trypanosoma cruzi, T. rhodesiense and L. donovani. One property that the tumor cells share with the trypanosomatids is rapid multiplication. Three organometallic complexes which have previously shown in vitro activity against the promastigote forms of L. donovani and have also shown a similar activity against the amastigote like forms, are Cis-Pt(DDH)(Ac.19 2,5-Dihydroxi-benzensulphonic)$_2$ and those of Rh(I): Rh(CO)$_2$Cl(5Cl-2-Methylbenzothiazole), Rh(CO)$_2$Cl(2-Aminobenzothiazole) were investigated by Mesa-Valle et al. (Mesa-Valle et al, 1996). In vitro toxicity of the complexes for the cells of the strain J-774 and the effect exerted on the parasite's biosynthesis of macromolecules were investigated. Only the Rh(I)(CO)$_2$Cl(2-Aminobenzothiazole) complex induced substantial toxicity in the cells. The Rh(I)(CO)$_2$Cl(5-Cl-2-Methylbenzothiazole) complex inhibited DNA, RNA, and protein synthesis. The best candidate, given its slight toxicity for mammal cells and its high activity against Leishmania by inhibiting the synthesis of macromolecules, is found as the complex Rh(I):Rh(CO)$_2$Cl(5-Cl-2-Methylbenzothiazole). Croft et al. investigated the effect of 27 Platinum, Rhodium and Iridium drug complexes against Leishmania donovani amastigotes in mouse peritoneal macrophages in vitro (Croft et al, 1992). Rh(III)-mepacrine, Ir(III) pyrrolidine dithiocarbamate and Ir(III) diethyl dithiocarbamate which showed antileishmanial activity had ED$_{50}$ values of less than 1 μM. The two Iridium complexes produced, respectively, a 50% and 39% suppression of L. donovani amastigotes in the liver of BALB/c mice following the subcutaneous administration of 200 mg/kg for 5 consecutive days. Ultrastructural studies suggest that the amastigote kinetoplast-mitochondrion complex is the primary site of action of the Ir and Rh complexes. Ir-(cycloocta-1,5-diene)-pentamidine tetraphenylborate which has previously been studied on promastigote forms of Leishmania, was investigated for its antileishmanial properties on Leishmania donovani and Leishmania major mouse models, compared with pentamidine used as reference compound in the year 2000 (Loiseau, et al, 2000). In vitro, the iridium complex had the same IC$_{50}$ value on intracellular forms of Leishmania as pentamidine (15 μM). In vivo, the compound could not be injected intravenously due to the DMSO excipient so that the treatments were performed intraperitoneally or subcutaneously. On the L. donovani LV9/Balb/C mouse model, the iridium complex was not toxic after intraperitoneal treatment at 232 mg/kg/day x 5 or

147 µmoles/kg/day x 5, whereas all the mice died within five days when treated at the same dose with pentamidine isethionate. However, only 23% of parasite suppression was observed with the iridium complex. On a L. major MON 74/Balb/C mouse model, susceptible to intravenously administered pentamidine at 6.7 µmoles/kg/day x 5 (54% of parasite suppression), the iridium complex exhibited 32% of parasite suppression after a treatment at 76 µmoles/kg/day x 5 administered subcutaneously. Transmission electron microscopy of amastigotes from infected and treated mice show aggregation of ribosomal material, distension of the nuclear membrane and kDNA depolymerization. The mechanism of action therefore involves several targets: membranes, ribosomes and kDNA. The researchers recommend the Iridium complex as a suitable candidate to be encapsulated in drug carriers such as liposomes or nanoparticles.

Organometallic complexes of Pt, Rh, Ir, Pd, Os, have been synthesized and their trypanocidal activity was studied in vitro and in vivo by Loiseau (Loiseau et al, 1992). Among these, the Ir-(cyclocta-1,5-diene)-pentamidine complex, showed in vitro activity at 60 µg/L on Tripanosoma brucei brucei. Moreover, all infected mice were cured by this compound subcutaneously administered in a single dose at 0.5 mg/kg (0.317 µmol/kg). In the same conditions, pentamidine cured all the mice at 5 µmol/kg. Ir-(cyclooca-1,5-diene)-pentamidine (or P1995) was 16 fold more efficient than pentamidine. Since the chemotherapeutic index of this molecule was 7.5 fold higher than those of pentamidine, the authors recommend P1995 to be considered as a potential trypanocidal drug of the future.

Scientists are looking for alternative approaches for the treatment of diabetes. Several trace elements, such as vanadium and zinc, exert insulin-mimetic effects in in vitro and in vivo systems (Hiromura & Sakurai, 2008). The complexes of these metals and small organic compounds (ligands) improved glucose utilization in both diabetic model animals and human diabetic patients . Both vanadyl and zinc complexes enhanced glucose uptake into the adipocytes without the addition of any hormones. Under the same experimental conditions, these complexes inhibited epinephrine-induced free fatty acid (FFA) release. Because of this insulin-mimetic activity, oxovanadium(IV) (vanadyl) and zinc(II) (zinc) complexes are proposed to be potent antidiabetic agents for both type 1 and type 2 Diabetes Mellitus therapy. New types of insulin-mimetic vanadyl and zinc complexes such as Bis(allixinato)oxovanadium(IV), [VO(alx)2], bis(allixinato)zinc(II) [Zn(alx)2], bis(thioallixin-N-methyl)zinc(II) [Zn(tanm)2] (Fig 21), were developed as the potent activators of the insulin signaling pathway. Although these complexes activate Akt/PKB, their critical action sites are slightly different from each other. Different action sites of the metal complexes may depend on the chemical characteristic of the vanadyl and zinc metal ions. The characteristic of ligand is important for the passing through the plasma membrane. $VO(alx)_2$, $Zn(alx)_2$, and $Zn(tanm)_2$ also play unique roles in cells; $VO(alx)_2$ regulates the activation of the FoxO1, while $Zn(alx)_2$ and $Zn(tanm)_2$ regulate the activation of HSL (hormone-sensitive lipase), resulting in the suppression of free fatty acid release. The common mechanism of action of $VO(alx)_2$, $Zn(alx)_2$, and $Zn(tanm)_2$ is their effect on the insulin signaling pathway; this in turn regulates gene transcription and suppresses lipolysis signaling.

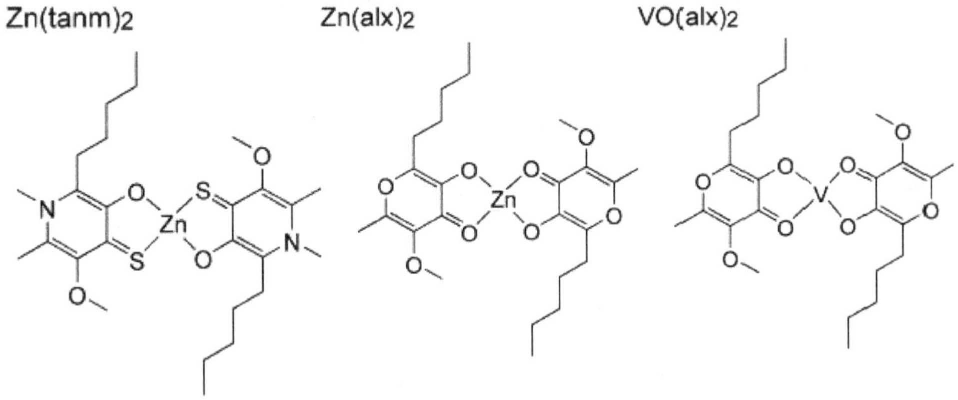

Zn(tanm)2   Zn(alx)2   VO(alx)2

Fig. 21. The molecular structures of VO(alx)₂, Zn(alx)₂, and Zn(tanm)₂ (Hiromura & Sakurai, 2008)

Another application of organometallic complexes is antiinflammatory therapy. Numerous Cu(II) complexes of NSAIDs with enhanced anti-inflammatory activity and reduced gastrointestinal (GI) toxicity compared with their uncomplexed parent drug, were developed (Hiromura & Sakurai, 2008). No Cu(II) anti-inflammatory drug is currently available for oral human use, although an ethanolic gel-base of Cu-salicylate (Alcusal®) is available for topical temporal relief of pain and inflammation in humans (Weder et al, 2002). A Cu(II) dimer of indomethacin (IndoH_/1- (4-chlorobenzoyl)-5-methoxy-2-methyl-1H-Indole-3-acetic acid) with low toxicity is commercially available in Australasia, South East Asia and South Africa in a variety of oral pharmaceutical dosage forms for veterinary use. These low toxicity Cu drugs are of enormous interest, because many of today's anti-inflammatory drug therapies, including the NSAIDs, remain either largely inadequate and/or are associated with problematic side effects, e.g. renal insufficiency and failure, GI ulceration, bleeding or perforation ('NSAID gastropathy'), exacerbation of hypertension and congestive heart failure (CHF). Sorenson reported that Cu(II)-complexes of these antiinflammatory drugs were more active in animal models than either their parent inorganic Cu(II) salt or the parent NSAID . The pharmacological activity was proposed to be due to the inherent physico-chemical properties of the complex itself rather than just that of its constituents, since the amount of Cu(II) in such complexes does not correlate with anti-inflammatory activity. Sorenson reported that a salicylate complex of Cu(II) was ≈30 times more effective than aspirin as an anti-inflammatory agent. In two previous reviews, Sorenson reported over 140 Cu(II) complexes with anti-inflammatory activity. However, limited information is available on the nature of the Cu complexes of NSAIDs in biological matrices and in pharmaceutical formulations. SOD activity, redox behavior, lipophilicity and stability constants may be useful parameters in evaluating the biological activity of these Cu compounds.

The proposed curative properties of Cu-based nonsteroidal anti-inflammatory drugs (NSAIDs) have led to the development of numerous Cu(II) complexes of NSAIDs with enhanced anti-inflammatory activity (Trinchero et al, 2004) Crystalline complexes, Cu(II)–

NSAID (ibuprofen, naproxen, tolmetin, and diclofenac), with a carboxylic function have been studied by means of infrared and Raman spectroscopy. All NSAIDs bind to the metal through the carboxylate group. The spectroscopic data support the formation of dimeric $[Cu_2L_4(H_2O)_2]$ complexes in which the COO^- group behaves as a bridging bidentate ligand. The preparation and properties of the Cu(II) complex $Cu(SAS)_2.H_2O$ are reported for the antiinflammatory drug Salsalate (SAS) (Underhill et al, 1989). The complex is reported to exhibit an increased superoxide dismutase activity compared with the parent drug molecule in the nitroblue tetrazolium assay. Weder and friends synthesized Cu(II) indomethacin complexes (Weder et al, 1999).

Drugs belonging to the non-steroidal anti-inflammatory drug group (NSAID) are not only used as anti-inflammatory and analgesic agents, but also exhibit chemopreventive and chemosuppressive effects on various cancer cell lines (Roy et al, 2006). They exert their anticancer effects by inhibiting both at the protein level and/or at the transcription level. Cu(II) complexes of these NSAIDs show better anti-cancer effects than the bare drugs. UV-Visible spectroscopy was used to characterize the complexation between Cu(II) and two NSAIDs belonging to the oxicam group, piroxicam and meloxicam, both of which exhibit anticancer properties. For the first time, this study shows that, Cu(II)-NSAID complexes can directly bind with the DNA backbone, and the binding constants and the stoichiometry or the binding site sizes have been determined. Thermodynamic parameters from van't Hoff plots showed that the interaction of these Cu(II)-NSAID complexes with ctDNA is an entropically driven phenomenon. Circular dichroism spectroscopy showed that the binding of these Cu(II)-NSAIDs with ctDNA result in DNA backbone distortions which is similar for both Cu(II)-piroxicam and Cu(II)-meloxicam complexes. Competitive binding with a standard intercalator like ethidium bromide (EtBr) investigated by circular dichroism spectroscopy as well as fluorescence measurements indicate that the Cu(II)-NSAID complexes could intercalate in the DNA.

Inspired from Sorenson's studies, new investigations on formation and synthesis of Cu(II) complexes with antiinflammatory drugs were carried out as well as Zn(II) complexes, where some of them are ternary complexes (Anılanmert et al, 2010). The formation conditions and constants of Cu(II)-tryptophan-aspirin and Zn(II)-tryptophan-aspirin ternary complexes in aqueous solutions were determined using potentiometric method to provide chemical data for the synthesis, considering the synergistic capability of aspirin, the antiinflammatory activity of Cu(II), the synergistic effect of tryptophan-aspirin combination in migraine and in diseases which cause immune activation, the stronger analgesic, antiinflammatory and antithrombotic effect of Cu(II)-aspirinate and Zn(II)-aspirinate than aspirin, decreased gastrointestinal toxicity of Cu(II)-aspirinate and Zn(II)-aspirinate than aspirin, the stronger analgesic and antiinflammatory effects of some Cu(II)-amino acid complexes than Cu(II)-aspirinate and the increased bioavailability of Zn(II)-amino acid complexes. The effects of leucine in cancer, wound healing and regulation of glucose in blood, anticancer activity and healing activity of Cu(II) on radiation effects, antiinflammatory effects of Cu(II)-aspirin and Cu(II)-amino acid compounds, sinergistic activity of aspirin and its anticancer effect which was proved in recent years are known (Anılanmert, 2006). Under the light of these effects, the formation of Cu(II)-leucine-aspirin was also investigated using potentiometric and spectrophotometric method. The anticancer action and wound healing effect on skin cancers topically and through injection into tumours should be investigated in the future. These ternary complexes have only been investigated using potentiometry, UV and IR spectrometry, synthesis studies are going on, yet no in vitro and in vivo study is performed, however they are recommended to be investigated for the above therapeutic effects.

3. Conclusion

In this chapter, clinical uses of organometallic complexes and some prominent studies on new therapeutic complexes were mentioned. Developments in explorations of organometallic compounds, in various therapeutic areas continue to be an active and productive area of research. Increasingly powerful tools, notably spectroscopic techniques like time-resolved infrared are used for identifying and structurally characterizing the solid complex, optical spectroscopic and potentiometric methods are used for monitoring intermediates and species in solution. Besides these preclinical and clinical studies are significantly enhancing our knowledge and understanding of the structure and mechanistic aspects of the therapeutic organometallic complexes.

4. References

Abu-Surrah, A.S., Kettunen, M., Leskelä, M., Al-Abed, Y. (2008), Platinum and Palladium Complexes Bearing New (1R,2R)-(-)-1,2-Diaminocyclohexane (DACH)-Based Nitrogen Ligands: Evaluation of the Complexes Against L1210 Leukemia, *Zeitschrift für anorganische und allgemeine Chemie*, Vol.634, No.14, (October 2008), 2655-2658, 1521-3749 DOI: 10.1002/zaac.200800281

Abu-Surrah, A.S., Kettunen, M. (2006), Platinum Group Antitumor Chemistry: Design and development of New Anticancer Drugs Complementary to Cisplatin, *Current Medicinal Chemistry*, Vol.13, 1337-1357, 0929-8673/06.

Allardyce, C. S., Dyson, P.J. (2006) Medicinal Properties of Organometallic Compounds, In: *Bioorganometallic Chemistry (Topics in Organometallic Chemistry)*, Gerard Simonneaux, Volume 17, pp.177-210, Springer-Verlag, 10 3-540-33047-9 , Berlin, Heidelberg DOI:10.1007/3418_001.

Anga, W. H., Casini, A., Sava, G., Dyson, P.J., (2011), Organometallic ruthenium-based antitumor compounds with novel modes of action, *Journal of Organometallic Chemistry*, Vol. 696, No.5, (March 2011), pp. 989-999, 0022-328X.

Anilanmert, B., Pekin, M., Apak, R. (2010), Investigation of the Formation of Copper(II)-Tryptophane-Aspirin Ternary Complexes, *Asian Journal of Chemistry*, Vol.22, No.10, (November-December 2010), 8060-8072, 0970-7077.

Anilanmert, B. (2006), *Determination of the stability constants of the ternary complexes that tryptophan-aspirin, leucine-aspirin ligands and Cu(II) and Zn(II) metals form, using potentiometric method*, doctorate thesis, Marmara University Institute of Health Sciences, 2006, Istanbul.

Antonarakis, E.S., Emadi, A., (2010), Ruthenium-based chemotherapeutics: are they ready for prime time?, *Cancer Chemotherapy and Pharmacology*, Vol.66, No.1, (March 2010), pp.1–9, 1432-0843.

Aston, K. Rath, N., Naik,A., Slomczynska, U., Schall,O. F., Riley, D.P.: Computer-Aided Design (CAD) of Mn(II) Complexes: Superoxide Dismutase Mimetics with Catalytic Activity Exceeding the Native Enzyme, Inorg. Chem. 2001, 40, 1779-1789, 0020-1669

Bharti, S.K., Singh, S.K. (2009) Recent Developments In The Field of Anticancer Metallopharmaceuticals, *International Journal of PharmTech Research*, Vol.1, No.4, (October-December 2009), pp. 1406-1420, 0974-4304.

Blackie, M.A.L., Chibale, K. (2008), Metallocene Antimalarials: The Continuing Quest, *Metal-Based Drugs*, Vol. 2008, Article ID 495123, doi:10.1155/2008/495123, 1687-5486.

Brabec V, Nováková O. DNA binding mode of ruthenium complexes and relationship to tumor cell toxicity. *Drug Resistance Updates*, Vol.9, No.3, (June 2006), pp. 111-22, 1368-7646.

Clarke, M.J., Zhu, F., Frasca, D.R., (1999) Non-Platinum Chemotherapeutic Metallopharmaceuticals, *Chemical Reviews*, Vol. 99, No.9, (July 1999), pp.2511-2533, 1520-6890.

Clarke, M.J. (2003) Ruthenium metallopharmaceuticals, *Coordination Chemistry Reviews*, Vol.236, No.1-2, (January 2010), pp.209-233, 0010-8545.

Croft, S.L., Neal, R.A., Craciunescu, D.G., Certad-Fombona, G. (1992), The activity of platinum, iridium and rhodium drug complexes against Leishmania donovani., *Tropical Medicine and Parasitology*, Vol. 43, No.1, (March 1992), pp.24-28, 0035-9203.

Dabrowiak, J.C. (2009), *Metals in Medicine*, pp.191-214, John Wiley and Sons, Ltd., Ist. Ed., West Sussex, 978-0-470-68196-1.

Dittrich, C., Hochhaus, A., Schaad, S., Salama, C., Jaehde, U., Jakupec, M. A., Hauses, M.,Gneist, M., Keppler, B. K. (2005) Phase I and pharmacokinetic study of the oral tris-(8-quinolinolato) gallium(III) complex (FFC11, KP46) in patients with solid tumors - a study of the CESAR Central European Society for Anticancer Drug Research – EWIV, *Journal of Clinical Oncology, Proceedings of ASCO Annual Meeting*. (June 2005), Vol 23, No. 16S, Part I of II, June 1 Supplement, pp.3205, 0732-183X.

Lentz, F., Drescher, A., Lindauer, A., Henke, M., Hilger, R.A., Hartinger, C.G., Scheulen, M.E., Dittrich, C., Keppler, B.K., Jaehde, U. (2009), Pharmacokinetics of a novel anticancer ruthenium complex (KP1019, FFC14A) in a phase I dose-escalation study, *Anti-Cancer Drugs*, Vol.20, No.2, (February 2009), pp. 97-103, 1473-5741.

Guo, Z., Sadler, P.J. (1999), Metals in Medicine *Angewandte Chemistry International Edition*, Vol.38, No.11, (June 1999), pp. 1512 – 1531, 1521-3773.

Gerlach, L.O., Jakobsen, J.S., Jensen, K.P., Rosenkilde, M.R., Skerlj, R.T., Ryde, U., Bridger, G.J., Schwartz, T.W. (2003), Metal Ion Enhanced Binding of AMD3100 to Asp262 in the CXCR4 Receptor, *Biochemistry*, Vol. 42, No.3, (January 2003),pp. 710-717, 1520-4995.

Hanif, M. (2010) *From Biomolecules to Organometallic Compounds with Tumor- Inhibiting Properties*, Supervisor: O. Univ.-Prof. Dr. Bernhard K. Kepler, Vienna.

Hannon, M.J., (2007), Metal-based anticancer drugs: From a past anchored in platinum chemistry to a post-genomic future of diverse chemistry and biology, *Pure and Applied Chemistry*, Vol.79, No.12, (January 2007), pp.2243–2261, 1365-3075.

Hiromura, M., Sakurai, H. (2008), Action mechanism of metallo-allixin complexes as antidiabetic agents, *Pure and Applied Chemistry*, Vol.80, No.12, pp. 2727–2733.

Jaouen, G., Top, S., Vessieres, A., (2006), Chap 3, Organometallics targeted to specific biological sites: The development of new therapies, In: *Bioorganometallics: Biomolecules, Labeling, Medicine*, Ed. Jaouen, G., pp 65-95, Wiley-VCH, 9783527607693, Weinheim.

Katsaros, N., Anagnostopoulou, A. (2002) Rhodium and its compounds as potential agents in cancer treatment., *Critical Reviews in Oncology/ Hematology*, Vol.42, No.3, (June 2002), pp. 297-308, 2002, 1040-8428.

Lee, S., Hille, A., Frias, C., Kater, B., Bonitzki, B., Wolf, S., Scheffler, H., Prokop, A., Gust, R. (2010), [NiII(3-OMe-salophene)]: A Potent Agent with Antitumor Activity, *Journal of Medicinal Chemistry*, Vol.53, No.16, (July 2010), pp 6064–6070, 1520-4804.

Liu, Z., Habtemariam, A., Pizarro, A.M., Fletcher, S.A., Kisova, A., Vrana, O., Salassa, L., Bruijnincx, P.C.A., Clarkson, G.J., Brabec, V., Sadler, P.J. (2011), Organometallic Half-Sandwich Iridium Anticancer Complexes, *Journal of Medicinal Chemistry*, Vol.54, No.8, (April 2011), pp.3011– 3026, 1520-4804.

Llorca, C.S.(2005): *New mono- and dinuclear ruthenium complexes containing the 3,5-bis(2-pyridyl)pyrazole ligand, synthesis, characterization and applications*, PhD dissertation, 84-689-2580-2, Girona.

Loiseau, P.M., Mbongo, N., Bories, C., Boulard, Y., Craciunescu, D.G. (2000), In vivo antileishmanial action of Ir-(COD)-pentamidine tetraphenylborate on Leishmania donovani and Leishmania major mouse models, *Parasite*, Vol. 7, No.2, (June 2000), pp.103-108, 1776-1042.

Loiseau, P.M., Craciunescu, D.G., Doadrio-Villarejo, J.C., Certad-Fombona, G., Gayral, P.(1992), Pharmacomodulations on new organometallic complexes of Ir, Pt, Rh, Pd, Os: in vitro and in vivo trypanocidal study against Trypanosoma brucei brucei., *Tropical Medicine and Parasitology*, Vol.43, No.2, (June 1992), pp.110-114, 0003-4983.

Maurel, J.C., Cudennec, C.A., (2009) *Manganese based organometallic complexes, pharmaceutical compositions and dietetic products*, Assignees: MEDESIS PHARMA S.A., IPC8 Class: AA61K3156FI, USPC Class: 514169, Publication date: 10/01/2009, Patent application number: 20090247492.

Meggers, E. (2007), Exploring biologically relevant chemical space with metal complexes, *Current Opinion in Chemical Biology*, Vol.11, No. 3, (June, 2007), pp. 287-292, 1367-5931.

Meng, X., Leyva, M.L., Jenny, M., Gross, I., Benosman, S., Fricker, B., Harlepp, S., He'braud, P., Boos, A., Wlosik, P., Bischoff, P., Sirlin, C., Pfeffer, M., Loeffler, J., Gaiddon, C. (2009) A Ruthenium-Containing Organometallic Compound Reduces Tumor Growth through Induction of the Endoplasmic Reticulum Stress Gene CHOP, *Cancer Research*, Vol.69 , No.13, (July 2009), 5458-5466, 1538-7445.

Mesa-Valle, C.M., Moraleda-Lindez,V., Craciunescu, D., Osuna, A. (1996), Antileishmanial action of organometallic complexes of Pt(II) and Rh(I), *Chemotherapy*, Vol. 91, No.5, (September/October 1996), pp. 625-633, 0009-3157.

New Indications for AMD-3100, In: *Drug Discovery Opinion, DDO Limited, Consultancy for Biotech and Pharma*, 2008, Available from: http://drugdiscoveryopinion.com/2008/08/new-indications-for-amd-3100/

Ogawa, K., Mukai, T., Asano, D., Kawashima, H., Kinuya, S., Shiba, K., Hashimoto, K., Mori, H., Saji, H., (2007), Therapeutic effects of a 186Re-complex-conjugated bisphosphonate for the palliation of metastatic bone pain in an animal model. *Journal of Nuclear Medicine*, Vol. 48, No.1, (January 2007), pp. 122-127, 2159-662X.

Ott, I., Gust R. (2007) Non platinum metal complexes as anti-cancer drugs, *Archive der Pharmazie*, Vol.340, No.3, (March 2007), pp.117-26, 0365-6233

Ott, I., Kircher, B., Bagowski, C.P., Vlecken, D.H.W., Ott, E.B., Will, J., Bensdorf, K., Sheldrick, W.S., Gust, R. (2009) Modulation of the Biological Properties of Aspirin by Formation of a Bioorganometallic Derivative *Angewandte Chemie International Edition*, Vol. 48, No. 6, (January 2009), pp. 1160–1163, 1521-3773

Palczewski, K., Kumasaka, T., Hori, T., Behnke, C. A., Motoshima, H., Fox, B. A., Le, T. I, Teller, D. C., Okada, T., Stenkamp, R. E. , Yamamoto, M., and Miyano, M. (2000) Crystal structure of rhodopsin: A G protein-coupled receptor, *Science*, Vol. 289 , No.5480, (August 2000), pp.739-745, 0036-8075.

Piacham, T., Isarankura-Na-Ayudhya, C., Nantasenamat, C., Yainoy, S., Ye, L., Bülow, L., Prachayasittikul, V. (2006) Metalloantibiotic Mn(II)-bacitracin complex mimicking manganese superoxide dismutase. *Biochemical and Biophysical Research Communications*, Vol.341, No. 4, (March 2006), pp.925-930, 0006-291X.

Rademaker-Lakhai, J.M., van den Bongard, D., Pluim, D., Beijnen, J.M., Schellens, J. H. M. (2004) A Phase I and Pharmacological Study with Imidazolium-trans-DMSO-imidazole-tetrachlororuthenate, a Novel Ruthenium Anticancer Agent, *Clinical Cancer Research*, Vol.10, No.11, (June 2004), pp. 3717-3727, 1557-3265.

Rafique, S., Idrees, M., Nasim, A., Akbar, H., Athar, A. (2010) Transition metal complexes as potential therapeutic Agents *Biotechnology and Molecular Biology Reviews*, Vol. 5, No. 2 (April 2010), pp.38-45, 1538-2273.

Roy S., Banerjee R., Sarkar, M. (2006), Direct binding of Cu(II)-complexes of oxicam NSAIDs with DNA backbone, *Journal of Inorganic Biochemistry*, Vol.100, No.8, (August 2006), pp.1320-1331, 0162-0134.

Rudrangi, S.R.S., Bontha, V.K., Bethi, S., Reddy, V., (2010), Ferrocenes: Legendary Magic Bullets In Organometallic Chemistry-An Overview, *International Journal of Pharma Research and Development*, Vol.2, No.8, (October 2010), pp.53-61, 0974-9446, Publication Ref No.: IJPRD/2010/PUB/ARTI/VOV-2/ISSUE-8/OCT/008

Sannella, A.R., Casini, A., Gabbiani, C., Messori, L., Bilia, A.R., Vincieri, F.R., Majori, G., Severini, C. (2008), New uses for old drugs. Auranofin, a clinically established antiarthritic metallodrug, exhibits potent antimalarial effects in vitro: mechanistic and pharmacological implications. *FEBS Letters*, Vol.582, No.6, (March 2008), pp.844–847, 0014-5793.

Sekhon, B.S., (2010), Metalloantibiotics and antibiotic mimics - an overview, *Journal of Pharmaceutical Education and Research*, Vol. 1, No. 1, (June 2010), pp.1-20, 0976 – 8238.

Snell, T.L. (2005), Synthesis and Characterization of Cross-Bridged AMD3100 Analogs, *Centaurus*, Vol. 13, pp.27-31, (May 2005), 0008-8994.

Tamamura, H., Ojida, A., Ogawa, T., Tsutsumi, H., Masuno, H., Nakashima, H., Yamamoto, N., Hamachi, I., Fujii, N., (2006), Identification of a New Class of Low Molecular Weight Antagonists against the Chemokine Receptor CXCR4 Having the Dipicolylamine-Zinc(II) Complex Structure, *Journal of Medicinal Chemistry*, Vol.49, No.11, (June 2006), pp. 3412-3415, 1520-4804.

Timerbaev, A.R., (2009), Advances in developing tris(8-quinolinolato)gallium(III) as ananticancer drug: critical appraisal and prospects., *Metallomics*, Vol.1, No.3, (April 2009), pp.193-198, 1756-5901.

T. Schilling, K. B. Keppler, M. E. Heim, G. Niebch, H. Dietzfelbinger, J. Rastetter, A. R. Hanauske (1995), Clinical phase I and pharmacokinetic trial of the new titanium complex budotitane, *Investigational New Drugs* , Vol. 13, No.4, (December 1995), pp.327-332, 1573-0646.

Top, S., Vessières, A., Cabestaing, C., Laios, I., Leclercq, G., Provot, C., Jaouen, G. (2001), Studies on organometallic selective estrogen receptor modulators. (SERMs) Dual activity in the hydroxy-ferrocifen series, *Journal of Organometallic Chemistry*, Vol. 637–639, (December 2001), pp.500-506, 2001, 0022-328X.

Trinchero, A., Bonora, S., Tinti, A., Fini, G. (2004), Spectroscopic behavior of copper complexes of nonsteroidal anti-inflammatory drugs, *Biopolymers*, Special Issue: Selected Papers from the 10th European Conference on the Spectroscopy of Biological Molecules (ECSBM 2003), Vol.74, No.1-2, (October, 2004), pp.120–124, 1097-0102.

Underhill, A.E., Bury, A., Odling, R.J., Fleet, M.B., Stevens, A., Gomm, P.S. (1989), Metal complexes of antiinflammatory drugs. Part VII: Salsalate complex of copper(II) , *Journal of Inorganic Biochemistry*, Vol.37, No.1, (September 1989), pp. 1-5, 0162-0134.

Vajragupta, O., Boonchoong, P., Sumanont, Y., Watanabe, H., Wongkrajang, Y., Kammasud, N. (2003), Manganese-Based Complexes of Radical Scavengers as Neuroprotective Agents, *Bioorganic Medicinal Chemistry*, Vol.11, No.10, (May 2003), pp.2329–2337, 0968-0896.

Valvassori, S.S., Cristiano, M.P., Cardoso, D.C., Santos, G.D., Martins, M.R., Quevedo, J., da Paula, M.M.S. (2006) Pharmacological Activity of Ruthenium Complexes trans-[RuCl$_2$(L)$_4$] (L = Nicotinic or i-Nicotinic acid) on Anxiety and Memory in Rats, *Neurochemical Research*, Vol.31, No.12, (December, 2006), pp.1457-1462, 0364-3190.

Weder, J.E., Dillon, C.T., Hambley, T.W., Kennedy, B.J, Lay, P.A., Biffin, J.R., Regtop, H.L., Davies, N.M. (2002), Copper complexes of non-steroidal anti-inflammatory drugs: an opportunity yet to be realized, *Coordination Chemistry Reviews*, Vol.232, No.1-2, (October, 2002), pp.95-126, 0010-8545.

Weder, J.E., Hambley, T.W., Kennedy, B.J., Lay, P.A., MacLachlan, D., Bramley, R., Delfs, C.D., Murray, K.S., Moubaraki, B., Warwick, B., Biffin, J.R., Regtop, H.L. (1999),

Anti-Inflammatory Dinuclear Copper(II) Complexes with Indomethacin. Synthesis, Magnetism and EPR Spectroscopy. Crystal Structure of the *N,N*-Dimethylformamide, *Adduct Inorganic Chemistry,* Vol.38 , No.8, (April 1999), pp.1736–1744, 1520-510X.

Zhang, C.X., Lippard, S.J. (2003) New metal complexes as potential therapeutics *Current Opinion in Chemical Biology,* Vol.7, No.4, (August, 2003),.481-489, 1367-5931.

Zhao, G., Lin, H. (2005), Metal complexes with aromatic N-containing ligands as potential agents in cancer tretment. *Current Medicinal Chemistry- Anticancer Agents.* Vol.5, No.2, (March 2005), 137-147, 1568-0118.

8

Aging: Drugs to Eliminate Methylglyoxal, a Reactive Glucose Metabolite, and Advanced Glycation Endproducts

Indu Dhar and Kaushik Desai

Department of Pharmacology, College of Medicine,
University of Saskatchewan, Saskatoon, SK,
Canada

1. Introduction

The aging process not only affects the whole body, but also affects individual cells. While the age-related changes in the body are popularly recognized as wrinkling of the skin, indicating alterations in basement membrane proteins, the processes of cellular aging are less well defined. The underlying common theme of cellular aging and whole body aging seems to be an increase in oxidative stress. Advanced glycation endproducts (AGEs), which are widely accepted to alter basement membrane proteins, also increase oxidative stress. Reactive dicarbonyls, such as methylglyoxal (MG), formed during glycolysis and other metabolic processes are precursors of AGEs formation and triggers of oxidative stress. MG, AGEs and oxidative stress are very likely to induce DNA damage and be at the root of cellular aging. Thus, a strategy to prevent an elevation of MG, formation of AGEs and the associated oxidative stress has great therapeutic potential to slow the aging process at the cellular and the whole body level.

2. The ageing process

The process of aging is accepted as an inevitable normal part of the life cycle of each and every living organism. Aging can be grossly defined as an overall decline in biological functions. Thus, aging involves gradual changes in the body such as reduced immunity, loss of muscle strength, stiffening of the arterial wall, loss of elasticity and wrinkling of the skin, and decline in memory, all of which result in increasing weakness, risk of developing diseases, and ultimately death. These changes take place at the cellular, organ and the whole organism level. The whole process of aging unfolds very clearly in species with a long life span such as human beings. Cellular aging ultimately translates into whole body aging.

Hayflick et al. [1] first described cellular senescence in the sixties when they showed that normal cells had a limited ability to proliferate in culture. Cellular senescence is believed to be initiated by increased cellular stress [2, 3]. Factors contributing to cellular stress and aging include dysfunctional telomeres (telomere length) [4, 5], DNA damage [6] and mitogenic or oncogenic stimuli and signals [2, 4, 5]. The factors such as age and oxidative stress affect telomere length and telomerase activity which in turn affects cellular senescence [4]. Oxidative stress has been shown to damage DNA and affect life span [7-10]. A controversial view of cellular senescence is that it is an important protective mechanism against transformation of the cell into a malignant phenotype, in which case it would affect only mitotically active cells [2, 3]. The molecular mechanisms involved in cellular senescence are still being unraveled and will not be considered further in this review. The focus of this review will be on MG, a reactive dicarbonyl metabolic intermediate produced in the body, AGEs, and oxidative stress, all of which are interrelated and affect cellular as well as whole body aging. We will discuss some compounds that can scavenge MG, prevent the formation of AGEs (inhibitors) or break the existing AGEs (AGE breakers).

3. Theories of aging

Aging has been attributed to a number of different causes which have been presented in the form of different theories. These theories are based broadly on two different ideas, one of which is programmed life processes (program theories, e.g. Biological Clock theory, Limited Number of Proliferation theory), and the other one is of errors, mainly at the DNA and gene level, in life processes (error theories, e.g. Disease theory, Cross-linking theory, Rate of living theory, Free radical theory). A number of theories of aging are based on the combination of these two ideas, i.e. program theories and error theories [11-14].

Changes at the cellular level ultimately affect the whole body. The cell is a dynamic centre of ongoing metabolic activity driven by almost constant use of oxygen. Reasonably, the metabolic activity may affect survival or the death of the cell. The 'Rate of living theory' implicates the role of metabolism in aging, which is based on the observation that animals with higher metabolic rates often have shorter life spans. Since the metabolic processes and oxygen consumption can also generate oxidative stress, an excess of which is deleterious for the cell, the 'Free radical theory' of aging has become one of the more popular theories. The free radical theory proposes a connection between the metabolic rate and aging through an increased oxidative stress generation.

4. Free radical theory of aging

Max Rubner proposed the 'rate of living theory' early in the 20th century [15]. He observed that larger animals, which generally have slower metabolic rates, live longer than smaller animals with faster metabolic rates [15]. Even though it is now common knowledge that metabolism is associated with the generation of free radicals, it was Commoner et al. [16] who discovered the formation of free radicals in vivo. Commoner et al. [16] found that an increase in an organism's metabolic activity can increase the concentration of endogenous free radicals. Free radicals are atoms or molecules with an unpaired electron in an orbit, making them highly reactive. The high reactivity of free radicals makes them deleterious for cells because they react with proteins, lipids, DNA and other biomolecules, and disrupt their structure and function. Free radicals can be derived from oxygen mainly in the form of superoxide anions ($O_2^{\bullet-}$) and hydroxyl radicals ($^{\bullet}OH$), which are known as reactive oxygen species (ROS). Free radicals can also be in the form of highly reactive non-radicals which do not have an unpaired electron in their orbit, such as hydrogen peroxide (H_2O_2). Normally, the cells and the body have adequate antioxidant defenses which can neutralize free radicals and prevent the generation of oxidative stress resulting from an excess of free radicals [17-22]. The formation of free radicals and the function of antioxidants have been nicely explained in reviews by Haliwell [20, 21].

The free radical theory of aging was proposed by Denham Harman in 1956 [23]. The free radical theory of aging attributes the aging process to cumulative cellular damage inflicted by the reaction of free radicals with key functional cellular and tissue constituents resulting in impaired function, disease and death [23]. The discovery of an antioxidant enzyme, superoxide dismutase (SOD) [24], which plays a key role to eliminate superoxide anion levels, provided some validity to the free radical theory, which was not initially accepted by many.

The mitochondrial respiratory chain is a major source of free radicals, mainly in the form of superoxide anions, which cause damage to the mitochondria and reduce life span [25, 26]. The damage inflicted by ROS, especially to DNA [7], rather than the metabolic rate, showed a greater correlation with life span [8]. Damage to DNA was formulated into the somatic mutation theory, which states that genetic mutations caused by an excess of free radicals could lead to accelerated aging [7, 9, 10].

The fact that increased production of ROS in the mitochondria can reduce life span was supported by several studies. Thus, Ku *et al.*, [27] showed that the rates of mitochondrial superoxide anion and hydrogen peroxide generation were inversely correlated to maximum life span potential when they compared seven different mammalian species with different life spans ranging from 3.5 to 30 years. Similarly, ROS production was higher in heart mitochondria of the rat, which has a life span of about 4 yrs, than in the long-lived pigeon, which has a longer life span of 35 yrs [28]. Theoretically, therefore, if the free radical production is diminished, the life span should increase. This has been demonstrated in several species. Thus, over expression of SOD and catalase in the worm *Caenorhabditis elegans* (*C. Elegans*) through *age-1* alleles, increases their oxidative defenses and life span by 65% longer on average [29, 30]. Increased activity of SOD and reduced oxidative stress in the transgenic *Drosophila* (*Drosophila melanogaster*) flies also slows the aging process and results in a longer life [31, 32]. Also, over expression of catalase in the peroxisome, the mitochondria or the nucleus in transgenic mice, reduced oxidative damage, hydrogen peroxide production, and delayed the development of cardiac pathology and cataract formation along with an average increase of 5.5 months in the life span [33]. The observation that long-lived animals have lower levels of antioxidant enzymes was explained as being due to a lower rate of production of oxygen radicals [34].

Interestingly, some of the studies in rodents did not produce the expected results. For example, the administration of antioxidants [35], or over expression of CuZn SOD and catalase in mice [36], or SOD in rats [37], did not increase their life spans. In rodents, one reason for the lack of additional protective effects, which are normally associated with an increase in antioxidants, could be their ability to synthesize vitamin C [38], which might already be providing the required protection. This was verified by knocking out the vitamin C synthesizing enzyme, L-gluconolactone oxidase (GLO) in mice, which then have to depend on dietary vitamin C [39]. GLO knockout mice had damaged aortic walls when they were fed a diet low in vitamin C, which underlined the importance of the constitutive antioxidant function of vitamin C in rodents [39]. Thus, studies in rodents do not provide unequivocal support for the free radical theory of aging [40].

Another way of increasing free radical production and oxidative stress is by increasing total caloric intake, which can be easily done be feeding an excess of glucose. A correlation between life span and dietary caloric intake was reported in rats and mice by McCay *et al.* [41]. One quantitative estimate was provided in the study by Weindruch and Walford [42] who showed that a 40% reduction in dietary caloric intake extended maximum life span by one third. A high dietary caloric intake causes an increased rate of DNA damage [43], due to a high metabolic rate which in turn results in higher amounts of superoxide anion, hydrogen peroxide and hydroxyl radical formation [44].

5. Methylglyoxal

Chemically, MG, or pyruvaldehyde, is a highly reactive electrophilic α,β-dicarbonyl compound [45, 46] (Fig. 1). MG has been proposed to be formed mainly during glycolysis, through spontaneous nonenzymatic transformation of triose phosphates [45, 47-49] (Fig. 2). MG synthase has been proposed to convert the triose phosphate intermediate, dihydroxyacetone phosphate (DHAP), into MG, especially when inadequate inorganic phosphate is available [50, 51]. Other sources of MG, which are believed to produce lower amounts of MG, include intermediates of protein and fatty acid metabolism, such as aminoacetone produced from L-threonine and glycine [52, 53], and acetone [54, 55], respectively (Fig. 2). Semicarbazide-sensitive amine oxidase (SSAO) catalyzes the breakdown of aminoacetone [52, 55, 56], while acetone and acetol mono-oxygenase (AMO) converts acetone to acetol and acetol to MG, respectively [54] (Fig. 2). SSAO is found in substantial amounts in the vascular smooth muscle cells and the plasma [55].

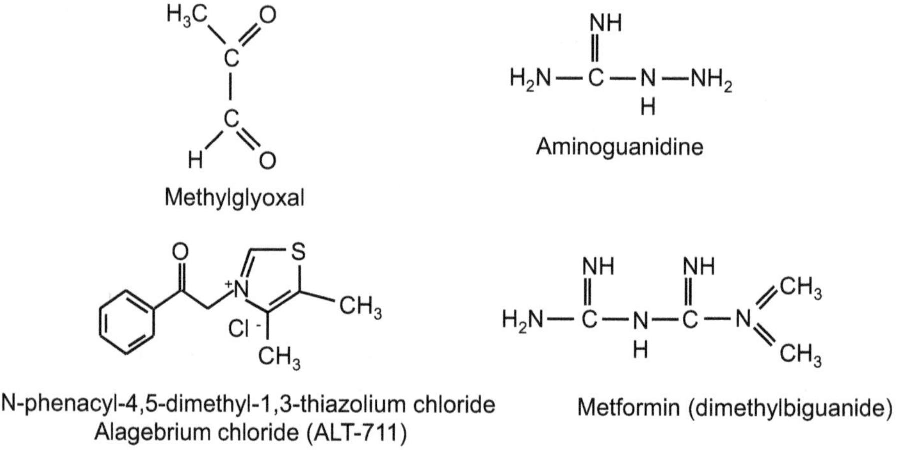

Fig. 1. Structure of methylglyoxal (MG) and three compounds with an ability to bind MG or inhibit the formation of advanced glycation endproducts (AGEs) or break formed AGEs. These compounds are discussed in this review.

After MG is formed, it is rapidly degraded to D-lactic acid by the highly efficient and ubiquitous glyoxalase system, which consists of two key enzymes, glyoxalase I (lactoylglutathione lyase) and glyoxalase II (hydroxyacylglutathione hydrolase) [57-59] (Fig. 2). Reduced glutathione (GSH) plays a key role by binding MG and presenting it to glyoxalase I. Thus, adequate availability of GSH is important in keeping MG levels low in the body. For this reason enzymes involved in the synthesis and recycling of GSH, such as glutathione peroxidase and glutathione reductase are also important in the metabolism of MG [60-62].

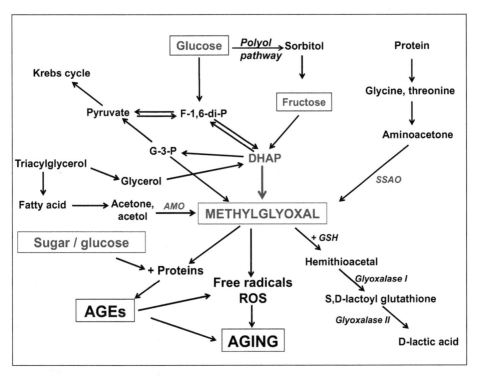

Fig. 2. A schematic of key sources and steps of methylglyoxal (MG) formation from intermediates of glucose, protein and fat metabolism, and its degradation by the glyoxalase enzymes. Abbreviations: AGEs – advanced glycation endproducts; AMO – amine oxidase; DHAP – dihydroxyacetone phosphate; FA – fatty acid; F-1-P – fructose-1-phosphate; F-1,6-di-P – fructose-1,6-diphosphate; F-6-P – fructose-6-phosphate; G-3-P – glyceraldehyde-3-phosphate; G-6-P – glucose-6-phosphate; ROS – reactive oxygen species; SSAO – semicarbazide-sensitive acetone/acetol mono-oxygenase; GSH, reduced glutathione.

Despite the efficient glyoxalase system, MG levels can increase significantly in the plasma and different organs such as the aorta and the kidneys [61, 63-66]. We have shown that MG levels are elevated in the plasma, aorta and kidney of fructose-fed Sprague-Dawley rats and spontaneously hypertensive rats (SHR) [61, 63-65]. Patients with type 1 and type 2 diabetes have 2-6 fold higher plasma levels of MG compared to healthy people [67, 68]. MG possibly plays a role in the pathogenesis of insulin resistance and type 2 diabetes as shown by several *in vitro* [69-71], and by our recent *in vivo* study in acute [66] and chronic MG-treated

Sprague-Dawley rats [72]. Elevated MG levels are linked to the development of micro-vascular complications of diabetes such as retinopathy and nephropathy, and other conditions such as atherosclerosis and neurodegenerative diseases [73-77]. MG levels are high in the cerebrospinal fluid of patients with Alzheimer's disease [76].

6. Advanced glycation endproducts

Unwanted chemical modification of physiologic constituent molecules of the body, which leads to the formation of harmful chemical entities, seems to be an unavoidable part of metabolic processes of the body. One type of modification, known as glycation, a nonenzymatic reaction, is a serious hazard of excess glucose availability in the body. The chemical interaction leading to the formation of AGEs starts when a reducing sugar condenses with the amino groups of proteins at their N terminus or on lysyl side chains (ε-amino groups) [78]. This nonenzymatic glycation involves a series of post-translational modifications. Glycation begins with the aldehyde or the ketone carbonyl group of the sugar combining with the protein to form an unstable aldimine intermediate or a Schiff base. Later on the Schiff base undergoes an Amadori rearrangement to form a stable Amadori product, a 1-amino-1-deoxyfructose derivative with a stable ketoamine linkage, which can get cyclized to form a ring structure [78-80]. The Amadori product can undergo oxidation, degradation or rearrangement and form AGEs, a heterogenous group of products. Auto oxidation of glucose (Wolff pathway) [81] or of the Schiff bases (Namiki pathway) [82] can lead to formation of reactive diacrbonyls, but these pathways which are readily observed at high glucose concentrations *in vitro*, are not predominant *in vivo* [83]. The Maillard reaction, also known as the "browning reaction", involves oxidation of the glycated product which forms a brown coloured product. Glucose, fructose and glucose-6-phosphate are all involved in glycation, albeit at different rates of reaction with glucose, the most important contributor, reacting at a comparatively slower rate than the other two [6]. Increased glucose levels, as seen in diabetic patients, causes more AGEs formation than in healthy people. These AGEs affect the normal function of several proteins and enzymes, and are responsible for aging [74, 80] and the complications of diabetes such as nephropathy and retinopathy [79]. Another way by which the glycation reaction causes damage is through the formation of reactive α-dicarbonyl compounds, such as MG, glyoxal and 3-deoxyglucosone (3-DG), when the sugar molecule undergoes fragmentation [78].

MG can also cause AGEs formation [78, 79]. In fact, MG and two other dicarbonyl metabolic intermediates, 3-DG and glyoxal, are believed to be major sources of intracellular and plasma AGEs formation [79, 84, 85], which are commonly implicated in the aging process. Any MG which is not degraded by the glyoxalase system or aldose reductase, reacts non-enzymatically with arginine or lysine residues of proteins [45] to form irreversible AGEs. This glycation is not random, but it depends on the structural configuration and (or) physical locations of the target proteins [86, 87]. The AGEs produced by the reaction between MG and arginine are hydroimidazolone Nε-(5-hydro-5-methyl-4-imidazolon-2-yl)-ornithine and argpyrimidine [88], whereas the AGE, Nε-carboxyethyllysine (CEL) [89, 90] is formed when MG reacts with lysine. Further crosslinking of these AGEs produces fluorescent products such as pentosidine and cross-line, and non-fluorescent ones such as argpyrimidine, methylglyoxal-lysine dimer (MOLD), glyoxal-lysine dimer (GOLD) and imidazolones [91, 92]. The presence of these AGEs can be detected immunohistochemically in tissues [93].

7. Methylglyoxal, AGEs, oxidative stress and aging

The damage inflicted by oxidative stress and the formation of intracellular AGEs likely contribute to cellular aging. From this point of view, both increased MG and AGEs would cause accelerated cellular aging. MG would be a double-edged sword because it is a potent inducer of oxidative stress [17, 62, 94, 95], as discussed below, and it is a major precursor of AGEs formation. AGEs also induce oxidative stress.

8. Methylglyoxal and oxidative stress

The role of MG in inducing oxidative stress is well established [17]. Several studies have helped to develop an integrated view of the multiple pathways activated by MG to increase oxidative stress (Fig. 3). The reader is referred to our earlier review on MG and oxidative stress [17]. MG increases the formation of superoxide [94, 96-99], hydrogen peroxide and peroxynitrite [94, 95, 98, 100], proinflammatory cytokines, such as interleukin 1β (IL-1β) [101], interleukin-6 (IL-6), interleukin-8 (IL-8) and tumor necrosis factor-α (TNF-α) [67, 101], in different cell types such as VSMCs [62, 94, 95], endothelial cells [102], rat kidney mesangial cells [97], rat hepatocytes [100], neutrophils [67, 98], platelets [99], cultured neural cells from rat hippocampus [101], cultured cortical neurons [103], and SH-SY5Y neuroblastoma cells [104].

MG has been shown to increase the activity of several prooxidant enzymes such as NADPH oxidase [94, 97] (Fig. 3), p38 MAPK [98, 102], and increase the of expression of JNK and PPAR-α [104].

Excess superoxide can react with nitric oxide (NO) to form peroxynitrite (ONOO-) [105] (Fig. 3). Peroxynitrite is a strong oxidant and nitrating agent. Because of its oxidizing properties, peroxynitrite can damage a wide range of molecules including DNA and proteins in cells [105].

Besides directly increasing free radical production, MG can increase oxidative stress by reducing antioxidants (Fig. 3) such as GSH [104, 106, 107], glutathione peroxidase [108], glutathione reductase [60, 62, 108, 109], and manganese superoxide dismutase (MnSOD) [96], in different cells such as erythrocytes [106, 107], VSMCs [62, 96], and endothelial cells [109]. Reduced antioxidants in turn impair the detoxification of MG, increase its half-life and set up a vicious cycle to cause further oxidant damage. Glutathione peroxidase removes hydrogen peroxide with the help of GSH which in turn is converted to oxidized glutathione (GSSG). Glutathione reductase recycles GSSG to GSH [62, 110] (Fig. 3).

An increased production of ROS was also observed in monocytes treated with MG-modified albumin [111]. Thus, MG induced thrombosis and inflammation by activating monocytes, induced apoptosis of neutrophils, and caused platelet-neutrophil aggregates [112].

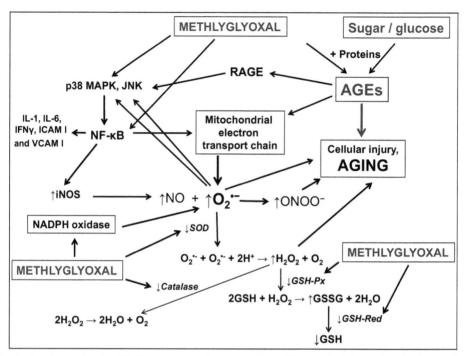

Fig. 3. A schematic of oxidative stress pathways activated by methylglyoxal and advanced glycation endproducts and their implication in aging. Abbreviations: AGEs, advanced glycation end products; GSH-Px, glutathione peroxidase; GSH-Red, glutathione reductase; GSH, reduced glutathione; GSSG, oxidized glutathione; H_2O_2, hydrogen peroxide; ICAM 1, intercellular adhesion molecule 1; IFNγ, interferon γ; IL1, interleukin 1; JNK, JUN N-terminal kinase; MG, methylglyoxal; NF-κB, nuclear factor-kappaB; NO, nitric oxide; $O_2^{\bullet-}$, superoxide anion; $ONOO^-$, peroxynitrite; p38 MAPK, p38 mitogen activated protein kinase; RAGE, receptor for advanced glycation endproduct; SOD, superoxide dismutase; VCAM 1, vascular cell adhesion molecule 1.

Metabolic activity in the mitochondria is at the centre of the free radical theory of aging. Mitochondria, which are the major sites of ATP and energy production in the cell, also generate about 85% of total intracellular superoxide when electrons escape, mainly from complex I and complex III, and react with oxygen [23, 113-116].

MG increases mitochondrial superoxide production [116, 117]. Treatment of rat aortic VSMCs (A-10 cells) with MG (30 μM) significantly increased mitochondrial superoxide production by 69.9% compared with untreated cells. The AGEs cross-link breaker, alagebrium (50 μM), and SOD mimetic 4-hydroxy-tempo (Tempol, 500 μM) significantly decreased MG-induced mitochondrial superoxide production by 57% and 85.8%, respectively. Mitochondrial nitrotyrosine formation was also increased by MG [96].

In *in vivo* studies elevated MG levels are associated with increased oxidative stress. For example, we have shown that in 13 wk old SHR with elevated blood pressure, significantly elevated plasma and aortic MG levels are associated with increased levels of superoxide, and significantly reduced GSH levels, glutathione peroxidase, and glutathione reductase activities, compared with age-matched Wistar Kyoto (WKY) rats [61]. Similarly, in diabetes mellitus and hypertension, increased MG levels are associated with increased oxidative stress [61, 65, 67, 68, 118].

An excess of MG, CEL and CML indicate carbonyl overload and are associated with oxidative stress [73, 79, 119-123].

Glycated proteins and AGEs also induce oxidative stress (Fig. 3) through several mechanisms. AGEs induce production of cytokines and growth factors [124-130]. AGEs bind to the receptor for AGEs (RAGE) and scavenger receptors to induce oxidative stress in various cells including VSMCs, endothelial cells, and mononuclear phagocytes [128, 131]. In endothelial cells AGEs increase expression of vascular cell adhesion molecule-1 (VCAM-1), intercellular adhesion molecule-1 (ICAM-1), and increase activity of NF-κB to increase oxidative stress [126, 132].

9. Methylglyoxal and aging

The accumulation of AGEs in extracellular tissue proteins, such as the basement membrane and matrix proteins of blood vessels and skin, is a well known phenomenon characteristic of aging and age-related diseases. Several studies demonstrate aging associated increase in AGEs. Thus, accumulation of AGEs in the vessel walls results in a gradual loss of elasticity, which makes older subjects more susceptible to cardiovascular diseases [133, 134]. MG-induced AGEs, such as CEL and CML, increased with age in human lens and cause cataract formation [90]. In a study on 172 subjects serum levels of CML, 8-isoprostanes and C-reactive protein, which are markers of oxidative stress, were higher in elderly people (>60 years old) compared with younger people (<45 years old) [135]. One reason why AGEs accumulate during the aging process could be due to an age-related decrease in antioxidant enzymes. Thus, Mailankot et al. [136] reported that the activity and expression of glyoxalase I protein, which is involved in MG degradation, decreased with age in the anterior epithelial cells of human lens, which causes an accumulation of MG. Similarly, an age-dependent decrease in catalase activity in the skin may be responsible for elevated MG and peroxynitrite production [137].

However, it is doubtful whether extracellular AGEs accumulation plays a causative role in aging. On the other hand AGEs formation inside the cell, such as AGE-nucleotides in DNA, may contribute to cellular senescence [6, 60, 74, 80]. DNA integrity is an important determinant of lifespan and errors in DNA repair would lead to substitutions, deletions, insertions, and transpositions of nucleotides, with increased risk of carcinogenesis and reduced life span. Animals with a longer lifespan and more efficient DNA repair have delayed carcinogenesis [80]. In this regard MG-induced DNA damage can have a more direct effect on aging.

Studies directly implicating MG in the aging process are very few and this is one area where there is a knowledge gap. The study by Morcos et al in the worm *C. elegans* highlights the role of MG, glyoxalase I and MG-induced ROS formation in aging and life span [138]. They showed that the activity of glyoxalase I was markedly reduced with age resulting in accumulation of MG-derived adducts and oxidative stress markers, which further inhibited the expression and the activity of glyoxalase I. Over expression of glyoxalase I decreased MG-induced modification of mitochondrial proteins and ROS production, and prolonged the lifespan of C. *elegans*; whereas CeGly knock-out produced the opposite effect [138].

Scheckhuber et al. studied the degradation of MG by the glyoxalase system enzymes and its effect on growth and lifespan in filamentous ascomycete and a model of aging, Podospora anserine (*P. anserina*) [139]. Using genetic manipulation of the two enzymes of the glyoxalase system, they found that up-regulation of both components of the glyoxalase system was effective in increasing lifespan in P. anserina.

Oxidative stress-induced cellular senescence was demonstrated in the study by Sejeresen and Rattan [140]. They treated human skin fibroblasts with MG (400 µM), or glyoxal (1.0 mM), and found the appearance of various senescent phenotypes within three days. These phenotypes showed growth arrest, had increased hydrogen peroxide and the glyoxal-induced AGE, Nε-carboxymethyl lysine (CML) protein levels, and altered SOD and catalase antioxidant enzyme activities [140]. Sejeresen and Rattan proposed this model to study cellular senescence *in vitro* [140].

In this review we have highlighted some important facts that oxidative stress is a major factor in the cellular and whole body aging processes, AGEs are strongly associated with aging and MG is a major precursor of AGEs formation, and both MG and AGEs are potent inducers of oxidative stress. Based on these facts, it is highly likely that MG may have a major role in the aging process through induction of oxidative stress as depicted in the scheme in Fig. 3. In fact, elevated MG levels may be responsible for causing accelerated aging in many tissues and organs of the cardiovascular system, nervous system, and other systems of the human body. A strategy to prevent aging should include targeting MG by reducing excessive formation, inhibit AGEs formation, and remove excessively formed MG and AGEs from the body.

10. Anti-MG and anti-AGEs compounds

The deleterious effects of MG and AGEs can be prevented by compounds that can do one or all of the following: (i) bind and neutralize reactive aldehydes, especially MG, (ii) prevent the formation of AGEs, (iii) neutralize formed AGEs, (iv) break down formed AGEs.

Considering these multiple ways of preventing the effects of MG or AGEs these compounds will be termed as "anti-MG" or "anti-AGE". Unfortunately, specific anti-MG or anti-AGE compounds are not yet available. The ones available are non-specific and have one or more other effects, which limits their usefulness. A number of the available compounds happen to have anti-MG as well as anti-AGE effects.

The possible sites at which anti-AGEs and anti-MG drugs can work are shown in Fig. 4, which outlines the various stages of AGEs formation.

Site 1. The first step in glycation is the binding of a sugar to the free amino groups of a protein. Drugs that bind to the amino group of proteins, such as aspirin, can prevent the binding of the sugar to the amino group. This group of compounds is likely to produce non-specific effects.

Site 2. Compounds can be used to bind aldose and ketose sugars to neutralize them and prevent them from reacting with proteins. E.g. Aminoguanidine reacts with the carbonyl group of glucose and prevents AGEs formation.

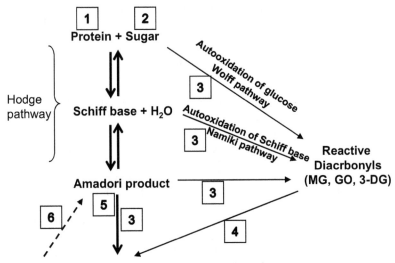

Fig. 4. Stages of formation of advanced glycation endproducts (AGEs) from glycation of proteins. Nonenzymatic glycation of protein leads to reversible formation of Schiff bases, which lead to further reversible formation of Amadori adducts and ultimate formation of stable irreversible AGEs. Solid vertical arrows show these steps which form the classical Hodge pathway of AGEs formation. Auto oxidation of glucose (Wolff pathway) or of the Schiff base (Namiki pathway) forms reactive dicarbonyls such as methylglyoxal (MG), glyoxal (GO) or 3-deoxyglucosone (3-DG) which is mostly seen *in vitro*, rather than *in vivo*. The dicarbonyls, which are also formed from other metabolic pathways, also contribute significantly to AGEs formation, as explained in the text. The various sites at which anti-AGEs and anti-MG compounds can act are indicated by numbers and discussed in the text. Based on the scheme proposed by Khalifah et al. [83]

Site 3. AGEs and reactive aldehydes also generate reactive oxygen species which adds to their damaging effects [17, 141, 142]. Antioxidants such as vitamin C or E [143] and metal chelators such as penicillamine [144] can be used to quench ROS and metal ions.

Site 4. Reactive aldehydes such as MG, glyoxal, glycoaldehyde and glucosones, which are formed during nutrient metabolism and AGEs formation, are a major source of AGEs formation. Reactive aldehydes can be neutralized by compounds such as aminoguanidine [145, 146] and metformin [147, 148].

Site 5. Amadori adducts, formed in the intermediate stages of AGEs formation can either be quenched by compounds such as aminoguanidine, or degraded enzymatically by enzymes such as amadoriase and human fructosamine-3-kinase, which belong to this group [149, 150]. Amadoriases have not been detected in higher organisms [151, 152].

Site 6. The final group of compounds acts on formed AGEs and are therefore, known as AGE breakers or cross-link breakers. E.g. phenacylthiazolium bromide (PTB) [153] and alagebrium (previously known as ALT-711), which are thiazolium compounds. AGEs which do not have cross-links such as pentosidine [154], GOLD and MOLD [155] will not be affected by these drugs.

Some of the more common compounds with anti-MG or anti-AGEs effects are described below.

Aminoguanidine is one of the popular and widely used AGEs inhibitor [145] and MG scavenger. Despite being a guanidine derivative it shares many common properties with hydrazine and is classified as a hydrazine [156]. As described above, aminoguanidine acts at site 2 as well as site 4 (Fig. 4) meaning that it prevents AGEs formation by combining with the carbonyl group of glucose as well as by scavenging reactive dicarbonyls formed during various metabolic processes [146]. The inhibitory effect of aminoguanidine is mainly at the Amadori stage [83]. Aminoguanidine is not a specific AGEs inhibitor or MG scavenger and it has other actions. Aminoguanidine potently inhibits histaminases [157, 158] and prevents deamination of histamine and putrescine. Aminoguanidine also inhibits nitric oxide synthase (NOS) [159, 160] and prevents the formation of nitric oxide (NO), a dynamic signaling molecule in the body [161], from L-arginine. Aminoguanidine also binds to the enzyme S-adenosylmethionine decarboxylase and increases synthesis of polyamines such as spermidine and spermine from ornithine [162]. Aminoguanidine can also bind pyridoxal and cause vitamin B6 deficiency, which in turn can result in adverse reactions to aminoguanidine [163]. A number of *in vitro* and *in vivo* studies have described the inhibitory effects of aminoguanidine on AGEs formation [145, 146, 164-167]. The doses used *in vivo* range from 25 mg/kg/day [145, 166] to 50 mg/kg/day [165] and up to 100 mg/kg/day [167]. Thus, aminoguanidine is far from an ideal MG scavenger and AGEs inhibitor. In clinical trials aminoguanidine was found to be too toxic for use in patients. Two double-masked, multiple-dose, placebo-controlled, randomized clinical trials, ACTION I and ACTION II [168, 169] investigated the therapeutic potential of aminoguanidine in preventing the progression of renal damage in patients with diabetic nephropathy. The ACTION I trial involving 690 participants did not show a statistically significant difference between the placebo group and the combined aminoguanidine dose groups, even though patients treated with aminoguanidine showed a tendency of having a lower risk of doubling of serum creatinine [168]. Due to safety concerns and an apparent lack of efficacy, the External Safety Monitoring Committee for the ACTION II trial involving 599 participants recommended early termination [169]. Patients with diabetes may have impaired red blood cell-deformability, which could cause microvascular and kidney damage. A one year trial with aminoguanidine and erythropoietin on 12 patients on dialysis restored red blood cell-deformability to near-normal levels, an effect attributed to inhibition of AGEs formation by aminoguanidine [170]. As mentioned earlier the toxic effects of aminoguanidine have limited its therapeutic potential. For example, like hydrazine, aminoguanidine may be associated with drug-induced systemic lupus erythematosus and abnormal liver function tests, and it can cause flu-like syndromes and vasculitis [169]. Aminoguanidine can also cause damage to DNA through hydroxyl- and hydrogen peroxide-formation in the presence of Fe^{+3} [171].

Metformin is an oral dimethylbiguanide antihyperglycemic agent, which can also inhibit AGEs formation [172], through its action in the post-Amadori stages [83, 173]. Metformin has also been proposed to have a MG scavenging effect attributed to its guanidino group, which binds with MG to form an inactive product, triazepinone [147, 148, 174, 175]. The MG-scavenging effect of metformin resulted in significantly reduced elevated MG levels in type 2 diabetes patients treated with high doses of metformin, between 1,500 and 2,500 mg/day [172]. We have shown that fructose-fed Sprague-Dawley rats had significantly elevated serum MG and blood pressure, and increased levels of MG, hydrogen peroxide and the MG-derived AGE, CEL, in the aorta, all of which were attenuated by metformin [65]. Metformin has been proposed to protect against MG-induced increased atherogenicity of low density lipoprotein (LDL) [176]. The use of metformin as a MG scavenger and AGEs inhibitor is limited, and hopefully more studies showing its anti-MG, anti-AGEs effectiveness will promote its use for this purpose. Metformin can be considered to have a good therapeutic potential in this regard since it is already in clinical use for type 2 diabetes as an insulin sensitizing agent.

Pioglitazone, a thiazolidinedione, is a peroxisome proliferator-activated receptor gamma (PPARγ) agonist which acts as an insulin sensitizer and is used in type 2 diabetes. Pioglitazone has been proposed to have anti-AGEs effect by inhibiting glycation, AGEs formation and protein cross-linking [177, 178]. Studies employing pioglitazone as an anti-MG or anti-AGEs compound are not forthcoming and more evidence is needed to make definitive statements about the therapeutic potential of pioglitazone in this regard.

N-acetylcysteine (NAC) is a MG scavenging and antioxidant compound [179, 180]. There are good reasons for using NAC as an anti-MG compound: NAC can increase GSH levels [181], which is an efficient MG scavenger and antioxidant [70, 179, 180], NAC is a cysteine containing thiol compound and MG binds with high affinity to cysteine [180, 181], and NAC is already used clinically for other conditions such as acetaminophen overdose [179, 181]. More studies employing NAC as an anti-MG drug should provide interesting results and may help to establish the potential of NAC in this regard.

A widely used class of antihypertensive drugs has been proposed to have anti-AGE effects. Angiotensin receptor blockers (ARBs) and angiotensin converting enzyme inhibitors (ACEIs) have been shown to protect against kidney damage, an effect claimed to be independent of their blood pressure lowering action [182-185], but proposed to be due to an anti-AGE effect. Clinical trials evaluating AGEs lowering effects of ARBs and ACEIs at blood pressure lowering doses can add to the therapeutic utility of these drugs.

A number of compounds have been investigated for anti-AGE effects in limited studies, but have not been widely used as such in experimental studies in animals or humans. These compounds include the cycloxygenase inhibitors, aspirin [186-188], ibuprofen [189], diclofenac [190], xanthine derivative, pentoxifylline [191, 192], which is used for claudication in peripheral vascular disease, metal chelators, D-penicillamine [144] and desferoxamine [83, 144], thiamine pyrophosphate and pyridoxamine [193-195]. Many more studies are necessary for these compounds in order to draw definitive conclusions about their anti-MG or anti-AGE effects.

A number of deglycating enzymes have been discovered, especially in microorganisms, which remove the sugar bound to the protein molecule, and possibly provide these bacteria with energy substrates derived from glycated products [196]. These enzymes, known as amadoriases, include fructosylamine oxidases [197, 198], fructosamine-3-kinase [149, 150], fructoselysine-6-kinase [199], fructoselysine-3-epimerase (FrlC) [200], and glucoselysine-6-

phosphate deglycase [201]. The use of these enzymes or development of stable analogues for deglycation therapy remains speculative .

A number of AGE inhibitors were synthesized and screened for their AGEs inhibitory effects by Rahbar et al. [173, 202, 203]. These are derivatives of aryl ureido and aryl carboxaminido phenoxy isobutyric acids and were derived from some known AGEs inhibitors. These compounds act at multiple stages of the AGEs formation process. Some of these compounds have AGEs breaking properties. More studies are needed for these compounds to establish their specificity and safety for therapeutic use.

11. AGEs breakers

The AGEs which have undergone cross-linking are very stable products and their concentration, especially in long-lived matrix proteins, increases with age. AGEs inhibitors are ineffective against formed AGEs and compounds which can break the cross-links are required. The AGEs breaker compounds can prove invaluable to slow down the aging process, and in the treatment of established stages of diseases such as diabetes, Alzheimer's, atherosclerosis and rheumatoid arthritis.

The first AGEs breaking compound reported was phenacylthiazolium bromide (PTB) in 1996. PTB breaks the covalent cross-links of AGEs [204]. Administration of PTB (10 mg/kg/day, intraperitoneal for 4 wks) reduced the amount of IgG bound to the surface of red blood cells in diabetic rats [153]. However, PTB is not stable.

The search for a stable derivative of PTB resulted in the synthesis of ALT 711 (4,5-dimethylthiazolium) [205]. ALT 711 (now known as alagebrium) reduced arterial stiffness in streptozotocin-induced diabetic rats [205]. In aging rats, ALA (10 mg/kg for 16 weeks) also increased glutathione peroxidase and superoxide dismutase activities and reduced oxidative stress [206]. Alagebrium improved impaired cardiovascular function in older rhesus monkeys [207]. Alagebrium demonstrated promising results and a good safety profile in phase 2 clinical trials. In a clinical study involving 93 subjects, 50 yrs and older, with evidence of vessel stiffness (pulse pressure ≥60 mm Hg, systolic blood pressure ≥140 mm Hg, and large artery compliance ≤1.25 mL/mm Hg), alagebrium (210 mg, once per day for 56 days) improved arterial compliance [208]. In another group of 13 patients aged 65±2 yrs with systolic hypertension (systolic blood pressure > 140 mmHg, diastolic blood pressure <90 mm Hg), alagebrium (210 mg/kg twice a day for 8 weeks) reduced vascular fibrosis and markers of inflammation [209]. Alagebrium (administered for 16 weeks) decreased left ventricular mass and improved left ventricular diastolic filling in another trial in 23 patients with diastolic heart failure [210, 211].

However, in a recent study [212] involving 102 patients (aged 62 ± 11 years) with heart failure (left ventricular ejection fraction (LVEF ≤0.45), alagebrium (400 mg/day/36 wks) did not improve exercise tolerance and systolic dysfunction, and no changes were observed in a number of secondary endpoints. Thus, the authors could not verify the claims that alagebrium has beneficial effects in systolic heart failure [212].

Alagebrium has been reported to be a weak inhibitor of thiamine diphosphokinase and is unlikely to interfere with thiamine metabolism at therapeutic concentrations [213]. However, the authors urge caution when new AGE-crosslink breakers based on thiamine are designed, to make sure they are not potent inhibitors of thiamine diphosphokinase.

In the studies described above alagebrium has been studied mainly for its chronic effects on AGEs as an AGEs breaker. We investigated whether alagebrium also has acute preventive effects against the reactive dicarbonyl, MG, in 12 wk old male Sprague-Dawley rats [66]. Our results showed that alagebrium also has acute (< 6 h) MG scavenging ability [66]. AGEs are formed slowly over a time ranging from 24 h to up to 7 days and more. Therefore, the attenuation of MG-induced acute effects (seen within 6 h of MG administration) is most likely due to scavenging of MG by alagebrium. Thus, alagebrium significantly attenuated the significant increases in MG levels in the plasma, and different organs (measured 2 h after administration), and also attenuated MG-induced impaired glucose tolerance and the reduced insulin-stimulated glucose uptake by adipose tissue. In an *in vitro* assay in which MG (10 μM) was incubated with or without alagebrium (100 μM) for different times at 37° C, alagebrium significantly reduced the amount of detectable MG [66]. Our results strongly indicate an acute MG scavenging effect of alagebrium which can add to its AGEs breaking ability. More direct evidence of interaction of alagebrium and MG using mass spectrometry would be very useful. We have also recently shown that alagebrium significantly attenuated the deleterious effects of chronic MG administration for 4 wks on glucose tolerance and pancreatic islet β-cell function in male Sprague-Dawley rats [72].

In conclusion, MG and AGEs are very likely to be involved in the initiation and or progression of the aging process. Commonly available pharmacological compounds to investigate these roles of MG and AGEs, such as aminoguanidine, are non-specific, whereas some of the newer compounds appear promising in inhibiting AGEs formation at multiple steps in the pathway in *in vitro* studies. However, more *in vivo* studies are required before their therapeutic potential can be established. A more dedicated effort is necessary to identify newer anti-MG and anti-AGEs compounds which are more specific and safer before more can be done about their therapeutic potential.

12. References

[1] Hayflick, L. The limited in vitro lifetime of human diploid cell strains. *Exp. Cell Res.* 37: 614-636; 1965.

[2] Kovacic, J. C.; Moreno, P.; Hachinski, V.; Nabel, E. G.; Fuster, V. Cellular senescence, vascular disease, and aging: Part 1 of a 2-part review. *Circulation* 123:1650-1660; 2011.

[3] Kovacic, J. C.; Moreno, P.; Nabel, E. G.; Hachinski, V.; Fuster, V. Cellular senescence, vascular disease, and aging: Part 2 of a 2-part review: Clinical vascular disease in the elderly. *Circulation* 123:1900-1910; 2011.

[4] Matthews, C.; Gorenne, I.; Scott, S.; Figg, N.; Kirkpatrick, P.; Ritchie, A.; Goddard, M.; Bennett, M. Vascular smooth muscle cells undergo telomere-based senescence in human atherosclerosis: Effects of telomerase and oxidative stress. *Circ. Res.* 99:156-164; 2006.

[5] Campisi, J.; d'Adda di Fagagna, F. Cellular senescence: When bad things happen to good cells. *Nat. Rev. Mol. Cell Biol.* 8:729-740; 2007.

[6] Bucala, R.; Model, P.; Cerami, A. Modification of DNA by reducing sugars: A possible mechanism for nucleic acid aging and age-related dysfunction in gene expression. *Proc. Natl. Acad. Sci. U. S. A.* 81:105-109; 1984.

[7] Beckman, K. B.; Ames, B. N. The free radical theory of aging matures. *Physiol. Rev.*78:547-581; 1998.

[8] Finkel, T.; Holbrook, N. J. Oxidants, oxidative stress and the biology of ageing. *Nature* 408:239-247; 2000.

[9] Barja, G.; Herrero, A. Oxidative damage to mitochondrial DNA is inversely related to maximum life span in the heart and brain of mammals. *FASEB J.* 14:312-318; 2000.

[10] Mandavilli, B. S.; Santos, J. H.; Van Houten, B. Mitochondrial DNA repair and aging. *Mutat. Res.* 509:127-151; 2002.

[11] Vina, J.; Borras, C.; Miquel, J. Theories of ageing. *IUBMB Life*59:249-254; 2007.

[12] Weinert, B. T.; Timiras, P. S. Invited review: Theories of aging. *J. Appl. Physiol.* 95:1706-1716; 2003.

[13] Semsei, I. On the nature of aging. *Mech. Ageing Dev.* 117:93-108; 2000.

[14] Medvedev, Z. A. An attempt at a rational classification of theories of ageing. *Biol. Rev. Camb. Philos. Soc.* 65:375-398; 1990.

[15] [Anonymous]. Max rubner--1854-1932. energy physiologist. *JAMA* 194:86-87; 1965.

[16] Commoner, B.; Townsend, J.; Pake, G. E. Free radicals in biological materials. *Nature* 174:689-691; 1954.

[17] Desai, K. M.; Wu, L. Free radical generation by methylglyoxal in tissues. *Drug Metabol. Drug Interact.* 23:151-173; 2008.

[18] McCord, J. M. The evolution of free radicals and oxidative stress. *Am. J. Med.* 108:652-659; 2000.

[19] Cadenas, E. Biochemistry of oxygen toxicity. *Annu. Rev. Biochem.* 58:79-110; 1989.

[20] Halliwell, B. Antioxidant defence mechanisms: From the beginning to the end (of the beginning). *Free Radic. Res.* 31:261-272; 1999.

[21] Halliwell, B. Reactive oxygen species in living systems: Source, biochemistry, and role in human disease. *Am. J. Med.* 91:14S-22S; 1991.

[22] Gilca, M.; Stoian, I.; Atanasiu, V.; Virgolici, B. The oxidative hypothesis of senescence. *J. Postgrad. Med.* 53:207-213; 2007.

[23] Harman, D. Aging: A theory based on free radical and radiation chemistry. *J. Gerontol.* 11:298-300; 1956.

[24] McCord, J. M.; Fridovich, I. Superoxide dismutase. an enzymic function for erythrocuprein (hemocuprein). *J. Biol. Chem.* 244:6049-6055; 1969.

[25] Harman, D. Aging: Overview. *Ann. N. Y. Acad. Sci.* 928:1-21; 2001.

[26] Gruber, J.; Schaffer, S.; Halliwell, B. The mitochondrial free radical theory of ageing--where do we stand? *Front. Biosci.* 13:6554-6579; 2008.

[27] Ku, H. H.; Brunk, U. T.; Sohal, R. S. Relationship between mitochondrial superoxide and hydrogen peroxide production and longevity of mammalian species. *Free Radic. Biol. Med.* 15:621-627; 1993.

[28] Herrero, A.; Barja, G. Sites and mechanisms responsible for the low rate of free radical production of heart mitochondria in the long-lived pigeon. *Mech. Ageing Dev.* 98:95-111; 1997.

[29] Johnson, T. E.; Tedesco, P. M.; Lithgow, G. J. Comparing mutants, selective breeding, and transgenics in the dissection of aging processes of caenorhabditis elegans. *Genetica* 91:65-77; 1993.

[30] Larsen, P. L. Aging and resistance to oxidative damage in caenorhabditis elegans. *Proc. Natl. Acad. Sci. U. S. A.* 90:8905-8909; 1993.

[31] Tower, J. Transgenic methods for increasing drosophila life span. *Mech. Ageing Dev.* 118:1-14; 2000.

[32] Arking, R.; Burde, V.; Graves, K.; Hari, R.; Feldman, E.; Zeevi, A.; Soliman, S.; Saraiya, A.; Buck, S.; Vettraino, J.; Sathrasala, K.; Wehr, N.; Levine, R. L. Forward and reverse selection for longevity in drosophila is characterized by alteration of antioxidant gene expression and oxidative damage patterns. *Exp. Gerontol.* 35:167-185; 2000.

[33] Schriner, S. E.; Linford, N. J.; Martin, G. M.; Treuting, P.; Ogburn, C. E.; Emond, M.; Coskun, P. E.; Ladiges, W.; Wolf, N.; Van Remmen, H.; Wallace, D. C.; Rabinovitch, P. S. Extension of murine life span by overexpression of catalase targeted to mitochondria. *Science* 308:1909-1911; 2005.

[34] Perez-Campo, R.; Lopez-Torres, M.; Cadenas, S.; Rojas, C.; Barja, G. The rate of free radical production as a determinant of the rate of aging: Evidence from the comparative approach. *J. Comp. Physiol. [B].*168:149-158; 1998.

[35] Huang, T. T.; Carlson, E. J.; Gillespie, A. M.; Shi, Y.; Epstein, C. J. Ubiquitous overexpression of CuZn superoxide dismutase does not extend life span in mice. *J. Gerontol. A Biol. Sci. Med. Sci.* 55:B5-9; 2000.

[36] Perez, V. I.; Van Remmen, H.; Bokov, A.; Epstein, C. J.; Vijg, J.; Richardson, A. The overexpression of major antioxidant enzymes does not extend the lifespan of mice. *Aging Cell.* 8:73-75; 2009.

[37] Mehlhorn, R. J. *Oxidants and antioxidanrs in aging. in: Physiological basis of aging and geriatrics.* Boca Raton, FL:CRC; 2003.

[38] Linster, C. L.; Van Schaftingen, E. Vitamin C. biosynthesis, recycling and degradation in mammals. *FEBS J.* 274:1-22; 2007.

[39] Maeda, N.; Hagihara, H.; Nakata, Y.; Hiller, S.; Wilder, J.; Reddick, R. Aortic wall damage in mice unable to synthesize ascorbic acid. *Proc. Natl. Acad. Sci. U. S. A.* 97:841-846; 2000.

[40] Muller, F. L.; Lustgarten, M. S.; Jang, Y.; Richardson, A.; Van Remmen, H. Trends in oxidative aging theories. *Free Radic. Biol. Med.* 43:477-503; 2007.

[41] McCay, C. M.; Crowell, M. F.; Maynard, L. A. The effect of retarded growth upon the length of life span and upon the ultimate body size. *J. Nutr.* 10:63-79; 1935.

[42] Weindruch, R.; Walford, R. L. *The retardation of aging and disease by dietary restriction.* Springfield IL: Charles C. Thomas.; 1988.

[43] Simic, M. G.; Bertgold, D. S. *Urinary biomarkers of oxidative DNA base damage and human caloric intake. in: Biological effects of dietary restriction.* New York: Springer-Verlag.; 1991.

[44] Szatrowski, T. P.; Nathan, C. F. Production of large amounts of hydrogen peroxide by human tumor cells. *Cancer Res.*51:794-798; 1991.

[45] Thornalley, P. J. Pharmacology of methylglyoxal: Formation, modification of proteins and nucleic acids, and enzymatic detoxification--a role in pathogenesis and antiproliferative chemotherapy. *Gen. Pharmacol.* 27:565-573; 1996.

[46] Kalapos, M. P. Methylglyoxal in living organisms: Chemistry, biochemistry, toxicology and biological implications. *Toxicol. Lett.* 110:145-175; 1999.

[47] Phillips, S. A.; Thornalley, P. J. The formation of methylglyoxal from triose phosphates. investigation using a specific assay for methylglyoxal. *Eur. J. Biochem.* 212:101-105; 1993.

[48] Sato, J.; Wang, Y. M.; van Eys, J. Methylglyoxal formation in rat liver cells. *J. Biol. Chem.* 255:2046-2050; 1980.

[49] Kalapos, M. P. The tandem of free radicals and methylglyoxal. *Chem. Biol. Interact.* 171:251-271; 2008.

[50] Hopper, D. J.; Cooper, R. A. The regulation of escherichia coli methylglyoxal synthase; a new control site in glycolysis? *FEBS Lett.* 13:213-216; 1971.

[51] Ray, S.; Ray, M. Isolation of methylglyoxal synthase from goat liver. *J. Biol. Chem.* 256:6230-6233; 1981.

[52] Lyles, G. A.; Chalmers, J. The metabolism of aminoacetone to methylglyoxal by semicarbazide-sensitive amine oxidase in human umbilical artery. *Biochem. Pharmacol.* 43:1409-1414; 1992.

[53] Deng, Y.; Yu, P. H. Simultaneous determination of formaldehyde and methylglyoxal in urine: Involvement of semicarbazide-sensitive amine oxidase-mediated deamination in diabetic complications. *J. Chromatogr. Sci.* 37:317-322; 1999.

[54] Casazza, J. P.; Felver, M. E.; Veech, R. L. The metabolism of acetone in rat. *J. Biol. Chem.* 259:231-236; 1984.

[55] Yu, P. H.; Wright, S.; Fan, E. H.; Lun, Z. R.; Gubisne-Harberle, D. Physiological and pathological implications of semicarbazide-sensitive amine oxidase. *Biochim. Biophys. Acta* 1647:193-199; 2003.

[56] Lyles, G. A.; Chalmers, J. Aminoacetone metabolism by semicarbazide-sensitive amine oxidase in rat aorta. *Biochem. Pharmacol.* 49:416-419; 1995.

[57] Vander Jagt D.L. *The glyoxalase system. in: Glutathione: Chemical, biochemical and medical aspects - part A.* John Wiley & Sons Inc.; 1989.

[58] Thornalley, P. J. Glyoxalase I--structure, function and a critical role in the enzymatic defence against glycation. *Biochem. Soc. Trans.* 31:1343-1348; 2003.

[59] Thornalley, P. J. The glyoxalase system in health and disease. *Mol. Aspects Med.* 14:287-371; 1993.

[60] Blakytny, R.; Harding, J. J. Glycation (non-enzymic glycosylation) inactivates glutathione reductase. *Biochem. J.* 288 (Pt 1):303-307; 1992.

[61] Wang, X.; Desai, K.; Chang, T.; Wu, L. Vascular methylglyoxal metabolism and the development of hypertension. *J. Hypertens.* 23:1565-1573; 2005.

[62] Wu, L.; Juurlink, B. H. Increased methylglyoxal and oxidative stress in hypertensive rat vascular smooth muscle cells. *Hypertension* 39:809-814; 2002.

[63] Wang, X.; Chang, T.; Jiang, B.; Desai, K.; Wu, L. Attenuation of hypertension development by aminoguanidine in spontaneously hypertensive rats: Role of methylglyoxal. *Am. J. Hypertens.* 20:629-636; 2007.

[64] Wang, X.; Desai, K.; Clausen, J. T.; Wu, L. Increased methylglyoxal and advanced glycation end products in kidney from spontaneously hypertensive rats. *Kidney Int.* 66:2315-2321; 2004.

[65] Wang, X.; Jia, X.; Chang, T.; Desai, K.; Wu, L. Attenuation of hypertension development by scavenging methylglyoxal in fructose-treated rats. *J. Hypertens.* 26:765-772; 2008.

[66] Dhar, A.; Desai, K. M.; Wu, L. Alagebrium attenuates acute methylglyoxal-induced glucose intolerance in sprague-dawley rats. *Br. J. Pharmacol.* 159:166-175; 2010.

[67] Wang, H.; Meng, Q. H.; Gordon, J. R.; Khandwala, H.; Wu, L. Proinflammatory and proapoptotic effects of methylglyoxal on neutrophils from patients with type 2 diabetes mellitus. *Clin. Biochem.* 40:1232-1239; 2007.

[68] McLellan, A. C.; Thornalley, P. J.; Benn, J.; Sonksen, P. H. Glyoxalase system in clinical diabetes mellitus and correlation with diabetic complications. *Clin. Sci. (Lond)* 87:21-29; 1994.

[69] Jia, X.; Olson, D. J.; Ross, A. R.; Wu, L. Structural and functional changes in human insulin induced by methylglyoxal. *FASEB J.* 20:1555-1557; 2006.

[70] Jia, X.; Wu, L. Accumulation of endogenous methylglyoxal impaired insulin signaling in adipose tissue of fructose-fed rats. *Mol. Cell. Biochem.*306:133-139; 2007.

[71] Riboulet-Chavey, A.; Pierron, A.; Durand, I.; Murdaca, J.; Giudicelli, J.; Van Obberghen, E. Methylglyoxal impairs the insulin signaling pathways independently of the formation of intracellular reactive oxygen species. *Diabetes* 55:1289-1299; 2006.

[72] Dhar, A.; Dhar, I.; Jiang, B.; Desai, K. M.; Wu, L. Chronic methylglyoxal infusion by minipump causes pancreatic beta-cell dysfunction and induces type 2 diabetes in sprague-dawley rats. *Diabetes* 60:899-908; 2011.

[73] Baynes JW Thorpe SR. Role of oxidative stress in diabetic complications: A new perspective on an old paradigm. *Diabetes* 48:1-9; 1999.

[74] Baynes, J. W. From life to death--the struggle between chemistry and biology during aging: The maillard reaction as an amplifier of genomic damage. *Biogerontology* 1:235-246; 2000.

[75] Baynes, J. W.; Thorpe, S. R. Glycoxidation and lipoxidation in atherogenesis. *Free Radic. Biol. Med.* 28:1708-1716; 2000.

[76] Kuhla, B.; Luth, H. J.; Haferburg, D.; Boeck, K.; Arendt, T.; Munch, G. Methylglyoxal, glyoxal, and their detoxification in alzheimer's disease. *Ann. N. Y. Acad. Sci.* 1043:211-216; 2005.

[77] Yu, P. H. Involvement of cerebrovascular semicarbazide-sensitive amine oxidase in the pathogenesis of alzheimer's disease and vascular dementia. *Med. Hypotheses* 57:175-179; 2001.

[78] Singh, R.; Barden, A.; Mori, T.; Beilin, L. Advanced glycation end-products: A review. *Diabetologia*44:129-146; 2001.

[79] Vlassara, H.; Bucala, R.; Striker, L. Pathogenic effects of advanced glycosylation: Biochemical, biologic, and clinical implications for diabetes and aging. *Lab. Invest.* 70:138-151; 1994.

[80] Baynes, J. W. The role of AGEs in aging: Causation or correlation. *Exp. Gerontol.* 36:1527-1537; 2001.

[81] Wolff, S. P.; Bascal, Z. A.; Hunt, J. V. "Autoxidative glycosylation": Free radicals and glycation theory. *Prog. Clin. Biol. Res.* 304:259-275; 1989.

[82] Glomb, M. A.; Monnier, V. M. Mechanism of protein modification by glyoxal and glycolaldehyde, reactive intermediates of the maillard reaction. *J. Biol. Chem.* 270:10017-10026; 1995.

[83] Khalifah, R. G.; Baynes, J. W.; Hudson, B. G. Amadorins: Novel post-amadori inhibitors of advanced glycation reactions. *Biochem. Biophys. Res. Commun.* 257:251-258; 1999.

[84] Kilhovd, B. K.; Giardino, I.; Torjesen, P. A.; Birkeland, K. I.; Berg, T. J.; Thornalley, P. J.; Brownlee, M.; Hanssen, K. F. Increased serum levels of the specific AGE-compound methylglyoxal-derived hydroimidazolone in patients with type 2 diabetes. *Metabolism* 52:163-167; 2003.

[85] Mostafa, A. A.; Randell, E. W.; Vasdev, S. C.; Gill, V. D.; Han, Y.; Gadag, V.; Raouf, A. A.; El Said, H. Plasma protein advanced glycation end products, carboxymethyl

cysteine, and carboxyethyl cysteine, are elevated and related to nephropathy in patients with diabetes. *Mol. Cell. Biochem.* 302:35-42; 2007.

[86] Jana, C. K.; Das, N.; Sohal, R. S. Specificity of age-related carbonylation of plasma proteins in the mouse and rat. *Arch. Biochem. Biophys.* 397:433-439; 2002.

[87] Poggioli, S.; Bakala, H.; Friguet, B. Age-related increase of protein glycation in peripheral blood lymphocytes is restricted to preferential target proteins. *Exp. Gerontol.* 37:1207-1215; 2002.

[88] Shipanova, I. N.; Glomb, M. A.; Nagaraj, R. H. Protein modification by methylglyoxal: Chemical nature and synthetic mechanism of a major fluorescent adduct. *Arch. Biochem. Biophys.* 344:29-36; 1997.

[89] Glomb, M. A.; Rosch, D.; Nagaraj, R. H. N(delta)-(5-hydroxy-4,6-dimethylpyrimidine-2-yl)-l-ornithine, a novel methylglyoxal-arginine modification in beer. *J. Agric. Food Chem.* 49:366-372; 2001.

[90] Ahmed, M. U.; Brinkmann Frye, E.; Degenhardt, T. P.; Thorpe, S. R.; Baynes, J. W. N-epsilon-(carboxyethyl)lysine, a product of the chemical modification of proteins by methylglyoxal, increases with age in human lens proteins. *Biochem. J.* 324 (Pt 2):565-570; 1997.

[91] Chellan, P.; Nagaraj, R. H. Protein crosslinking by the maillard reaction: Dicarbonyl-derived imidazolium crosslinks in aging and diabetes. *Arch. Biochem. Biophys.* 368:98-104; 1999.

[92] Konishi, Y.; Hayase, F.; Kato, K. Novel imidazolones compound formed by the advanced maillard reaction of 3-deoxyglucosone and arginine residues in proteins. *Biosci Biotechnol Biochem* 58:1953-1955; 1994.

[93] Uchida, K.; Khor, O. T.; Oya, T.; Osawa, T.; Yasuda, Y.; Miyata, T. Protein modification by a maillard reaction intermediate methylglyoxal. immunochemical detection of fluorescent 5-methylimidazolone derivatives in vivo. *FEBS Lett.* 410:313-318; 1997.

[94] Chang, T.; Wang, R.; Wu, L. Methylglyoxal-induced nitric oxide and peroxynitrite production in vascular smooth muscle cells. *Free Radic. Biol. Med.* 38:286-293; 2005.

[95] Dhar, A.; Desai, K.; Kazachmov, M.; Yu, P.; Wu, L. Methylglyoxal production in vascular smooth muscle cells from different metabolic precursors. *Metabolism* 57:1211-1220; 2008.

[96] Wang, H.; Liu, J.; Wu, L. Methylglyoxal-induced mitochondrial dysfunction in vascular smooth muscle cells. *Biochem. Pharmacol.* In press; 2009.

[97] Ho, C.; Lee, P. H.; Huang, W. J.; Hsu, Y. C.; Lin, C. L.; Wang, J. Y. Methylglyoxal-induced fibronectin gene expression through ras-mediated NADPH oxidase activation in renal mesangial cells. *Nephrology (Carlton)* 12:348-356; 2007.

[98] Ward, R. A.; McLeish, K. R. Methylglyoxal: A stimulus to neutrophil oxygen radical production in chronic renal failure? *Nephrol. Dial. Transplant.* 19:1702-1707; 2004.

[99] Leoncini, G.; Poggi, M. Effects of methylglyoxal on platelet hydrogen peroxide accumulation, aggregation and release reaction. *Cell Biochem. Funct.* 14:89-95; 1996.

[100] Kalapos, M. P.; Littauer, A.; de Groot, H. Has reactive oxygen a role in methylglyoxal toxicity? A study on cultured rat hepatocytes. *Arch. Toxicol.* 67:369-372; 1993.

[101] Di Loreto, S.; Caracciolo, V.; Colafarina, S.; Sebastiani, P.; Gasbarri, A.; Amicarelli, F. Methylglyoxal induces oxidative stress-dependent cell injury and up-regulation of interleukin-1beta and nerve growth factor in cultured hippocampal neuronal cells. *Brain Res.* 1006:157-167; 2004.

[102] Akhand, A. A.; Hossain, K.; Mitsui, H.; Kato, M.; Miyata, T.; Inagi, R.; Du, J.; Takeda, K.; Kawamoto, Y.; Suzuki, H.; Kurokawa, K.; Nakashima, I. Glyoxal and methylglyoxal trigger distinct signals for map family kinases and caspase activation in human endothelial cells. *Free Radic. Biol. Med.* 31:20-30; 2001.

[103] Kikuchi, S.; Shinpo, K.; Moriwaka, F.; Makita, Z.; Miyata, T.; Tashiro, K. Neurotoxicity of methylglyoxal and 3-deoxyglucosone on cultured cortical neurons: Synergism between glycation and oxidative stress, possibly involved in neurodegenerative diseases. *J. Neurosci. Res.*57:280-289; 1999.

[104] Amicarelli, F.; Colafarina, S.; Cattani, F.; Cimini, A.; Di Ilio, C.; Ceru, M. P.; Miranda, M. Scavenging system efficiency is crucial for cell resistance to ROS-mediated methylglyoxal injury. *Free Radic. Biol. Med.* 35:856-871; 2003.

[105] Pacher, P.; Beckman, J. S.; Liaudet, L. Nitric oxide and peroxynitrite in health and disease. *Physiol. Rev.* 87:315-424; 2007.

[106] Nicolay, J. P.; Schneider, J.; Niemoeller, O. M.; Artunc, F.; Portero-Otin, M.; Haik, G.,Jr; Thornalley, P. J.; Schleicher, E.; Wieder, T.; Lang, F. Stimulation of suicidal erythrocyte death by methylglyoxal. *Cell. Physiol. Biochem.* 18:223-232; 2006.

[107] Beard, K. M.; Shangari, N.; Wu, B.; O'Brien, P. J. Metabolism, not autoxidation, plays a role in alpha-oxoaldehyde- and reducing sugar-induced erythrocyte GSH depletion: Relevance for diabetes mellitus. *Mol. Cell. Biochem.* 252:331-338; 2003.

[108] Park, Y. S.; Koh, Y. H.; Takahashi, M.; Miyamoto, Y.; Suzuki, K.; Dohmae, N.; Takio, K.; Honke, K.; Taniguchi, N. Identification of the binding site of methylglyoxal on glutathione peroxidase: Methylglyoxal inhibits glutathione peroxidase activity via binding to glutathione binding sites arg 184 and 185. *Free Radic. Res.* 37:205-211; 2003.

[109] Paget, C.; Lecomte, M.; Ruggiero, D.; Wiernsperger, N.; Lagarde, M. Modification of enzymatic antioxidants in retinal microvascular cells by glucose or advanced glycation end products. *Free Radic. Biol. Med.* 25:121-129; 1998.

[110] Juurlink, B. H. Management of oxidative stress in the CNS: The many roles of glutathione. *Neurotox Res.* 1:119-140; 1999.

[111] Rondeau, P.; Singh, N. R.; Caillens, H.; Tallet, F.; Bourdon, E. Oxidative stresses induced by glycoxidized human or bovine serum albumin on human monocytes. *Free Radic. Biol. Med.* 45:799-812; 2008.

[112] Gawlowski, T.; Stratmann, B.; Stirban, A. O.; Negrean, M.; Tschoepe, D. AGEs and methylglyoxal induce apoptosis and expression of mac-1 on neutrophils resulting in platelet-neutrophil aggregation. *Thromb. Res.* 121:117-126; 2007.

[113] Chance, B.; Oshino, N.; Sugano, T.; Mayevsky, A. Basic principles of tissue oxygen determination from mitochondrial signals. *Adv. Exp. Med. Biol.* 37A:277-292; 1973.

[114] Turrens, J. F.; Boveris, A. Generation of superoxide anion by the NADH dehydrogenase of bovine heart mitochondria. *Biochem. J.*191:421-427; 1980.

[115] Turrens, J. F. Superoxide production by the mitochondrial respiratory chain. *Biosci. Rep.* 17:3-8; 1997.

[116] Rosca, M. G.; Mustata, T. G.; Kinter, M. T.; Ozdemir, A. M.; Kern, T. S.; Szweda, L. I.; Brownlee, M.; Monnier, V. M.; Weiss, M. F. Glycation of mitochondrial proteins from diabetic rat kidney is associated with excess superoxide formation. *Am. J. Physiol. Renal Physiol.* 289:F420-30; 2005.

[117] Rabbani, N.; Thornalley, P. J. Dicarbonyls linked to damage in the powerhouse: Glycation of mitochondrial proteins and oxidative stress. *Biochem. Soc. Trans.* 36:1045-1050; 2008.

[118] Vander Jagt, D. L. Methylglyoxal, diabetes mellitus and diabetic complications. *Drug Metabol. Drug Interact.* 23:93-124; 2008.

[119] Ando, K.; Beppu, M.; Kikugawa, K.; Nagai, R.; Horiuchi, S. Membrane proteins of human erythrocytes are modified by advanced glycation end products during aging in the circulation. *Biochem. Biophys. Res. Commun.* 258:123-127; 1999.

[120] Li, Y. M.; Steffes, M.; Donnelly, T.; Liu, C.; Fuh, H.; Basgen, J.; Bucala, R.; Vlassara, H. Prevention of cardiovascular and renal pathology of aging by the advanced glycation inhibitor aminoguanidine. *Proc. Natl. Acad. Sci. U. S. A.*93:3902-3907; 1996.

[121] Kilhovd, B. K.; Giardino, I.; Torjesen, P. A.; Birkeland, K. I.; Berg, T. J.; Thornalley, P. J.; Brownlee, M.; Hanssen, K. F. Increased serum levels of the specific AGE-compound methylglyoxal-derived hydroimidazolone in patients with type 2 diabetes. *Metabolism* 52:163-167; 2003.

[122] Degenhardt, T. P.; Thorpe, S. R.; Baynes, J. W. Chemical modification of proteins by methylglyoxal. *Cell. Mol. Biol. (Noisy-Le-Grand)* 44:1139-1145; 1998.

[123] Sugimoto, K.; Nishizawa, Y.; Horiuchi, S.; Yagihashi, S. Localization in human diabetic peripheral nerve of N(epsilon)-carboxymethyllysine-protein adducts, an advanced glycation endproduct. *Diabetologia* 40:1380-1387; 1997.

[124] Lo, T. W.; Westwood, M. E.; McLellan, A. C.; Selwood, T.; Thornalley, P. J. Binding and modification of proteins by methylglyoxal under physiological conditions. A kinetic and mechanistic study with N alpha-acetylarginine, N alpha-acetylcysteine, and N alpha-acetyllysine, and bovine serum albumin. *J. Biol. Chem.* 269:32299-32305; 1994.

[125] Oya, T.; Hattori, N.; Mizuno, Y.; Miyata, S.; Maeda, S.; Osawa, T.; Uchida, K. Methylglyoxal modification of protein. chemical and immunochemical characterization of methylglyoxal-arginine adducts. *J. Biol. Chem.* 274:18492-18502; 1999.

[126] Kikuchi, S.; Shinpo, K.; Takeuchi, M.; Yamagishi, S.; Makita, Z.; Sasaki, N.; Tashiro, K. Glycation--a sweet tempter for neuronal death. *Brain Res. Brain Res. Rev.* 41:306-323; 2003.

[127] Westwood, M. E.; Thornalley, P. J. Induction of synthesis and secretion of interleukin 1 beta in the human monocytic THP-1 cells by human serum albumins modified with methylglyoxal and advanced glycation endproducts. *Immunol. Lett.* 50:17-21; 1996.

[128] Wautier, M. P.; Chappey, O.; Corda, S.; Stern, D. M.; Schmidt, A. M.; Wautier, J. L. Activation of NADPH oxidase by AGE links oxidant stress to altered gene expression via RAGE. *Am. J. Physiol. Endocrinol. Metab.* 280:E685-94; 2001.

[129] Basta, G.; Lazzerini, G.; Massaro, M.; Simoncini, T.; Tanganelli, P.; Fu, C.; Kislinger, T.; Stern, D. M.; Schmidt, A. M.; De Caterina, R. Advanced glycation end products activate endothelium through signal-transduction receptor RAGE: A mechanism for amplification of inflammatory responses. *Circulation* 105:816-822; 2002.

[130] Chen, J.; Brodsky, S. V.; Goligorsky, D. M.; Hampel, D. J.; Li, H.; Gross, S. S.; Goligorsky, M. S. Glycated collagen I induces premature senescence-like phenotypic changes in endothelial cells. *Circ. Res.* 90:1290-1298; 2002.

[131] Thornalley, P. J. Cell activation by glycated proteins. AGE receptors, receptor recognition factors and functional classification of AGEs. *Cell. Mol. Biol. (Noisy-Le-Grand)* 44:1013-1023; 1998.

[132] Bierhaus, A.; Chevion, S.; Chevion, M.; Hofmann, M.; Quehenberger, P.; Illmer, T.; Luther, T.; Berentshtein, E.; Tritschler, H.; Muller, M.; Wahl, P.; Ziegler, R.; Nawroth, P. P. Advanced glycation end product-induced activation of NF-kappaB is suppressed by alpha-lipoic acid in cultured endothelial cells. *Diabetes* 46:1481-1490; 1997.

[133] Asif, M.; Egan, J.; Vasan, S.; Jyothirmayi, G. N.; Masurekar, M. R.; Lopez, S.; Williams, C.; Torres, R. L.; Wagle, D.; Ulrich, P.; Cerami, A.; Brines, M.; Regan, T. J. An advanced glycation endproduct cross-link breaker can reverse age-related increases in myocardial stiffness. *Proc. Natl. Acad. Sci. U. S. A.* 97:2809-2813; 2000.

[134] Scuteri, A. Slowing arterial aging: How far have we progressed? *J. Hypertens.* 25:509-510; 2007.

[135] Uribarri, J.; Cai, W.; Peppa, M.; Goodman, S.; Ferrucci, L.; Striker, G.; Vlassara, H. Circulating glycotoxins and dietary advanced glycation endproducts: Two links to inflammatory response, oxidative stress, and aging. *J. Gerontol. A Biol. Sci. Med. Sci.* 62:427-433; 2007.

[136] Mailankot, M.; Padmanabha, S.; Pasupuleti, N.; Major, D.; Howell, S.; Nagaraj, R. H. Glyoxalase I activity and immunoreactivity in the aging human lens. *Biogerontology* 2009.

[137] Corstjens, H.; Declercq, L.; Hellemans, L.; Sente, I.; Maes, D. Prevention of oxidative damage that contributes to the loss of bioenergetic capacity in ageing skin. *Exp. Gerontol.* 42:924-929; 2007.

[138] Morcos, M.; Du, X.; Pfisterer, F.; Hutter, H.; Sayed, A. A.; Thornalley, P.; Ahmed, N.; Baynes, J.; Thorpe, S.; Kukudov, G.; Schlotterer, A.; Bozorgmehr, F.; El Baki, R. A.; Stern, D.; Moehrlen, F.; Ibrahim, Y.; Oikonomou, D.; Hamann, A.; Becker, C.; Zeier, M.; Schwenger, V.; Miftari, N.; Humpert, P.; Hammes, H. P.; Buechler, M.; Bierhaus, A.; Brownlee, M.; Nawroth, P. P. Glyoxalase-1 prevents mitochondrial protein modification and enhances lifespan in caenorhabditis elegans. *Aging Cell.* 7:260-269; 2008.

[139] Scheckhuber, C. Q.; Mack, S. J.; Strobel, I.; Ricciardi, F.; Gispert, S.; Osiewacz, H. D. Modulation of the glyoxalase system in the aging model podospora anserina: Effects on growth and lifespan. *Aging (Albany NY)* 2:969-980; 2010.

[140] Sejersen, H.; Rattan, S. I. Dicarbonyl-induced accelerated aging in vitro in human skin fibroblasts. *Biogerontology* 10:203-211; 2009.

[141] Chappey, O.; Dosquet, C.; Wautier, M. P.; Wautier, J. L. Advanced glycation end products, oxidant stress and vascular lesions. *Eur. J. Clin. Invest.*27:97-108; 1997.

[142] Gillery, P. Advanced glycation end products (AGEs), free radicals and diabetes. *J. Soc. Biol.* 195:387-390; 2001.

[143] Kutlu, M.; Naziroglu, M.; Simsek, H.; Yilmaz, T.; Sahap Kukner, A. Moderate exercise combined with dietary vitamins C and E counteracts oxidative stress in the kidney and lens of streptozotocin-induced diabetic-rat. *Int. J. Vitam. Nutr. Res.* 75:71-80; 2005.

[144] Wondrak, G. T.; Cervantes-Laurean, D.; Roberts, M. J.; Qasem, J. G.; Kim, M.; Jacobson, E. L.; Jacobson, M. K. Identification of alpha-dicarbonyl scavengers for cellular protection against carbonyl stress. *Biochem. Pharmacol.* 63:361-373; 2002.

[145] Brownlee, M.; Vlassara, H.; Kooney, A.; Ulrich, P.; Cerami, A. Aminoguanidine prevents diabetes-induced arterial wall protein cross-linking. *Science* 232:1629-1632; 1986.

[146] Edelstein, D.; Brownlee, M. Mechanistic studies of advanced glycosylation end product inhibition by aminoguanidine. *Diabetes* 41:26-29; 1992.

[147] Beisswenger, P.; Ruggiero-Lopez, D. Metformin inhibition of glycation processes. *Diabetes Metab.* 29:6S95-103; 2003.

[148] Ruggiero-Lopez, D.; Lecomte, M.; Moinet, G.; Patereau, G.; Lagarde, M.; Wiernsperger, N. Reaction of metformin with dicarbonyl compounds. possible implication in the inhibition of advanced glycation end product formation. *Biochem. Pharmacol.* 58:1765-1773; 1999.

[149] Szwergold, B. S.; Kappler, F.; Brown, T. R. Identification of fructose 3-phosphate in the lens of diabetic rats. *Science* 247:451-454; 1990.

[150] Delpierre, G.; Rider, M. H.; Collard, F.; Stroobant, V.; Vanstapel, F.; Santos, H.; Van Schaftingen, E. Identification, cloning, and heterologous expression of a mammalian fructosamine-3-kinase. *Diabetes* 49:1627-1634; 2000.

[151] Saxena, A. K.; Saxena, P.; Monnier, V. M. Purification and characterization of a membrane-bound deglycating enzyme (1-deoxyfructosyl alkyl amino acid oxidase, EC 1.5.3) from a pseudomonas sp. soil strain. *J. Biol. Chem.* 271:32803-32809; 1996.

[152] Takahashi, M.; Pischetsrieder, M.; Monnier, V. M. Isolation, purification, and characterization of amadoriase isoenzymes (fructosyl amine-oxygen oxidoreductase EC 1.5.3) from aspergillus sp. *J. Biol. Chem.* 272:3437-3443; 1997.

[153] Vasan, S.; Zhang, X.; Zhang, X.; Kapurniotu, A.; Bernhagen, J.; Teichberg, S.; Basgen, J.; Wagle, D.; Shih, D.; Terlecky, I.; Bucala, R.; Cerami, A.; Egan, J.; Ulrich, P. An agent cleaving glucose-derived protein crosslinks in vitro and in vivo. *Nature* 382:275-278; 1996.

[154] Grandhee, S. K.; Monnier, V. M. Mechanism of formation of the maillard protein cross-link pentosidine. glucose, fructose, and ascorbate as pentosidine precursors. *J. Biol. Chem.* 266:11649-11653; 1991.

[155] Frye, E. B.; Degenhardt, T. P.; Thorpe, S. R.; Baynes, J. W. Role of the maillard reaction in aging of tissue proteins. advanced glycation end product-dependent increase in imidazolium cross-links in human lens proteins. *J. Biol. Chem.* 273:18714-18719; 1998.

[156] Nilsson, B. O. Biological effects of aminoguanidine: An update. *Inflamm. Res.* 48:509-515; 1999.

[157] SCHULER, W. The inhibition of histaminase. *Experientia* 8:230-232; 1952.

[158] Ivy, A. C.; Ivy, E. K.; Karvinen, E.; Lin, T. M. Effect of an histaminase inhibitor (aminoguanidine) on the gastric secretory response to exogenous histamine. *Am. J. Physiol.* 186:231-238; 1956.

[159] Corbett, J. A.; Tilton, R. G.; Chang, K.; Hasan, K. S.; Ido, Y.; Wang, J. L.; Sweetland, M. A.; Lancaster, J. R.,Jr; Williamson, J. R.; McDaniel, M. L. Aminoguanidine, a novel inhibitor of nitric oxide formation, prevents diabetic vascular dysfunction. *Diabetes* 41:552-556; 1992.

[160] Laszlo, F.; Evans, S. M.; Whittle, B. J. Aminoguanidine inhibits both constitutive and inducible nitric oxide synthase isoforms in rat intestinal microvasculature in vivo. *Eur. J. Pharmacol.* 272:169-175; 1995.

[161] Moncada, S.; Palmer, R. M.; Higgs, E. A. Nitric oxide: Physiology, pathophysiology, and pharmacology. *Pharmacol. Rev.* 43:109-142; 1991.

[162] Stjernborg, L.; Persson, L. Stabilization of S-adenosylmethionine decarboxylase by aminoguanidine. *Biochem. Pharmacol.* 45:1174-1176; 1993.

[163] Miyata, T.; van Ypersele de Strihou, C. Angiotensin II receptor blockers and angiotensin converting enzyme inhibitors: Implication of radical scavenging and transition metal chelation in inhibition of advanced glycation end product formation. *Arch. Biochem. Biophys.* 419:50-54; 2003.

[164] Sajithlal, G. B.; Chithra, P.; Chandrakasan, G. Advanced glycation end products induce crosslinking of collagen in vitro. *Biochim. Biophys. Acta* 1407:215-224; 1998.

[165] Corman, B.; Duriez, M.; Poitevin, P.; Heudes, D.; Bruneval, P.; Tedgui, A.; Levy, B. I. Aminoguanidine prevents age-related arterial stiffening and cardiac hypertrophy. *Proc. Natl. Acad. Sci. U. S. A.* 95:1301-1306; 1998.

[166] Seyer-Hansen, M.; Andreassen, T. T.; Oxlund, H.; Jorgensen, P. H. The influence of aminoguanidine on borohydride reducible collagen cross-links and wound strength. *Connect. Tissue Res.* 26:181-186; 1991.

[167] Ino-ue, M.; Ohgiya, N.; Yamamoto, M. Effect of aminoguanidine on optic nerve involvement in experimental diabetic rats. *Brain Res.* 800:319-322; 1998.

[168] Bolton, W. K.; Cattran, D. C.; Williams, M. E.; Adler, S. G.; Appel, G. B.; Cartwright, K.; Foiles, P. G.; Freedman, B. I.; Raskin, P.; Ratner, R. E.; Spinowitz, B. S.; Whittier, F. C.; Wuerth, J. P.; ACTION I Investigator Group. Randomized trial of an inhibitor of formation of advanced glycation end products in diabetic nephropathy. *Am. J. Nephrol.* 24:32-40; 2004.

[169] Freedman, B. I.; Wuerth, J. P.; Cartwright, K.; Bain, R. P.; Dippe, S.; Hershon, K.; Mooradian, A. D.; Spinowitz, B. S. Design and baseline characteristics for the aminoguanidine clinical trial in overt type 2 diabetic nephropathy (ACTION II). *Control. Clin. Trials* 20:493-510; 1999.

[170] Brown, C. D.; Zhao, Z. H.; Thomas, L. L.; deGroof, R.; Friedman, E. A. Effects of erythropoietin and aminoguanidine on red blood cell deformability in diabetic azotemic and uremic patients. *Am. J. Kidney Dis.* 38:1414-1420; 2001.

[171] Suji, G.; Sivakami, S. DNA damage by free radical production by aminoguanidine. *Ann. N. Y. Acad. Sci.* 1067:191-199; 2006.

[172] Beisswenger, P. J.; Howell, S. K.; Touchette, A. D.; Lal, S.; Szwergold, B. S. Metformin reduces systemic methylglyoxal levels in type 2 diabetes. *Diabetes*48:198-202; 1999.

[173] Rahbar, S.; Figarola, J. L. Novel inhibitors of advanced glycation endproducts. *Arch. Biochem. Biophys.* 419:63-79; 2003.

[174] Baynes, J. W. Role of oxidative stress in development of complications in diabetes. *Diabetes* 40:405-412; 1991.

[175] Ota, K.; Nakamura, J.; Li, W.; Kozakae, M.; Watarai, A.; Nakamura, N.; Yasuda, Y.; Nakashima, E.; Naruse, K.; Watabe, K.; Kato, K.; Oiso, Y.; Hamada, Y. Metformin prevents methylglyoxal-induced apoptosis of mouse schwann cells. *Biochem. Biophys. Res. Commun.* 357:270-275; 2007.

[176] Rabbani, N.; Godfrey, L.; Xue, M.; Shaheen, F.; Geoffrion, M.; Milne, R.; Thornalley, P. J. Glycation of LDL by methylglyoxal increases arterial atherogenicity: A possible contributor to increased risk of cardiovascular disease in diabetes. *Diabetes* 60:1973-1980; 2011.

[177] Rahbar, S.; Natarajan, R.; Yerneni, K.; Scott, S.; Gonzales, N.; Nadler, J. L. Evidence that pioglitazone, metformin and pentoxifylline are inhibitors of glycation. *Clin. Chim. Acta* 301:65-77; 2000.

[178] Hirasawa, Y.; Matsui, Y.; Ohtsu, S.; Yamane, K.; Toyoshi, T.; Kyuki, K.; Sakai, T.; Feng, Y.; Nagamatsu, T. Involvement of hyperglycemia in deposition of aggregated protein in glomeruli of diabetic mice. *Eur. J. Pharmacol.* 601:129-135; 2008.

[179] Millea, P. J. N-acetylcysteine: Multiple clinical applications. *Am. Fam. Physician* 80:265-269; 2009.

[180] Vasdev, S.; Ford, C. A.; Longerich, L.; Parai, S.; Gadag, V.; Wadhawan, S. Aldehyde induced hypertension in rats: Prevention by N-acetyl cysteine. *Artery* 23:10-36; 1998.

[181] Lauterburg, B. H.; Corcoran, G. B.; Mitchell, J. R. Mechanism of action of N-acetylcysteine in the protection against the hepatotoxicity of acetaminophen in rats in vivo. *J. Clin. Invest.* 71:980-991; 1983.

[182] Forbes, J. M.; Cooper, M. E.; Thallas, V.; Burns, W. C.; Thomas, M. C.; Brammar, G. C.; Lee, F.; Grant, S. L.; Burrell, L. M.; Jerums, G.; Osicka, T. M. Reduction of the accumulation of advanced glycation end products by ACE inhibition in experimental diabetic nephropathy. *Diabetes* 51:3274-3282; 2002.

[183] Izuhara, Y.; Nangaku, M.; Inagi, R.; Tominaga, N.; Aizawa, T.; Kurokawa, K.; van Ypersele de Strihou, C.; Miyata, T. Renoprotective properties of angiotensin receptor blockers beyond blood pressure lowering. *J. Am. Soc. Nephrol.* 16:3631-3641; 2005.

[184] Miyata, T.; van Ypersele de Strihou, C.; Ueda, Y.; Ichimori, K.; Inagi, R.; Onogi, H.; Ishikawa, N.; Nangaku, M.; Kurokawa, K. Angiotensin II receptor antagonists and angiotensin-converting enzyme inhibitors lower in vitro the formation of advanced glycation end products: Biochemical mechanisms. *J. Am. Soc. Nephrol.* 13:2478-2487; 2002.

[185] Nangaku, M.; Miyata, T.; Sada, T.; Mizuno, M.; Inagi, R.; Ueda, Y.; Ishikawa, N.; Yuzawa, H.; Koike, H.; van Ypersele de Strihou, C.; Kurokawa, K. Anti-hypertensive agents inhibit in vivo the formation of advanced glycation end products and improve renal damage in a type 2 diabetic nephropathy rat model. *J. Am. Soc. Nephrol.* 14:1212-1222; 2003.

[186] Rao, G. N.; Lardis, M. P.; Cotlier, E. Acetylation of lens crystallins: A possible mechanism by which aspirin could prevent cataract formation. *Biochem. Biophys. Res. Commun.* 128:1125-1132; 1985.

[187] Lin, P. P.; Barry, R. C.; Smith, D. L.; Smith, J. B. In vivo acetylation identified at lysine 70 of human lens alphaA-crystallin. *Protein Sci.* 7:1451-1457; 1998.

[188] Ajiboye, R.; Harding, J. J. The non-enzymic glycosylation of bovine lens proteins by glucosamine and its inhibition by aspirin, ibuprofen and glutathione. *Exp. Eye Res.* 49:31-41; 1989.

[189] Raza, K.; Harding, J. J. Non-enzymic modification of lens proteins by glucose and fructose: Effects of ibuprofen. *Exp. Eye Res.* 52:205-212; 1991.

[190] van Boekel, M. A.; van den Bergh, P. J.; Hoenders, H. J. Glycation of human serum albumin: Inhibition by diclofenac. *Biochim. Biophys. Acta* 1120:201-204; 1992.

[191] Regensteiner, J. G.; Stewart, K. J. Established and evolving medical therapies for claudication in patients with peripheral arterial disease. *Nat. Clin. Pract. Cardiovasc. Med.* 3:604-610; 2006.

[192] Rahbar, S.; Natarajan, R.; Yerneni, K.; Scott, S.; Gonzales, N.; Nadler, J. L. Evidence that pioglitazone, metformin and pentoxifylline are inhibitors of glycation. *Clin. Chim. Acta* 301:65-77; 2000.

[193] Booth, A. A.; Khalifah, R. G.; Hudson, B. G. Thiamine pyrophosphate and pyridoxamine inhibit the formation of antigenic advanced glycation end-products: Comparison with aminoguanidine. *Biochem. Biophys. Res. Commun.* 220:113-119; 1996.

[194] Nagaraj, R. H.; Sarkar, P.; Mally, A.; Biemel, K. M.; Lederer, M. O.; Padayatti, P. S. Effect of pyridoxamine on chemical modification of proteins by carbonyls in diabetic rats: Characterization of a major product from the reaction of pyridoxamine and methylglyoxal. *Arch. Biochem. Biophys.* 402:110-119; 2002.

[195] Stitt, A.; Gardiner, T. A.; Alderson, N. L.; Canning, P.; Frizzell, N.; Duffy, N.; Boyle, C.; Januszewski, A. S.; Chachich, M.; Baynes, J. W.; Thorpe, S. R. The AGE inhibitor pyridoxamine inhibits development of retinopathy in experimental diabetes. *Diabetes* 51:2826-2832; 2002.

[196] Monnier, V. M. Bacterial enzymes that can deglycate glucose- and fructose-modified lysine. *Biochem. J.*392:e1-3; 2005.

[197] Horiuchi, T.; Kurokawa, T.; Saito, N. Purification and properties of fructosylamino acid oxidase from corynebacterium sp. 2-4-1. *Agri Biol Chem* 53:103-110; 1989.

[198] Horiuchi, T.; Kurokawa, T. Purification and properties of fructosylamine oxidase from aspergillus sp. 1005. *Agri Biol Chem* 55:333-338; 1991.

[199] Wiame, E.; Delpierre, G.; Collard, F.; Van Schaftingen, E. Identification of a pathway for the utilization of the amadori product fructoselysine in escherichia coli. *J. Biol. Chem.* 277:42523-42529; 2002.

[200] Wiame, E.; Van Schaftingen, E. Fructoselysine 3-epimerase, an enzyme involved in the metabolism of the unusual amadori compound psicoselysine in escherichia coli. *Biochem. J.*378:1047-1052; 2004.

[201] Wiame, E.; Lamosa, P.; Santos, H.; Van Schaftingen, E. Identification of glucoselysine-6-phosphate deglycase, an enzyme involved in the metabolism of the fructation product glucoselysine. *Biochem. J.* 392:263-269; 2005.

[202] Rahbar, S.; Kumar Yernini, K.; Scott, S.; Gonzales, N.; Lalezari, I. Novel inhibitors of advanced glycation endproducts. *Biochem. Biophys. Res. Commun.* 262:651-656; 1999.

[203] Rahbar, S.; Yerneni, K. K.; Scott, S.; Gonzales, N.; Lalezari, I. Novel inhibitors of advanced glycation endproducts (part II). *Mol. Cell Biol. Res. Commun.* 3:360-366; 2000.

[204] Ulrich, P.; Zhang, X. Pharmacological reversal of advanced glycation end-product-mediated protein crosslinking. *Diabetologia* 40 Suppl 2:S157-9; 1997.

[205] Wolffenbuttel, B. H.; Boulanger, C. M.; Crijns, F. R.; Huijberts, M. S.; Poitevin, P.; Swennen, G. N.; Vasan, S.; Egan, J. J.; Ulrich, P.; Cerami, A.; Levy, B. I. Breakers of advanced glycation end products restore large artery properties in experimental diabetes. *Proc. Natl. Acad. Sci. U. S. A.* 95:4630-4634; 1998.

[206] Guo, Y.; Lu, M.; Qian, J.; Cheng, Y. L. Alagebrium chloride protects the heart against oxidative stress in aging rats. *J. Gerontol. A Biol. Sci. Med. Sci.* 2009.

[207] Vaitkevicius, P. V.; Lane, M.; Spurgeon, H.; Ingram, D. K.; Roth, G. S.; Egan, J. J.; Vasan, S.; Wagle, D. R.; Ulrich, P.; Brines, M.; Wuerth, J. P.; Cerami, A.; Lakatta, E. G. A cross-link breaker has sustained effects on arterial and ventricular properties in older rhesus monkeys. *Proc. Natl. Acad. Sci. U. S. A.* 98:1171-1175; 2001.

[208] Kass, D. A.; Shapiro, E. P.; Kawaguchi, M.; Capriotti, A. R.; Scuteri, A.; deGroof, R. C.; Lakatta, E. G. Improved arterial compliance by a novel advanced glycation end-product crosslink breaker. *Circulation* 104:1464-1470; 2001.

[209] Zieman, S. J.; Melenovsky, V.; Clattenburg, L.; Corretti, M. C.; Capriotti, A.; Gerstenblith, G.; Kass, D. A. Advanced glycation endproduct crosslink breaker (alagebrium) improves endothelial function in patients with isolated systolic hypertension. *J. Hypertens.* 25:577-583; 2007.

[210] Little, W. C.; Zile, M. R.; Kitzman, D. W.; Hundley, W. G.; O'Brien, T. X.; Degroof, R. C. The effect of alagebrium chloride (ALT-711), a novel glucose cross-link breaker, in the treatment of elderly patients with diastolic heart failure. *J. Card. Fail.* 11:191-195; 2005.

[211] Bakris, G. L.; Bank, A. J.; Kass, D. A.; Neutel, J. M.; Preston, R. A.; Oparil, S. Advanced glycation end-product cross-link breakers. A novel approach to cardiovascular pathologies related to the aging process. *Am. J. Hypertens.* 17:23S-30S; 2004.

[212] Hartog, J. W.; Willemsen, S.; van Veldhuisen, D. J.; Posma, J. L.; van Wijk, L. M.; Hummel, Y. M.; Hillege, H. L.; Voors, A. A.; for the BENEFICIAL investigators. Effects of alagebrium, an advanced glycation endproduct breaker, on exercise tolerance and cardiac function in patients with chronic heart failure. *Eur. J. Heart Fail.* 13:899-908; 2011.

[213] Krautwald, M.; Leech, D.; Horne, S.; Steele, M. L.; Forbes, J.; Rahmadi, A.; Griffith, R.; Munch, G. The advanced glycation end product-lowering agent ALT-711 is a low-affinity inhibitor of thiamine diphosphokinase. *Rejuvenation Res.* 14:383-391; 2011.

9

The Involvement of Purinergic System in Pain: Adenosine Receptors and Inosine as Pharmacological Tools in Future Treatments

Francisney Pinto Nascimento[1,2],
Sérgio José Macedo Jr.[2] and Adair Roberto Soares Santos[1,2]
[1]Department of Pharmacology;
[2]Laboratory of Neurobiology of Pain and Inflammation,
Department of Physiological Sciences; Universidade Federal de Santa Catarina
Brazil

1. Introduction

During the recent years, the interest in the purinergic system has been gaining importance, and this interest is not accidental. The purinergic system is so far known to be involved in several physiological conditions in mammals, becoming a potential therapeutic target for the treatment of many pathologies and disorders. One of the physiological roles is the control of pain. This chapter will emphasize adenosine receptors (P1) and its activation and inhibition by adenosine and by specific agonists or antagonists in the treatment of pain. Although most of the studies quoted in this chapter were performed in animals, in this chapter we will use the expression *analgesia* instead of *antinociception* (term used to report pain in animals) to simplify our communication. Some drugs that act on adenosine receptors have presented interesting results in clinical studies of pain and other drugs are under investigation. Of note, it has recently been shown that inosine, a metabolite of adenosine, has significant analgesic effects in several pre-clinical models of pain. Thus, the inosine can be an important tool in this area of study or even a molecule of interest for future pharmacological approaches, knowing that such as adenosine, it is produced endogenously and devoid of side effects in normal doses. In addition, new approaches using enzyme inhibitors of the purinergic system or supplies of adenosine suggest alternatives to potentiate and lasting analgesic effects of adenosine or analogs. Moreover, the release of purines and the adenosine A_1 receptor activation are essential to analgesia by acupuncture in mice. Thus, purinergic system will be the target of many future pain-treatment researches. After all, it is indispensable to students and biomedical professionals to know and understand basic concepts about this endogenous system.

2. Involvement of purinergic system in pain

2.1 Purinergic receptors: History and involvement in pain

Purinergic receptors history began when Drury and Szent-Györgi described the potent actions of purines adenine and adenosine on the heart and blood vessels (Drury & Szent-

Györgi, 1929). Later, in 1970 Burnstock presented evidence that ATP acted as a neurotransmitter in nonadrenergic noncholinergic (NANC) nerves supplying the gut, and finally, in 1972, the purinergic neurotransmission hypothesis was proposed (Burnstock, 1972). With these discoveries, the number of publications involving ATP and its metabolites grew quickly and continues to do so (Figure 1).

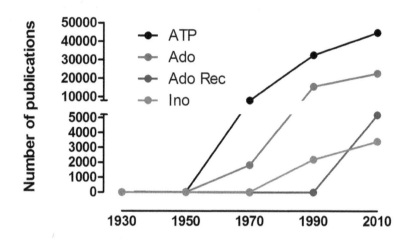

Fig. 1. Total of publications with keywords ATP, Adenosine (Ado), Adenosine Receptors (Ado Rec) and Inosine (Ino) from 1930 until 2010. Source: Pubmed

Afterwards, it was established that the ATP acted as a cotransmitter with classical transmitters in both the peripheral nervous system and in the central and that purines are also powerful extracellular messengers to non-neuronal cells (Burnstock & Knight, 2004). Burnstock, in 1978, provided the basis for the distinction of two classes of purinergic receptors; adenosine-sensitive P1 and ATP-sensitive P2 receptor classes. In 1985, Burnstock and Kennedy proposed a basis for distinguishing two types of P2 purinoceptors, namely, P2X and P2Y. Afterwards, in 1994 Abbracchio and Burnstock through studies of transduction mechanisms and cloning of both P2X and P2Y receptors put forward a new nomenclature system, naming them, P2X ionotropic ligand-gated ion channel receptors and P2Y metabotropic G protein-coupled receptors, respectively. Currently, seven subtypes of P2X receptors (P2X$_1$, P2X$_2$, P2X$_3$, P2X$_4$, P2X$_5$, P2X$_6$, P2X$_7$) and eight subtypes of P2Y receptors (P2Y$_1$, P2Y$_2$, P2Y$_4$, P2Y$_6$, P2Y$_{11}$, P2Y$_{12}$, P2Y$_{13}$, P2Y$_{14}$) are clearly established. P2X and P2Y receptor activation by ATP stimulates cellular excitability, augments the release of excitatory amino acids, and consequently initiates pain responses (Burnstock, 2007; Burnstock & Williams, 2000). In the context of pain neurotransmission, preclinical studies show us that activation of P1 receptors by adenosine decreases pain, inflammation, and cellular excitability (McGaraughty & Jarvis, 2006). During the 80's and 90's research evaluating purinergic system in pain rocketed (Figure 2).

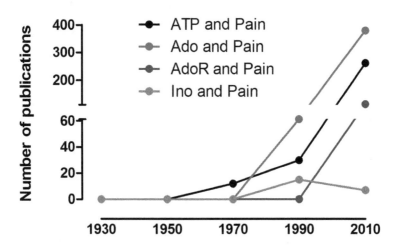

Fig. 2. Total of publications with keywords ATP, Adenosine (Ado), Adenosine Receptors
(AdoR) and Inosine (Ino) plus Pain from 1930 until 2010. Source: Pubmed

3. Adenosine receptors and pain

3.1 Adenosine receptors

Adenosine is the natural ligand of P1 receptors, also called adenosine receptors. All these
receptors are G-protein coupled and are divided according to pharmacological, biochemical
and molecular properties into four subtypes: A_1, A_{2A}, A_{2B} and A_3. Each receptor has a
distinct distribution and due to its special features, has distinct roles as well (Burnstock et
al., 2011; Fredholm et al., 2011; Ralevic & Burnstock, 1998; Ribeiro et al., 2002; Sawynok &
Liu, 2003). Adenosine receptors were cloned and characterized in several mammal species
(Burnstock, 2008).

3.2 Distribution of adenosine receptors

Adenosine receptors are present in several species and in distinct tissues. However, their
distribution is quite irregular and different among species and mainly among tissues
(Fredholm et al., 2011). A_1 receptor (A_{1R}) is a ubiquitous receptor. In the central nervous
system, it is distributed in the cerebellum, cerebral cortex, hippocampus, thalamus, spinal
cord (substantia gelatinosa), brain stem, olfactory bulb and other central sites. Peripherally
A_{1R} distribution is less wide than centrally, but there is a considerable density of A_{1R} in
sensory afferent fibers, mainly on C-fibers which are responsible for receiving and
conducting the painful stimuli (Dixon et al., 1996; Sawynok, 2009). A_{2A} receptor (A_{2AR})has an
even distribution between central and peripheral nervous system, but mainly in central
structures as nucleus accumbens, putamen, caudate and in immune tissues, vascular smooth
muscle, endothelium, platelets and sensory neurons (Dixon et al., 1996; Fredholm, 1995;
Ralevic & Burnstock, 1998; Sawynok, 2009). A_{2B} receptor (A_{2BR}) is also a ubiquitous receptor
and it has been found either in many central or peripheral tissues. However, A_{2BR} density is

very low and it has been found in great density only in bowel and bladder. A_3 receptors (A_{3R})are widely distributed in several mammals, however, few studies have indicated specific roles for this receptor (Dixon et al., 1996; Ralevic & Burnstock, 1998; Salvatore et al., 1993).

3.3 General adenosine receptor signaling

All adenosine receptors are coupled to G-protein. Nevertheless there are many kinds of G-protein and each one may activate a distinct pathway. Thus, the four adenosine receptors can stimulate or inhibit several pathways and consequently exert many physiological actions (Jacobson & Gao, 2006; Ralevic & Burnstock, 1998). We show below the main signaling characteristics of each adenosine receptor.

3.3.1 A₁ receptor signaling

A_{1R} is coupled to Gi/0 protein family which is pertussis toxin-sensitive. Most of the biological effects induced by A_{1R} activation are due to inhibition of cAMP second messenger (Burnstock, 2007; Jacobson & Gao, 2006; Ralevic & Burnstock, 1998; Sawynok, 1998) (Figure 3 and Table 1).

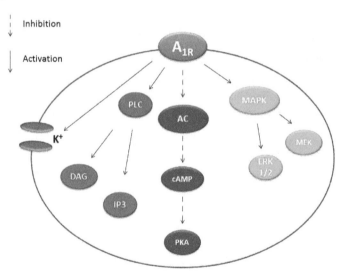

Fig. 3. Adenosine A₁ receptors and its main pathways. A_{1R}, adenosine A₁ receptor; AC, adenylate cyclase; cAMP, cyclic adenosine monophosphate; DAG, diacylglicerol; ERK1/2, extracellular signal-regulated kinases 1 and 2; IP₃, inositol triphosphate; K⁺, potassium channels; MAPK, mitogen-activated protein kinase; MEK, MAPK and ERK kinase; PKA, protein kinase; PLC, phospholipase C.

Beta and gamma subunities of A_{1R}, when activated stimulate phospholipase C (PLC). Activation of PLC cleaves phosphatidylinositol 4,5-bisphosphate (PIP_2) into diacylglycerol (DAG) and inositol 1,4,5-trisphosphate (IP_3) leading to increased levels Ca^{+2}. Moreover, the enhancement of intracellular calcium can induce some enzymes such as protein kinase C

(PKC), phospholipase D (PLD), phospholipase A_2 (PLA_2) and others. Furthermore, adenosine or adenosine agonists can activate K^+ channels (Jacobson & Gao, 2006; Megson et al., 1995; Ralevic & Burnstock, 1998). A_{1R} activation can also activate PI3K and MAPK pathways, more specifically ERK1/2 and MEK inducing gene expression changes and glial cell protection (Boison et al., 2010; Shulte & Fredholm, 2003).

3.3.2 A_{2A} receptor signaling

$A_{2A}R$ is coupled to Gs (the most part) and Golf protein (mainly in striatum). The main intracellular event after activation of these proteins is adenylate cyclase activation followed by cAMP production enhancement (Table 1).

Receptor	Adenosine affinity (EC50;nm)	G-protein	cAMP	PKA	PLC	Ca^{+2} channels	K^+ channels
A_1	~ 70	Gi/Go	Decrease	Inhibits	Activates	Inhibits	Activates
A_{2A}	~ 150	Gs/Golf	Increase	Activates		Inhibits or Activates	Activates
A_{2B}	~ 5100	Gs/Gq	Decrease	Activates	Activates		
A_3	~ 6500	Gi/Go	Increase	Inhibits	Activates		

Table 1. Adenosine receptors signaling. Adapted from Ralevic and Burnstock, 1998; Sawynok and Liu, 2003; Jacobson and Guao, 2006.

The increasing of cAMP stimulates cAMP-dependent kinase (PKA). Thus, PKA becomes able to activate several pathways through PKC, calcium channels, potassium channels, cAMP responsive element-binding (CREB), MAPK, PLC activation (Burnstock, 2007; Cunha et al., 2008; Fredholm et al., 2003, 2007; Jacobson & Gao, 2006; Ralevic & Burnstock, 1998).

3.3.3 A_{2B} receptor signaling

Through Gs and Gq activation A_{2B} receptor induces adenylate cyclase and PLC. In humans, $A_{2B}R$ can increase intracellular calcium by IP_3 activation. Moreover, the arachidonic acid pathway is also involved in $A_{2B}R$ signaling (Feoktistov & Biaggioni, 2011; Jacobson & Gao, 2006; Peakman and Hill, 1994).

3.3.4 A_3 receptor signaling

A_3R like A_{1R} is coupled to Gi/0 and also to Gq/11 protein. Its main signaling transduction is the inhibition of adenylate cyclase and stimulation of PLC, IP_3, DAG, PKC and PLD. Also, like other adenosine receptors, A_3R activates MAPK pathway, mainly ERK1/2 (Abbracchio et al., 1995; Armstrong & Ganote, 1994; Palmer et al., 1995; Shneyvays et al., 2004).

3.4 A₁ receptors and pain

A_{1R} is the main responsible for inducing analgesia among the adenosine receptors (Burnstock et al., 2011; Sawynok, 1998; Sawynok & Liu, 2003). It has been shown that A_{1R} is widely distributed in the dorsal spinal cord, mainly in lamina II (substantia gelatinosa) (Choca et al., 1988; Horiuchi et al., 2010; Sawynok, 1998). In this site, many afferent sensory nerve have connections with post-synaptic neurons. Also, A_{1R} are localized in the descending projection within dorsal horn (Choca et al., 1988).

3.4.1 Effects of A₁ receptor activation in acute pain

There are several published data showing the important effect of A_{1R} in controlling acute pain (review see Jacobson & Gao, 2006; Sawynok, 1998). Moreover, it has been shown that systemic administration of various A_{1R} agonists can produce analgesic effect in several models of acute pain in animals (Gong et al., 2010; Sawynok, 1998). Probably, these effects are caused by peripheral, supraspinal and mostly by spinal A_{1R}. In mice lacking A_{1R} (knockout animals) a lower pain threshold was observed in hyperalgesia tests (Wu et al., 2005). Further, analgesic effect induced by intrathecal adenosine was abolished as well as the increase of thermal hyperalgesia in A_{1R} knockout mice (Johansson et al., 2001).

Several studies published show that intrathecal injection of A_{1R} agonists cause analgesia in various animal models of acute pain, including tail flick, tail immersion, hot-plate, formalin, acetic acid, capsaicin models and others (Nascimento et al., 2010; Song et al., 2011; Zahn et al., 2007).

A_{1R} is also found in primary afferent neurons and in the cell body and the dorsal root ganglia (Lima et al., 2010; Sawynok, 2009), then it has an important role in modulation of peripheral pain. Many studies have shown that administration of A_{1R} agonists into the paw of animals causes an analgesic effect in several animal models of pain. It has been shown that A_{1R} activation in the periphery inhibits formalin-induced pain and reduces hyperalgesia induced by PGE_2 (Karlsten et al., 1992; Taiwo & Levine, 1990). Further, when the peripheral adenosine A_{1R} is activated, it triggers the $NO/cGMP/PKG/K_{ATP}$ intracellular signaling pathway and then inhibits pain (Lima et al., 2010). Moreover, A_{1R} agonists reduce the thermal hyperalgesia, but not mechanical allodynia, caused by sciatic nerve injury. The thermal hyperalgesia is mediated by C fibers and mechanical allodynia, in turn, is mediated by A fibers, which demonstrates the presence of A_{1R} in C but not in A fibers (Sawynok, 2009).

3.4.2 A₁ receptor and chronic pain

Several authors have shown that different agonists of A_{1R} are able to reduce distinct kinds of chronic pain. The agonist R-PIA inhibits mechanical allodynia induced by spinal nerve ligation in rats (Hwang et al., 2005; Song et al., 2011). In addition, R-PIA also reduces thermal pain threshold in rats that underwent an injury in the spinal cord (Horiuchi et al., 2010). Moreover, other mechanisms are generally involved in analgesic effect in chronic pain induced by A_{1R} activation, such as inhibition of glutamate release. Another A_{1R} agonist, CPA, when given to rats, inhibits pain induced by arthritis and pain induced by neuropathy (Curros-Criado & Herrero, 2005). Also, in experiments with A_{1R} knockout mice it has been observed that these animals present a lower pain threshold than wild-type animals in inflammatory and neuropathic pain models (Wu et al., 2005).

3.4.3 Interactions between A_1 receptor and opioid system

There is a strong relationship between opioidergic and adenosinergic systems in pain modulation. Morphine and other opioids are able to release adenosine (Sawynok et al., 1989; Sweeney et al., 1987a,b; Sweeney et al., 1989). Adenosine or analog administration combined with opioids enhances the analgesic effect of the latter (DeLander & Hopkins, 1986). However, administration of methylxanthines, adenosine receptor antagonists, can augment, decrease or have no effect on analgesic activity of opioids (Sawynok, 2011). In addition, A_{1R} can undergo dimerization with μ receptor in afferents neurons and induce the decrease of cAMP production (Sawynok, 1998).

3.4.4 Interactions among A_1 receptor and other receptors in pain mechanisms

A_{1R} is able to dimerize with alpha-2-adrenergic receptor. Also, it has been shown that serotonin releases adenosine from primary afferents and that A_{1R} receptor antagonist blocks serotonin analgesic actions, suggesting a close involvement between adenosinergic and serotoninergic systems in pain modulation (Sawynok, 1998).

3.4.5 A_1 agonists/antagonists

Methylxanthines (caffeine included) are natural antagonists of adenosine A_{1R} and A_{2AR}. However, the main selective agonists/antagonists to A_{1R} are synthetics. Some of them are listed in Table 2.

Role of drugs	Drug	Chemical name
Agonists A_{1R}	R-PIA	(−)-N^6-(2-Phenylisopropyl)adenosine
	CHA	N6-ciclohexyladenosine
	CPA	N6-cyclopentyladenosine
	CCPA	2-chloro-N6-cyclopentyladenosine
Antagonists A_{1R}	CPT	8-cyclopentyl-1,3-dimethylxanthine
	DPCPX	8-Cyclopentyl-1,3-dipropylxanthine
	8-PT	8-phenyltheophylline

Table 2. Principal adenosine A_1 receptor agonists and antagonists.

3.5 A_{2A} receptors and pain

Taiwo & Levine (1990) demonstrated clear distinct effects of A_{1R} and A_{2AR} activation in peripheral pain. They showed that, in peripheral sites, A_{1R} mediates analgesia while A_{2AR} facilitates painful perception. In addition, other studies also showed that peripheral A_{2AR} activation induced pain (Doak & Sawynok, 1995; Li et al., 2010; Taiwo & Levine, 1990). However, systemically and spinally, the role of A_{2AR} is not entirely clear. Some publications have demonstrated that A_{2AR} activation induces pain (Bastia et al., 2002; Hussey et al., 2007). On the other hand, other authors have showed a reduction of pain when A_{2AR} is activated (By et al., 2011; Borghi et al., 2002; Yoon et al., 2005). These controversial results might be associated with A_{2AR} intracellular signaling. A_{2AR} activation induces cAMP increased production (it can cause pain) and also K^+ channels opening (it can inhibit pain) (Jacobson & Gao, 2006; Regaya et al., 2004; Sawynok, 1998).

A_{2AR} knockout animals are less sensitive to pain, suggesting that A_{2AR} is a pain facilitator in acute (Hussey et al., 2007) and chronic pain (Bura et al., 2008). Bura and coworkers (2008) also demonstrated that microglia and astrocytes expression was higher in wild-type A_{2AR} animals than in A_{2AR} knockout animals. Also, A_{2AR} located in glial cells is responsible for the release of inflammatory mediators that induce and maintain chronic pain (Boison et al., 2010). Thus, A_{2AR} blockade might be an interesting approach for future treatments of neuropathic and chronic pain. Meantime, also in chronic pain exists distinct results about A_{2AR}. A report showed that only one spinal injection of A_{2AR} agonist was able to induce analgesia during several days in rats undergoing neuropathic pain (Loram et al., 2009). After all, it is clear that A_{2AR} is involved in pain modulation. However, more studies are necessary to precisely explain how this receptor works in distinct situations, only then it will be possible to make clinical approaches.

3.6 A_{2B} receptors and pain

Few studies have been evaluating the A_{2BR} role in pain. Most part of these studies showed that A_{2BR} facilitates pain transmission, because A_{2BR} antagonists have reduced pain (Abo-Salem et al., 2004; Bilkei-Gorzo et al., 2008; GodFrey et al., 2006). A_{2BR} antagonist reduced thermal hyperalgesia and was able to potentiate the analgesic effect caused by morphine and acetaminophen (Abo-Salem et al., 2004; Godfrey et al., 2006). Also, the blockade of A_{2BR} presented an analgesic effect in inflammatory pain (Bilkei-Gorzo et al., 2008).

3.7 A_3 receptors and pain

Similar to A_{2BR}, adenosine A_{3R} is not an interesting target to pain relief. However, A_{3R} is implicated in pathological conditions such as ischemic diseases and in inflammation (for review see Borea et al., 2009). Regarding pain, there are few studies evaluating A_{3R} role. Sawynok and colleagues (1997) showed that A_{3R} activation causes pain and paw oedema through release of histamine and serotonin. A_{3R} knockout animals presented an increased pain threshold in some models of pain but not difference in others (Fedorova et al., 2003; Wu et al., 2002). A_{3R} might be an interesting target to inflammatory and autoimmune diseases, but not to pain states.

3.8 Novel approaches in pain management involving adenosine receptors

3.8.1 Management of adenosine receptors by metabolism modulation

The first report showing that adenosine kinase (AK) inhibition reduces behaviour associated to pain was published by Keil and DeLander, 1992. AK inhibitors are able to decrease pain levels when given peripherally or sistemically (Kowaluk et al., 1999; Lynch et al., 1999; Sawynok, 1998). Moreover, these inhibitors are efficacious against acute and chronic pain (Kowaluk et al., 2000; Lynch et al., 1999; McGaraughty et al., 2005; Poon & Sawynok, 1998, 1999; Suzuki et al., 2001). Another enzyme that regulates adenosine level is adenosine deaminase (ADA), that converts adenosine to inosine (Sawynok, 1998). However, the analgesic effect caused by ADA inhibition is not so clear yet. It has been showed that

The Involvement of Purinergic System in Pain: Adenosine Receptors and Inosine as
Pharmacological Tools in Future Treatments

217

inhibitors of ADA itself are able to cause analgesia in determined animal models (Poon & Sawynok, 1999), but not in others (Keil & DeLander, 1992, 1994).

Coadministration of AK and ADA inhibitors potentiates the analgesic effect of the former (Poon & Sawynok, 1999). Also, adenosine effect is synergically augmented by coadministration of ADA inhibitor (Keil & DeLander, 1994). Distinct effects between AK inhibitors and ADA inhibitors might be because adenosine has a higher affinity by AK than ADA (Arch & Newsholme, 1978). In this point of view, AK seems to be the most important enzyme to regulate adenosine endogenous levels.

3.8.2 Analgesic effect by supply of purinergic substrates

Ecto-5′-nucleotidase (NT5E) is an enzyme located in the cell membrane that catalyzes the extracellular conversion of adenosine monophosphate (AMP) into adenosine in several tissues, included dorsal root ganglia (DRG) and substantia gelatinosa (Zylka, 2011). Recent studies have demonstrated that the analgesic effect of AMP combined with an AK inhibitor halved in NT5E knockout animals and is totally reversed in A_{1R} knockout animals (Sowa et al., 2010a). These results inspired another study that evaluated whether exogenous supply of NT5E (increases supply of adenosine) could induce a long lasting analgesic effect. NT5E presented effects that lasted for 2 days in models of inflammatory and chronic pain. Both effects were dependent on A_{1R} (Sowa, 2010b). Hence, the supply of enzymes that generate adenosine is a new interesting approach that may be used in studies to treat chronic pain.

3.8.3 Involvement of adenosine receptors in acupuncture pain relief

In an elegant study published in 2010, Goldman and colleagues showed that analgesia induced by acupuncture depends on purine release, such as ATP, ADP, AMP and adenosine. In addition, it has been showed that A_{1R} agonist replicates the acupuncture effect. Also, in A_{1R} knockout animals, acupuncture did not present analgesia. Moreover, inhibition of adenosine deaminase prolonged the analgesic effect of acupuncture in mice (Goldman et al., 2010). It is interesting to mention that caffeine, the most widely used drug across the world in beverages such as teas, coffee, *mate*, soft drinks, energy drinks and others is an antagonist of adenosine receptors. Therefore, patients in treatment with acupuncture should not drink these caffeine beverages, because caffeine might reduce the acupuncture analgesic effect (for review see Zylka, 2010).

4. Inosine and pain

4.1 Inosine within of purinergic system

ATP is the main molecule of purinergic system. Inside the cell, ATP may be bi-directionally converted into AMP. AMP is broken down into adenosine. Adenosine may be converted back into AMP through phosphorylation by AK. Moreover, adenosine might leave the cell by nucleoside transporter (NT). Inside the cell, adenosine deaminase is responsible for the conversion from adenosine to inosine. Outside the cell, this conversion is performed by ecto-adenosine kinase or even adenosine deaminase. Inosine is a substrate to purine nucleoside phosphorylase (PNP), leading to hypoxanthines as its products. Hypoxanthines are converted into xanthines and afterwards to uric acid by xanthine oxidase (Figure 4) (See review Sawynok & Liu, 2003).

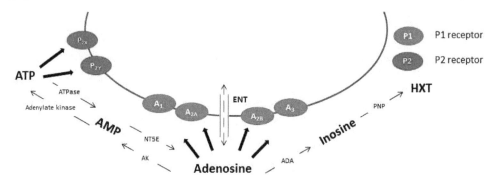

Fig. 4. Purinergic metabolism and its main molecules and enzymes. A_1, adenosine A_1 receptor; A_{2A}, adenosine A_{2A} receptor; A_{2B}, adenosine A_{2B} receptor; A_3, adenosine A_3 receptor ADA, adenosine deaminase; AK, adenosine kinase; AMP, adenosine monophosphate; ATP, adenosine triphosphate; ENT, equilibrative nucleoside transporter; HXT, hypoxanthines; *NT5E, ecto-5'nucleotidase*; P2X, purine P_{2X} receptor; P_{2Y}, purine P_{2Y} receptor; PNP, purine nucleoside phosphorilase.

Thus, inosine is one among many molecules in purinergic system. However, inosine has specific roles in several physiological states, we will show some functions and discuss the role of inosine in pain control in next sections.

4.2 Inosine physiological roles

In recent decades, many physiological roles for inosine have been shown. During the 70's, Aviado demonstrated that inosine exerts cardiotonic actions, such as preventing negative inotropic effect and increasing coronary vasodilatation (Aviado, 1978). Also, inosine presents several effects on axonal growth, such as axon growth induction and damaged neurons stimulation (Benowitz et al., 1999, 2002; Chen et al., 2002). Inosine also induces a regrowth in axotomized retinal ganglion cells in rats (Wu et al., 2003). These data indicate that inosine may constitute a new approach to treat the injured or degenerated nerves in central or peripheral nervous system. Despite of cardiovascular and axonal growth effects, the inflammatory effects of inosine are the most studied. Inosine has significant anti-inflammatory effects in several *in vivo* and *in vitro* models of inflammation (Gomez & Sitkovsky, 2003; Haskó et al., 2000; Marton et al., 2001; Schneider et al., 2006). These effects seem to be mediated by A_{1R}, A_{2R} and A_{3R} (Gomez & Sitkovsky, 2003; Haskó et al., 2000, 2004).

4.3 Inosine effect on acute pain

Inosine has analgesic action when administered by different routes (i.e. intraperitoneal, oral, intrathecal or intracerebroventricular) against pain induced by acetic acid (Nascimento et al., 2010). Of note, inosine also inhibits pain induced by formalin. Formalin test induces 2 distinct types of pain, neurogenic phase (acute pain) and inflammatory phase (inflammatory pain). Inosine is not able to relieve pain in neurogenic phase. However, inosine reduces nearly totally the inflammatory pain in formalin test (Nascimento et al., 2010). The effects of inosine in this model of pain extended the acetic acid data because formalin is a more

The Involvement of Purinergic System in Pain: Adenosine Receptors and Inosine as
Pharmacological Tools in Future Treatments

219

specific model. Therefore, these results indicate that inosine is able to prevent and reduce pain induced by inflammatory mediators. In this way, inosine may be inhibiting the synthesis or release of several neurotransmitters and mediators involved in pain conditions (Nascimento et al., 2010). We can also conclude that inosine is able to inhibit pain induced by central facilitation. Therefore, inosine increases pain threshold and it may be useful to treat some kinds of pain injury that result from a central sensitization. Adenosine receptors distribution on substantia gelatinosa, mainly A_{1R} and A_{2AR} could explain how inosine acts in this case (Sawynok, 1998; Sawynok & Liu, 2003). Inosine also presents a significant and dose-related inhibition of pain induced by glutamate (acute pain model) injection into the paw of mice (Nascimento et al., 2010).

4.4 Inosine effects on chronic pain

The data described in literature strongly suggests that inosine may have an important effect in controlling chronic pain, since it has anti-inflammatory effect and can reduce acute pain. In fact, Nascimento and colleagues (2010) demonstrated that acute administration of inosine, intraperitoneally, was able to inhibit chronic inflammatory pain induced by CFA in mice, being effective up to 4 hours after administration. The CFA is responsible for inducing chronic inflammation by stimulating the body's immune response, this response is mediated by the synthesis and release of cytokines and inflammatory mediators (Zhang et al., 2011).

In the study published by Nascimento and colleagues (2010), inosine was effective against mechanical and thermal allodynia induced by partial sciatic nerve ligation (PSNL) up to 4 hours after treatment by intraperitoneal route. Further, in another experiment, inosine was given daily for until 22 days and it also presented significant analgesic effect. Pain induced by PSNL is very strong and may last for weeks (Ueda, 2006). Animal models of neuropathic pain induce many functional and biochemical changes in local injury site. After the surgery there is the release of multiple inflammatory and pain mediators which in turn, may also be present in other areas involved and affected by sciatic nerve, as spinal cord and brain (Bridges et al., 2001; Ji & Woolf, 2001; Inoue et al., 2004; Ueda, 2006). Inosine activity in this kind of pain may indicate a promising molecule to new studies, because inosine might have a longer half-life than adenosine and admittedly does not have toxic or side effects.

4.5 Adenosine receptors involved in analgesic effects of inosine

A_{1R} has been considered the main receptor responsible for analgesic effect among adenosine receptors (Burnstock, 2007; Sawynok, 1998). A_{1R} is also the main receptor involved in inosine analgesic effect. Both A_{1R} antagonists DPCPX and 8-PT were able to reverse the inosine action. Inosine in a direct or indirect way activates A_{1R} to induce analgesia (Nascimento et al., 2010). Other studies have showed that adenosine receptor antagonists block *in vivo* and *in vitro* inosine effects (Haskó et al., 2000) and adenosine receptor knockout animals do not present immunoprotective effects of inosine (Gomez & Sitkovsky, 2003). Thus, it is clear that the A_{1R} activation is essential for inosine to exert its effect (Figure 5).

Involvement of A_{2AR} in pain is quite controversial. Some studies show that A_{2AR} blockade leads to analgesic effect (Borghi et al., 2002; Yoon et al., 2005) while other studies demonstrate that the blockade or deletion of A_{2AR} causes pain relief (Bastia et al., 2002; Ledent et al., 1997). Inosine activates A_{2AR} to induce analgesia, at least in the acetic acid model (Nascimento et al., 2010). However, the participation of A_{2AR} receptor in inosine analgesia in other pain animal models might be different or does not exist. Moreover, the A_{2AR} involvement on inosine effect can occur due to its anti-inflammatory profile (Milne & Palmer, 2011) and due to activation of the K^+ channels (Regaya et al., 2004).

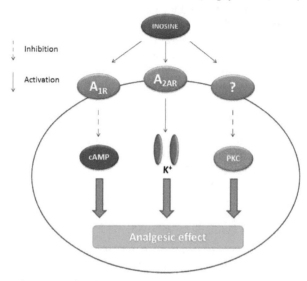

Fig. 5. Principal mechanisms of inosine antinociception. A_{1R}, adenosine A_1 receptor; A_{2AR}, adenosine A_{2A} receptor, cAMP, cyclic adenosine monophosphate; K^+, potassium channels; PKC, protein kinase C.

A_{2BR} and A_{3R} adenosine receptors do not have significant role in pain transmission or modulation (Sawynok, 1998). Although it has been shown that inosine binds to A_{3R}, it seems that A_{2BR} and A_{3R} receptors are not involved in inosine analgesic effect (Nascimento et al., 2010).

4.5.1 Does inosine binds to adenosine receptor?

Few studies have evaluated if inosine binds to adenosine receptor. Jin and co-workers demonstrated that inosine binds to A_{3R} in mast cells, but not to A_{1R} or A_{2AR} (Jin et al., 1997). In 2001, Fredholm's group observed that inosine weakly bound to A_{1R} and A_{3R}, but not to A_{2R} (Fredholm et al., 2001). Fredholm concluded that inosine could not be considered a natural ligand of adenosine receptors. However, because of these few studies and considering *in vivo* studies where adenosine antagonists are able to block inosine effects, it is not is possible to affirm whether inosine is or not a natural ligand or a partial agonist of adenosine receptors. More studies are necessary to elucidate this issue.

4.6 Intracellular signalling involved in analgesic effects of inosine

The intracellular signaling involved in analgesic action of inosine is yet not entirely elucidated. Assuming that inosine effects depend on adenosine receptors, A_{1R} and A_{2AR}, we can consider that adenosine receptors signaling pathways are the major effectors of this

The Involvement of Purinergic System in Pain: Adenosine Receptors and Inosine as
Pharmacological Tools in Future Treatments

221

effect. As fully mentioned previously, A_{1R} is coupled to Gi/0 protein. A_{1R} signaling causes downstream inhibition of adenylyl cyclase and induction of PLC activity. Further, when A_{1R} is activated it causes potassium channel opening, PI3K and MAPK stimulation. All these pathways might participate in the inosine analgesic effect (Ansari et al., 2009; Jacobson & Gao, 2006; Sawynok, 1998; Schulte & Fredholm, 2003). Inosine inhibits the pain caused by PKC activator. Thus, at least in part, the analgesic action of inosine depends on PKC inhibition (Nascimento et al., 2010), even though it is not clear yet how it happens (Figure 5). Costenla and coworkers showed that an adenosine analog that has preference for A_{2AR} is able to inhibit sodium current in NMDA receptors (Costenla et al., 1999). This signaling occurring *in vivo* could partially explain how A_{2AR} works in analgesia induced by inosine.

4.7 Perspectives

As previously described in this chapter, purinergic system is an important endogenous modulator of pain. Hundreds of pre-clinical studies targeting the adenosine receptors showed analgesic effect in distinct pain models. Inosine, an endogenous modulator of several physiological functions also presents a role in pain transmission. Inosine might be a natural activator of adenosine receptors. Also, it can indirectly increase the release or reduce the uptake of adenosine, potentiating the effect of its precursor. Thus, understanding how inosine acts to induce analgesia may help discover new ways to inhibit pain or new therapeutic targets. Moreover, inosine may be a potential molecule to treat pain, and it has a great advantage to be devoid of toxic or side effects because it has been used clinically for many years for other purposes. Another interesting approach would be to attempt to prolong and potentiate the effect of inosine. For this, a great understanding of purinergic metabolism is necessary in order to correctly and effectively approach this matter.

5. Active drugs on adenosine receptors and their clinical applications

Nowadays there is increasing interest in the therapeutic potential of adenosinergic compounds (including receptor agonists and antagonists, enzyme inhibitors and others), and many adenosine compounds have been evaluated.

5.1 Adenosine receptor ligands and their potential as novel drugs

Adenosine itself, for a long time, was the only adenosine agonist used in humans. It is widely used in the treatment of paroxysmal supraventricular tachycardia (Adenocard®) due to its activation of A_{1R}, and as a diagnostic for myocardial perfusion imaging (Adenoscan®) utilizing its A_{2AR}-activating effects resulting in vasodilation (Müller & Jacobson, 2011). However, other A_{1R}-selective agonists such as Selodenoson, Capadenoson e Tecadenoson have been clinically evaluated for the treatment of paroxysmal supraventricular tachycardia, atrial fibrillation, or angina pectoris (Müller & Jacobson, 2011). Still talking about cardiovascular disorders, selective A_{2AR} agonist, Apadenoson, Binodenoson and Sonedenoson appears as candidates for clinical use (Awad et al., 2006; Desai et al., 2005; Udelson et al. 2004). These agonists are of interest as vasodilator agents in cardiac imaging (Cerqueira, 2006) and inflammation suppressors. Accordingly, Regadenoson is already approved for diagnostic imaging (Iskandrian et al., 2007). A_{3R} selective agonists are also currently in clinical trials and exhibit nanomolar affinity at the receptor, CF101 (Can-Fite Biopharma) and Cl-IB-MECA (CF102) are in trials for autoimmune inflammatory disorders and for liver cancer, respectively. Two other A_{3R} agonists CP-608,039 and its N6-(2,5-dichlorobenzyl) analogue CP-532,903 were previously under development for cardioprotection. MRS3558 (CF502) is in preclinical development for the treatment of autoimmune disease (Avni et al., 2010; Wan et al., 2008).

5.2 Adenosinergic drugs in pain clinical studies and practical

Clinical studies confirm the pre-clinical trials showing that in neuropathic pain patients, adenosine was able to alleviate spontaneous pain, tactile and thermal allodynia, as well as thermal hyperalgesia (Qu et al., 1997). In addition, intravenous infusion of adenosine during breast surgery reduced the postoperative pain (Lynch et al., 2003; Sollevi et al., 1995). Spinal administration of adenosine and adenosine analogs in humans also exhibited analgesic effect. A phase I clinical safety study in healthy volunteers demonstrated that 1000 µg of adenosine given intrathecally lacked side effects and led to a significant decrease in mustard oil-induced inflammatory pain, in tourniquet induced ischemic pain, and decreased areas of secondary allodynia after skin inflammation (Rane et al., 1998).

In another study, a single dose of 0.1 – 0.5 mg/kg of SDZ WAG 994 (adenosine A_{1R} agonist), was evaluated in a phase I clinical study, and this compound was well tolerated. A dose of 1 mg/kg was used in a randomized double-blind clinical trial to determine its efficacy in postoperative dental pain after third molar surgery. However, SDZ WAG 994 did not show significant difference from placebo and was not effective in attenuating postoperative pain after third molar surgery. On the other hand, at higher doses, the compound showed dose-dependent adverse events (Seymour et al., 1999; Wagner et al., 1995; Yan et al., 2003).

Another full high-affinity A_{1R} agonists, GR79236X, was also evaluated in patients with dental pain after third molar extraction. Patients received a 15-min double-blind infusion containing 10 µg/kg of GR79236X, unfortunately, no evidence of efficacy of GR79236X was observed with this compound compared with placebo (Sneyd et al., 2007). Another A_{1R} agonist GW493838 developed by GlaxoSmithKline, was evaluated in phase II clinical trials to determine its analgesic effect in patients with postherpetic neuralgia or peripheral nerve injury caused by trauma or surgery. However, further development of GW493838 has been discontinued (Nelsen et al., 2004; as cited in Elzein & Zablocki, 2008).

Allosteric modulation of A_{1R} function may also be an interesting tool. Accordingly, the A_{1R}-selective allosteric enhancer T-62, given orally was also shown to reduce hypersensitivity in carrageenan-inflamed rats, in addition, phase I clinical trials of T62 have been completed as a treatment for neuropathic pain (Childers et al., 2005). Therewithal, the A_{2AR} agonist BVT.115959 from Biovitrum completed the clinical trials for diabetic neuropathic pain and it was well tolerated but did not significantly improve pain symptoms (Biovitrum, 2005; Zylka, 2011).

6. Conclusion and future directions

This chapter presented a general and updated review about the purinergic system with emphasis in adenosine receptors (P1) and pain. It is possible to conclude that the modulation of this system and its receptors is quite important and interesting for the control of pain. Recent studies have approached this system in new ways and contributed to the development of this research field. Some clinical studies have been carried out with

The Involvement of Purinergic System in Pain: Adenosine Receptors and Inosine as
Pharmacological Tools in Future Treatments

223

purinergic drugs (adenosine analogs) and some studies have showed quite satisfactory effects, although others haven't showed statistical difference between treated and non-treated groups. Finally, the possibility of new drugs targeting the purinergic system to treat distinct kinds of pain reaching clinical trials in the next years is clear.

7. References

Abbracchio, MP. & Burnstock, G. (1994). Purinoceptores: are there families of P2X and P2Y purinoceptores? *Pharmacology & Therapeutics,* Vol. 64, No.3, pp. (445-475)

Abbracchio, MP., Brambilla, R., Ceruti, S., Kim, HO., von Lubitz, DK., Jacobson, KA. & Cattabeni, F. (1995). G protein-dependent activation of phospholipase C by adenosine A3 receptors in rat brain. *Molecular Pharmacology,* Vol.48, No. 6, (December, 1995), pp.(1038-1045), ISSN 1038-1045.

Abo-Salem, OM., Hayallah, AM., Bilkei-Gorzo, A., Filipek, B., Zimmer, A. & Müller, CE. (2004). Antinociceptive effects of novel A2B adenosine receptor antagonists. *The Journal of Pharmacology Experimental Therapeutics,* Vol 308, No. 1, (January, 2004), pp. (358-66), ISSN 1521-0103.

Ansari, HR., Teng, B., Nadeem, A., Roush, KP., Martin, KH., Schnermann, J., & Mustafa, SJ. (2009). A(1) adenosine receptor-mediated PKC and p42/p44 MAPK signaling in mouse coronary artery smooth muscle cells. *American Journal of Physiology. Heart and Circulatory Physiology,* Vol. 297, No 3, (September, 2009), pp. (H1032-H1039), ISSN 1522-1539.

Arch, JR. & Newsholme, EA. (1978). Activities and some properties of 5'-nucleotidase, adenosine kinase and adenosine deaminase in tissues from vertebrates and invertebrates in relation to the control of the concentration and the physiological role of adenosine. *The Biochemical Journal,* Vol. 174, No 3, (September, 1978), pp. (965-977).

Armstrong, SC. & Ganote, E. (1994). Adenosine receptor specificity in preconditioning of isolated rabbit cardiomyocytes: evidence of A3 receptor involvement. *Cardiovascular Research,* Vol. 28, No. 7, (July, 1994) pp. (1049-1056).

Aviado, DM. (1978). Effects of fluorocarbons, chlorinated solvents, and inosine on the cardiopulmonary ystem. *Environmental Health Perspectives,* Vol. 26, No. 1, (October, 1978), pp. (207-215).

Avni, HJ., Garzozi, IS., Barequet, F., Segev, F., Varssano, D., Sartani, G., Chetrit, N., Bakshi, E., Zadok, D., Tomkins, O., Litvin, G., Jacobson, KA., Fishman, S., Harpaz, Z., Farbstein, M., Yehuda, SB., Silverman, MH., Kerns, WD., Bristol, DR., Cohn, I. & Fishman, P. (2010). Treatment of dry eye syndrome with orally-administered CF101: data from a phase 2 clinical trial, *Ophthalmology,* Vol. 117, No. 7, (July, 2010), pp. (1287–1293).

Awad, AS., Huang, L., Ye, H., Duong, ET., Bolton, WK., Linden, J. & Okusa, MD. (2006). Adenosine A2A receptor activation attenuates inflammation and injury in diabetic nephropathy. *American Journal of Physiology. Renal Physiology,* Vol. 290, No. 4, (April, 2006), pp. (F828–F837).

Bastia, E., Varani, K., Monopoli, A. & Bertorelli R (2002). Effects of A(1) and A(2A) adenosine receptor ligands in mouse acute models of pain. *Neuroscience Letters,* Vol. 328, No. 3, (August, 2002), pp. (241-244).

Benowitz, LI., Goldberg, DE. & Irwin, N. (2002). Inosine stimulates axon growth in vitro and in the adult CNS. *Progress in Brain Research,* Vol. 137, No. 1, pp. (389-399).

Benowitz, LI., Goldberg, DE., Madsen, JR., Soni, D. & Irwin, N. (1999). Inosine stimulates extensive axon collateral growth in the rat corticospinal tract after injury. *Proceedings of the National Academy Sciences of the United States of America,* Vol. 96, No. 23, (November, 1999), pp. (13486-13490).

Bilkei-Gorzo, A., Abo-Salem, OM., Hayallah, AM., Michel, K., Müller, CE. & Zimmer, A. (2008). Adenosine receptor subtype-selective antagonists in inflammation and hyperalgesia. *Naunyn- Schmiedebergs Archives of Pharmacology,* Vol. 377, No. 1, (March, 2008), pp. (65-76).

Biovitrum, (January, 2008). A Double-Blind, Placebo-Controlled, Randomized, Parallel-Group Study Evaluating the Efficacy and Tolerability of Oral BVT.115959, a Novel A2A Agonist, Versus Placebo in the Treatment of Diabetic Neuropathic Pain, 08.25.2011, Available from
http://www.clinicaltrials.gov/ct2/show/NCT00452777?term=Efficacy+and+tolerability+of+novel+A2A+agonist+in+treatment+of+diabetic+neuropathic+pain&rank=1

Boison, D., Chen, JF. & Fredholm, BB. (2010). Adenosine signaling and function in glial cells. *Cell Death Differentiation,* Vol. 17, No. 7, (July, 2010), pp. (1071-1082).

Borea, PA., Gessi, S., Bar-Yehuda, S. & Fishman, P. (2009). A3 adenosine receptor: pharmacology and role in disease. *Handbook of Experimental Pharmacology,* Vol. 193, No. 1, pp. (297-327).

Borghi, V., Przewlocka, B., Labuz, D., Maj, M., Ilona, O. & Pavone, F. (2002). Formalin-induced pain and mu-opioid receptor density in brain and spinal cord are modulated by A1 and A2a adenosine agonists in mice. *Brain Research,* Vol. 956, No. 2, (November, 2002), pp. (339-348).

Bridges, D., Thompson SW. & Rice, AS. (2001). Mechanisms of neuropathic pain. *British Journal of Anaesthesia,* Vol. 87, No. 1, (July, 2001), pp. (12-26), ISSN 1471-67

Bura, SA., Nadal, X., Ledent, C., Maldonado, R. & Valverde, O. (2008). A2A adenosine receptor regulates glia proliferation and pain after peripheral nerve injury. *Pain,* Vol. 140, No. 1, (November, 2008), pp. (95-103).

Burnstock, G. (1972). Purinergic nerves. *Pharmacological Reviews,* Vol. 24, No. 3, (September, 1972), pp. (509–581), ISSN: 1521-0081

Burnstock, G. (1978). A basis for distinguishing two types of purinergic receptor, In: *Cell Membrane Receptors for Drugs and Hormones: A Multidisciplinary Approach,* Straub, RW. & Bolis L., pp. (107–118), Raven Press, New York.

Burnstock, G. (2007). Purine and pyrimidine receptors. *Cellular and Molecular Life Sciences,* Vol. 64, No. 12, (June, 2007), pp. (1471-1483).

Burnstock, G. (2008). Purinergic signalling and disorders of the central nervous system. *Nature Reviews. Drug Discovery,* Vol. 7, No. 7, (July, 2008), pp. (575-590), ISSN: 1474-1784

Burnstock, G. & Kennedy, C. (1985). Is there a basis for distinguishing two types of P2-purinoceptor? *General Pharmacology,* Vol. 16, No. 5, pp. (433–440).

Burnstock, G. & Knight, GE. (2004). Cellular distribution and functions of P2 receptor subtypes in different systems. *International Review of Cytology,* Vol. 240, No.1, pp. (31–304).

The Involvement of Purinergic System in Pain: Adenosine Receptors and Inosine as
Pharmacological Tools in Future Treatments

225

Burnstock, G. & Williams, M. (2000). P2 purinergic receptors: modulation of cell function and therapeutic potential. *The Journal of Pharmacology and Experimental Therapeutics*, Vol. (295), No. 3, (December, 2000), pp. (862–869), ISSN 1521-0103

Burnstock, G., Fredholm, BB. & Verkhratsky, A. (2011). Adenosine and ATP receptors in the brain. *Current Topics in Medicinal Chemistry*, Vol.11, No.8, (April, 2011), pp. (973-1011), ISSN: 1568-0266

By, Y., Condo, J., Durand-Gorde, JM., Lejeune, PJ., Mallet, B., Guieu, R. & Ruf, J. (2011). Intracerebroventricular injection of an agonist-like monoclonal antibody to adenosine A(2A) receptor has antinociceptive effects in mice. *Journal of Neuroimmunology*, Vol. 230, No. 1-2, (January, 2011), pp. (178-182).

Cerqueira, MD. (2006). Advances in pharmacologic agents in imaging: new A2A receptor agonists. *Current Cardiology Reports*, Vol. 8, No. 2, (March, 2006), pp. (119–122).

Chen, P., Goldberg, DE., Kolb, B., Lanser, M. & Benowitz, LI. (2002). Inosine induces axonal rewiring and improves behavioral outcome after stroke. *Proceedings of the National Academy of Sciences of the United States of America*, Vol. 99, No. 13, (June, 2002), pp. (9031-9036).

Childers, SR., Li, X., Xiao, R. & Eisenach, JC. (2005). Allosteric modulation of adenosine A1 receptor coupling to G-proteins in brain. *Journal of Neurochemistry*, Vol. 93, No.3, (May, 2005), pp. (715 -723).

Choca, JI., Green, RD. & Proudfit, HK. (1988). Adenosine A1 and A2 receptors of the substantia gelatinosa are located predominantly on intrinsic neurons: an autoradiography study. *Journal of Pharmacology and Experimental Therapeutics*, Vol. 247, No. 2, (November, 1988), pp. (757-764), ISSN: 1521-0103

Costenla, AR., De Mendonca, A., Sebastião, A. & Ribeiro, JA. (1999). An adenosine analogue inhibits NMDA receptor-mediated responses in bipolar cells of the rat retina. *Experimental Eye Research*, Vol. 68, No. 3, (March, 1999), pp. (367-70).

Cunha, RA., Ferre, S., Vaugeois, JM. & Chen, JF. (2008). Potential therapeutic interest of adenosine A2A receptors in psychiatric disorders. *Current Pharmaceutical Design*, Vol. 14, No. 15, (May, 2008), pp. (1512-1524), ISSN: 1381-6128

Curros-Criado, MM. & Herrero, JF. (2005). The antinociceptive effects of the systemic adenosine A1 receptor agonist CPA in the absence and in the presence of spinal cord sensitization. *Pharmacology, Biochemistry and Behaviour*, Vol. 82, No. 4, (December, 2005), pp. (721-726).

DeLander, GE. & Hopkins, CJ. (1986). Spinal adenosine modulates descending antinociceptive pathways stimulated by morphine. *Journal of Pharmacology and Experimental Therapeutics*, Vol.239, No. 1, (October, 1986), pp. (88-93), ISSN 1521-0103

Desai, C., Victor-Veja, S., Gadangi, S., Montesinos, MC., Chu, CC. & Cronstein, BN. (2005). Adenosine A2A receptor stimulation increases angiogenesis by down-regulating production of the antiangiogenic matrix protein thrombospondin 1. *Molecular Pharmacology*, Vol. 67, No. 5, (May, 2005), pp. (1406–1413), ISSN: 1521-0111

Dixon, AK., Gubitz, AK., Sirinathsinghji, DJ., Richardson, PJ. & Freeman, TC. (1996). Tissue distribution of adenosine receptor mRNAs in the rat. *British Journal of Pharmacology*, Vol. 118, No. 6, (July, 1996), pp. (1461-1468).

Doak, GJ. & Sawynok, J. (1995). Complex role of peripheral adenosine in the genesis of the response to subcutaneous formalin in the rat. *European Journal of Pharmacology*, Vol. 281, No. 3, (August, 1995), pp. (311-318).

Drury, AN. & Szent-Györgyi, A. (1929). The physiological activity of adenine compounds with special reference to their action upon the mammalian heart. *The Journal of Physiology*, Vol. 68, No. 3, (November, 1929), pp. (213-237).

Elzein, E. & Zablocki, J. (2008). A1 adenosine receptor agonists and their potential therapeutic applications. *Expert Opinion on Investigational Drugs*, Vol. 17, No. 12, (December, 2008), pp. (1901-1910).

Fedorova, IM., Jacobson, MA., Basile, A. & Jacobson, KA. (2003). Behavioral characterization of mice lacking the A3 adenosine receptor: sensitivity to hypoxic neurodegeneration. *Cellular and Molecular Neurobiology*, Vol. 23, No. 3, (June, 2003), pp. (431-447).

Feoktistov, I. & Biaggioni, I. (2011). Role of adenosine A(2B) receptors in inflammation. *Advaces in Pharmacology*, Vol. 61, No. 1, pp. (115-144).

Fredholm, BB. (1995). Purinoceptors in the nervous system. *Pharmacology & Toxicology*, Vol. 76, No. 4, (April, 1995), pp. (228-239).

Fredholm, BB., Cunha, RA. & Svenningsson, P. (2003). Pharmacology of adenosine A2A receptors and therapeutic applications. *Current Topics in Medicinal Chemistry*, Vol. 3, No. 4, (February, 2003), pp. (413-426), ISSN 1568-0266

Fredholm, BB., Chern, Y., Franco, R. & Sitkovsky, M. (2007). Aspects of the general biology of adenosine A2A signaling. *Progress in Neurobiology*, Vol. 83, No 5, (December, 2007), pp. (263-276).

Fredholm, BB., IJzerman, AP., Jacobson, KA., Linden, J. and Muller, CE. (2011). International Union of Basic and Clinical Pharmacology. LXXXI. Nomenclature and classification of adenosine receptors- an update. *Pharmacological Reviews*, Vol.63, No. 1, (March, 2011), pp. (1-34), ISSN 1521-0081

Fredholm, BB., Irenius, E., Kull, B. & Schulte, G. (2001). Comparison of the potency of adenosine as an agonist at human adenosine receptors expressed in Chinese hamster ovary cells. *Biochemical Pharmacology*, Vol. 61, No. 4, (February, 2001), pp. (443-448).

Godfrey, L., Yan, L., Clarke, GD., Ledent, C., Kitchen, I. & Hourani, SM. (2006). Modulation of paracetamol antinociception by caffeine and by selective adenosine A2 receptor antagonists in mice. *European Journal of Pharmacology*, Vol. 531, No.1-3, (February, 2006), pp. (80-86).

Goldman, N., Chen, M., Fujita, T., Xu, Q., Peng, W., Liu, W., Jensen, TK., Pei, Y., Wang, F., Han, X., Chen, JF., Schnermann, J., Takano, T., Bekar, L., Tieu, K. & Nedergaard, M. (2010). Adenosine A1 receptors mediate local anti-nociceptive effects of acupuncture. *Nature Neuroscience*, Vol. 13, No. 7, (July, 2010), pp. (883-888), ISSN 1546-1726

Gomez, G. & Sitkovsky, MV. (2003). Differential requirement for A2a and A3 adenosine receptors for the protective effect of inosine in vivo. *Blood*, Vol. 102, No. 13, (December, 2003), pp. (4472-4478), ISSN 1528-0020

Gong, QJ., Li, YY., Xin, WJ., Wei, XH., Cui, Y., Wang, J., Liu, Y., Liu, CC., Li, YY. & Liu, XG. (2010). Differential effects of adenosine A1 receptor on pain-related behavior in

The Involvement of Purinergic System in Pain: Adenosine Receptors and Inosine as
Pharmacological Tools in Future Treatments

227

normal and nerve-injured rats. *Brain Research*, Vol. 1361, (November, 2010), pp. (23-30).

Haskó, G., Kuhel, DG., Németh, ZH., Mabley, JG., Stachlewitz, RF., Virág, L., Lohinai, Z., Southan, GJ., Salzman, AL. & Szabó, C. (2000). Inosine inhibits inflammatory cytokine production by a posttranscriptional mechanism and protects against endotoxin-induced shock. *Journal of Immunology*, Vol. 164, No. 2, (January, 2000), pp. (1013-1019), ISSN 1550-6606

Haskó, G., Sitkovsky, MV. & Szabó, C. (2004). Immunomodulatory and neuroprotective effects of inosine. *Trends in Pharmacological Science*, Vol. 25, No. 3, (March, 2004), pp. (152-157).

Horiuchi, H., Ogata, T., Morino, T. & Yamamoto, H. (2010). Adenosine A1 receptor agonists reduce hyperalgesia after spinal cord injury in rats. *Spinal Cord*, Vol. 48, No. 9, (September, 2010), pp. (685-690), ISSN 1476-5624

Hussey, MJ., Clarke, GD., Ledent, C., Hourani, SM. & Kitchen, I. (2007). Reduced response to the formalin test and lowered spinal NMDA glutamate receptor binding in adenosine A2A receptor knockout mice. *Pain*, Vol. 129, No. 3, (June, 2007), pp. (287-294).

Hwang, JH., Hwang, GS., Cho, SK. & Han, SM. (2005). Morphine can enhance the antiallodynic effect of intrathecal R-PIA in rats with nerve ligation injury. *Anesthesia & Analgesia*, Vol. 100, No 2, (February, 2005), pp. (461-468), ISSN 1526-7598

Inoue, M., Rashid, MH., Fujita, R., Contos, JJ., Chun, J. & Ueda, H. (2004). Initiation of neuropathic pain requires lysophosphatidic acid receptor signaling. *Nature Medicine*, Vol. 10, No. 7, (July, 2004), pp. (712-718), ISSN 1546-170X

Iskandrian, AE., Bateman, TM., Belardinelli, L., Blackburn, B., Cerqueira, MD., Hendel, RC., Lieu, H., Mahmarian, JJ., Olmsted, A., Underwood, SR., Vitola, J. & Wang, W. (2007). Adenosine versus regadenoson comparative evaluation in myocardial perfusion imaging: results of the ADVANCE phase 3 multicenter international trial. *Journal of Nuclear Cardiology*, Vol. 14, No. 5, (September, 2007) pp. (645–658).

Jacobson, KA. & Gao, GZ. (2006). Adenosine receptors as therapeutic targets. *Nature Reviews. Drug Discovery*, Vol. 5, No. 3, (March, 2006), pp. (247-264), ISSN 1474-1784

Ji, RR. & Woolf, CJ. (2001). Neuronal plasticity and signal transduction in nociceptive neurons: implications for the initiation and maintenance of pathological pain. Neurobiology of Disease, Vol. 8, No. 1, (February, 2001), pp. (1-10).

Jin, X., Shepherd, RK., Duling, BR. & Linden, J. (1997). Inosine binds to A3 adenosine receptors and stimulates mast cell degranulation. *The Journal of Clinical Investigation*, Vol. 100, No. 11, pp. (2849-2857).

Johansson, B., Halldner, L., Dunwiddie, TV., Masino, SA., Poelchen, W., Giménez-Llort, L., Escorihuela, RM., Fernández-Teruel, A., Wiesenfeld-Hallin, Z., Xu, XJ., Hardemark, A., Betsholtz, C., Herlenius, E. & Fredholm, BB. (2001). Hyperalgesia, anxiety, and decreased hypoxic neuroprotection in mice lacking the adenosine A1 receptor. *Proceedings of the National Academy of Sciences of the United States of America*, Vol. 98, No. 16, (July, 2001), pp. (9407-9412).

Karlsten, R., Gordh, T. & Post, C. (1992). Local antinociceptive and hyperalgesic effects in the formalin test after peripheral administration of adenosine analogues in mice. *Pharmacology & Toxicology*, Vol. 70, No. 6 Pt 1, (June, 1992), pp. (434-438).

Keil, GJ 2nd. & DeLander, GE. (1992). Spinally-mediated antinociception is induced in mice by an adenosine kinase-, but not by an adenosine deaminase-, inhibitor. *Life Sciences*, Vol. 51, No. 19, pp. (PL171 - PL176).

Keil, GJ 2nd. & DeLander, GE. (1994). Adenosine kinase and adenosine deaminase inhibition modulate spinal adenosine- and opioid agonist-induced antinociception in mice. *European Journal of Pharmacology*, Vol. 271, No. 1, (December, 1994), pp. (37-46).

Kowaluk, EA., Mikusa, J., Wismer, CT., Zhu, CZ., Schweitzer, E., Lynch, JJ., Lee, CH., Jiang, M., Bhagwat, SS., Gomtsyan, A., McKie, J., Cox, BF., Polakowski, J., Reinhart, G., Williams, M. & Jarvis, MF. (2000). ABT-702 (4-amino-5-(3-bromophenyl)-7-(6-morpholino-pyridin- 3-yl)pyrido[2,3-d]pyrimidine), a novel orally effective adenosine kinase inhibitor with analgesic and anti-inflammatory properties. II. In vivo characterization in the rat. *Journal of Pharmacology and Experimental Therapeutics*, Vol. 295, No. 3, (December, 2000), pp. (1165-1174).

Kowaluk, EA., Kohlhaas, KL., Bannon, A., Gunther, K., Lynch, JJ 3rd. & Jarvis, MF. (1999). Characterization of the effects of adenosine kinase inhibitors on acute thermal nociception in mice. *Pharmacology, Biochemitry & Behaviour*, Vol. 63, No. 1, (May, 1999), pp. (83-91).

Ledent, C., Vaugeois, JM., Schiffmann, SN., Pedrazzini, T., El Yacoubi, M., Vanderhaeghen, JJ., Costentin, J., Heath, JK., Vassart, G. & Parmentier, M. (1997). Aggressiveness, hypoalgesia and high blood pressure in mice lacking the adenosine A2a receptor. *Nature*, Vol. 388, No. 6643, pp. (674-678), ISSN 1476-4687

Li, X., Conklin, D., Pan, HL. & Eisenach, JC. (2003). Allosteric adenosine receptor modulation reduces hypersensitivity following peripheral inflammation by a central mechanism. *The Journal of Pharmacology and Experimental Therapeutics*, Vol. 305, No. 3, (June, 2003), pp. (950-955), ISSN 1521-0103

Lima, FO., Souza, GR., Verri, WA Jr., Parada, CA., Ferreira, SH., Cunha, FQ. & Cunha, TM. (2010). Direct blockade of inflammatory hypernociception by peripheral A1 adenosine receptors: involvement of the NO/cGMP/PKG/KATP signaling pathway. *Pain*, Vol. 151, No. 2, (November, 2009), pp. (506-515).

Loram, LC., Harrison, JA., Sloane, EM., Hutchinson, MR., Sholar, P., Taylor, FR., Berkelhammer, D., Coats, BD., Poole, S., Milligan, ED., Maier, SF., Rieger, J. & Watkins, LR. (2009). Enduring reversal of neuropathic pain by a single intrathecal injection of adenosine 2A receptor agonists: a novel therapy for neuropathic pain. *The Journal of Neuroscience*, Vol. 29, No. 44, (November, 2009), pp. (14015-14025), ISSN 1529-2401

Lynch, JJ 3rd., Jarvis, MF. & Kowaluk, EA. (1999). An adenosine kinase inhibitor attenuates tactile allodynia in a rat model of diabetic neuropathic pain. *European Journal of Pharmacology*, Vol. 364, No.2-3, (January, 1999), pp. (141-146).

Lynch, ME., Clark, AJ. & Sawyonk, J. (2003). Intravenous adenosine alleviates neuropathic pain: a double blind placebo controlled crossover trial using an enriched enrollment design. *Pain*, Vol. 103, No. (1-2), (May, 2003), pp. (111 -117).

Marton, A., Pacher, P., Murthy, KG., Németh, ZH., Haskó, G. & Szabó, C. (2001). Anti-inflammatory effects of inosine in human monocytes, neutrophils and epithelial cells in vitro. *International Journal of Molecular Medicine*, Vol. 8, No. 6, (December, 2001), pp. (617-621).

The Involvement of Purinergic System in Pain: Adenosine Receptors and Inosine as
Pharmacological Tools in Future Treatments

229

McGaraughty, S. & Jarvis, MF. (2006). Purinergic control of neuropathic pain. *Drug Development Research*, Vol. 67, No. 4, (April, 2006), pp. (376–388).

McGaraughty, S., Cowart, M., Jarvis, MF. & Berman, RF. (2005). Anticonvulsant and antinociceptive actions of novel adenosine kinase inhibitors. *Current Topics Medicinal Chemistry*, Vol. 5, No. 1, pp. (43-58). ISSN: 1568-0266

Megson, AC., Dickenson, JM., Townsend-Nicholson, A. & Hill, SJ. (1995). Synergy between the inositol phosphate responses to transfected human adenosine A1-receptors and constitutive P2-purinoceptors in CHO-K1 cells. *British Journal of Pharmacology*, Vol. 115, No. 8, (August, 1995), pp. (1415-14124).

Milne, GR. & Palmer, TM. (2011). Anti-inflammatory and immunosuppressive effects of the A2A adenosine receptor. *The Scientific World Journal*, Vol. 11, No. 1, (February, 2011), pp. (320-339).

Müller, CE. & Jacobson, KA. (2011). Recent developments in adenosine receptor ligands and their potential as novel drugs. *Biochimica et Biophysica Acta*, Vol. 1808, No. 5, (May, 2011), pp. (1290-1308).

Nascimento, FP., Figueredo, SM., Marcon, R., Martins, DF., Macedo, SJ Jr., Lima, DA., Almeida, RC., Ostroski, RM., Rodrigues, AL. & Santos, ARS. (2010). Inosine reduces pain-related behavior in mice: involvement of adenosine A1 and A2A receptor subtypes and protein kinase C pathways. *The Journal of Pharmacology and Experimental Therapeutics*, Vol. 334, No. 2, (May, 2010), pp. (590-598), ISSN: 1521-0101

Palmer, TM., Benovic, JL. & Stiles, GL. (1995). Agonist-dependent phosphorylation and desensitization of the rat A3 adenosine receptor. Evidence for a G-protein-coupled receptor kinase-mediated mechanism. *The Journal of Biological Chemistry*, Vol. 270, No. 49, (December, 1995), pp. (29607-29613), ISSN: 1083-351-X

Peakman, MC. & Hill, SJ. (1994). Adenosine A2B-receptor-mediated cyclic AMP accumulation in primary rat astrocytes. *British Journal of Pharmacology*, Vol. 111, No. 1, (January, 1994), pp. (191-198)

Poon, A. & Sawynok, J. (1999). Antinociceptive and anti-inflammatory properties of an adenosine kinase inhibitor and an adenosine deaminase inhibitor. *European Journal of Pharmacology*, Vol. 384, No. 2-3, (November, 1999), pp. (123-38)

Poon, A. & Sawynok, J. (1998). Antinociception by adenosine analogs and inhibitors of adenosine metabolism in an inflammatory thermal hyperalgesia model in the rat. *Pain*, Vol. 74, No. 2-3, (January, 1998), pp. (235-245)

Qu, X., Cooney, G. & Donnelly, R. (1997). Short-term metabolic and haemodynamic effects of GR79236 in normal and fructose-fed rats. *European Journal of Pharmacology*, Vol. 338, No. 3, (November, 1997), pp. (269 -276)

Ralevic, V. & Burnstock, G. (1998). Receptors for purines and pyrimidines. *Pharmacological Reviews*, Vol. 50, No. 3, (September, 1998), pp. (413-492). ISSN: 1521-0081

Rane, K., Segerdahl, M., Goiny, M. & Sollevi, A. (1998). Intrathecal adenosine administration, a phase 1 clinical safety study in healthy volunteers, with additional evaluation of its influence on sensory thresholds and experimental pain. *Anesthesiology*, Vol. 89, No. 5, (November, 1998), pp. (1108–1115).

Regaya, I., Pham, T., Andreotti, N., Sauze, N., Carrega, L., Martin-Eauclaire, MF., Jouirou, B., Peragut, JC., Vacher, H., Rochat, H., Devaux, C., Sabatier, JM. & Guieu, R. (2004). Small conductance calcium-activated K+ channels, SkCa, but not voltage-gated K+ (Kv) channels, are implicated in the antinociception induced by

CGS21680, a A2A adenosine receptor agonist. *Life Sciences*, Vol. 76, No. 4, (December, 2004), pp. (367-377).

Ribeiro, JA., Sebastiao, AM. & de Mendonça, A. (2002). Adenosine receptors in the nervous system: pathophysiological implications. *Progress in Neurobiology*, Vol. 68, No. 6, (December, 2002), pp. (377-392).

Salvatore, CA., Jacobson, MA., Taylor, HE., Linden, J. & Johnson, RG. (1993). Molecular cloning and characterization of the human A3 adenosine receptor. *Proceedings of the National Academy of Sciences of the United States of America*, Vol. 90, No. 21, (November, 1993), pp. (10365-10369).

Sawynok, J. (1998). Adenosine receptor activation and nociception. *European Journal of Pharmacology*, Vol. 347, No. 1, (April, 1998), pp. (1-11).

Sawynok, J. (2009). Adenosine Receptors, In: *Peripheral Receptor Targets for Analgesia: Novel Approaches to Pain Management*, Brian E Cairns, pp. (137-152), John Wiley and Sons, Inc, ISBN: 978-0-470-25131-7, New Jersey, USA

Sawynok, J. (2011). Methylxanthines and pain, In: *Methylxanthines - Handbook Experimental Pharmacology*, Bertil B Fredholm, Vol. 200, pp. (311-329), Springer Berlin Heidelberg, ISBN: 3642-134424, Berlin, Germany

Sawynok, J. & Liu, XJ. (2003). Adenosine in the spinal cord and periphery: release and regulation of pain. *Progress in Neurobiology*, Vol. 69, No. 5, (April, 2003), pp. (313-340)

Sawynok, J., Sweeney, MI. & White, TD. (1989). Adenosine release may mediate spinal analgesia by morphine. *Trends in Pharmacological Sciences*, Vol. 10, No. 5, (May, 1989), pp. (186-189)

Sawynok, J., Zarrindast, MR., Reid, AR. & Doak, GJ. (1997). Adenosine A3 receptor activation produces nociceptive behaviour and edema by release of histamine and 5-hydroxytryptamine. *European Journal of Pharmacology*, Vol. 333, No. 1, (August, 1997), pp. (1-7)

Schneider, L., Pietschmann, M., Hartwig, W., Marcos, SS., Hackert, T., Gebhard, MM., Uhl, W., Büchler, MW. & Werner, J. (2006). Inosine reduces microcirculatory disturbance and inflammatory organ damage in experimental acute pancreatitis in rats. *American Journal of Surgery*, Vol. 191, No. 4, (April, 2006), pp. (510-514)

Schulte, G. & Fredholm, BB. (2003). Signalling from adenosine receptors to mitogen-activated protein kinases. *Cell Signalling*, Vol 15, No. 9, (September, 2003), pp. (813-827)

Seymour, RA., Hawkesford, JE., Hill, CM., Frame, J. & Andrews, C. (1999). The efficacy of a novel adenosine agonist (WAG 994) in postoperative dental pain. *British Journal of Clinical Pharmacology*, Vol. 47, No. 6, (June, 1999), pp. (675-680)

Shneyvays, V., Zinman, T. & Shainberg, A. (2004). Analysis of calcium responses mediated by the A3 adenosine receptor in cultured newborn rat cardiac myocytes. *Cell Calcium*, Vol. 36, No. 5, (November, 2004), pp. (387-396)

Sneyd, JR., Langton, JA., Allan, LG., Allan, LG., Peacock, JE. & Rowbotham, DJ. (2007). Multicenter evaluation of the adenosine agonist GR79236X in patients with dental pain after third molar extraction. *British Journal of Anaesthesia*, Vol. 98, No. 5, (May, 2007), pp. (672 -676)

Sollevi, A., Belfrage, M., Lundeberg, T., Segerdahl, M. & Hansen, P. (1995). Systemic adenosine infusion: a new treatment modality to alleviate neuropathic pain. *Pain*, Vol. 61, No. 1, (April, 1995), pp. (155-158)

The Involvement of Purinergic System in Pain: Adenosine Receptors and Inosine as
Pharmacological Tools in Future Treatments

231

Song, JG., Hahm, KD., Kim, YK., Leem, JG., Lee, C., Jeong, SM., Park, PH. & Shin, JW. (2011). Adenosine triphosphate-sensitive potassium channel blockers attenuate the antiallodynic effect of R-PIA in neuropathic rats. *Anesthesia & Analgesia*, Vol. 112, No. 6, (June, 2011), pp. (1494-1499)

Sowa, NA., Taylor-Blake, B. & Zylka, MJ. (2010a). Ecto-5'-nucleotidase (CD73) inhibits nociception by hydrolyzing AMP to adenosine in nociceptive circuits. *The Journal of Neurosci*, Vol. 30, No. 6, (February, 2010), pp. (2235-2244), ISSN: 1529-2401

Sowa, NA., Voss, MK. & Zylka, MJ. (2010b). Recombinant ecto-5'-nucleotidase (CD73) has long lasting antinociceptive effects that are dependent on adenosine A1 receptor activation. *Molecular Pain*, Vol. 6, No. 20, (April, 2010)

Suzuki, R., Stanfa, LC., Kowaluk, EA., Williams, M., Jarvis, MF. & Dickenson, AH. (2001). The effect of ABT-702, a novel adenosine kinase inhibitor, on the responses of spinal neurones following carrageenan inflammation and peripheral nerve injury. *British Journal of Pharmacology*, Vol. 132, No. 7, (April, 2001), pp. (1615-1623).

Sweeney, MI., White, TD., Jhamandas, KH. & Sawynok, J. (1987b). Morphine releases endogenous adenosine from the spinal cord in vivo. *European Journal of Pharmacology*, Vol. 141, No. 1, (September, 1987), pp.(169-170)

Sweeney, MI., White, TD. & Sawynok, J. (1987a). Involvement of adenosine in the spinal antinociceptive effects of morphine and noradrenaline. *The Journal of Pharmacology and Experimental Therapeutics*, Vol. 243, No. 2, (November, 1987) pp. (657-665)

Sweeney, MI., White, TD. & Sawynok, J. (1989). Morphine, capsaicin and K+ release purines from capsaicin-sensitive primary afferent nerve terminals in the spinal cord. *The Journal of Pharmacology and Experimental Therapeutics*, Vol. 248, No. 1, (January, 1989), pp. (447-454)

Taiwo, YO. & Levine, JD. (1990). Direct cutaneous hyperalgesia induced by adenosine. *Neuroscience*, Vol. 38, No. 3, (March, 1990), pp. (757-762)

Udelson, JE., Heller, GV., Wackers, FJ., Chai, A., Hinchman, D., Coleman, PS., Dilsizian, V., DiCarli, M., Hachamovitch, R., Johnson, JR., Barrett, RJ. & Gibbons, RJ. (2004). Randomized, controlled dose-ranging study of the selective adenosine A2A receptor agonist binodenoson for pharmacological stress as an adjunct to myocardial perfusion imaging. *Circulation*, Vol. 109, No. 4, (February, 2004), pp. (457–464), ISSN: 1524-4539

Ueda, H. (2006). Molecular mechanisms of neuropathic pain-phenotypic switch and initiation mechanisms. *Pharmacology & Therapeutics*, Vol. 109, No. 1-2, (January, 2006), pp. (57-77)

Wagner, H., Milavec-Krizman, M., Gadient, F., Menninger, K., Schoeffter, P., Tapparelli, C., Pfannkuche, HJ. & Fozard, JR. (1995). General pharmacology of SDZ WAG 994, a potent selective and orally active adenosine A1 receptor agonist. *Drug Development Research*, Vol. 34, No. 3, (March, 1995), pp. (276 – 288).

Wan, TC., Ge, ZD., Tampo, A., Mio, Y., Bienengraeber, MW., Tracey, WR., Gross, JG., Kwok, WM. & Auchampach, JA. (2008). The A3 adenosine receptor agonist CP-532,903 [N6-(2,5-dichlorobenzyl)-3'-aminoadenosine-5'-N-methylcarboxamide] protects against myocardial ischemia/reperfusion injury via the sarcolemmal ATPsensitive potassium channel. *The Journal of Pharmacology and Experimental Therapeutics*, Vol. 324, No. 1, (September, 2007), pp. (234–243), ISSN: 1521-0103

Wu, WP., Hao, JX., Halldner, L., Lövdahl, C., DeLander, GE., Wiesenfeld-Hallin, Z., Fredholm, BB. & Xu, XJ. (2005). Increased nociceptive response in mice lacking the adenosine A1 receptor. *Pain*, Vol. 113, No. 3, (February, 2005), pp. (395-404).

Wu, MM., You, SW., Hou, B., Jiao, XY., Li, YY. & Ju, G. (2003). Effects of inosine on axonal regeneration of axotomized retinal ganglion cells in adult rats. *Neuroscience Letters*, Vol. 341, No. 1, (April, 2003), pp. (84-86).

Wu, WP., Hao, JX., Halldner-Henriksson, L., Xu, XJ., Jacobson, MA., Wiesenfeld-Hallin, Z. & Fredholm, BB. (2002). Decreased inflammatory pain due to reduced carrageenan-induced inflammation in mice lacking adenosine A3 receptors. *Neuroscience*, Vol. 114, No. 3, (October, 2002), pp. (523-527)

Yan, L., Burbiel, JC., Maass, A. & Muller, CE. (2003). Adenosine receptor agonists from basic medicinal chemistry to clinical development. *Expert Opinion on Emerging Drugs*, Vol. 8, No. 2, (November, 2003), pp. (537 -576), ISSN: 1472-8214

Yoon, MH., Bae, HB. & Choi, JI. (2005). Antinociception of intrathecal adenosine receptor subtype agonists in rat formalin test. *Anesthesia & Analgesia*, Vol. 101, No. 5, (November, 2005), pp. (1417-1421), ISSN: 1526-7598

Zahn, PK., Straub, H., Wenk, M. & Pogatzki-Zahn, EM. (2007). Adenosine A1 but not A2a receptor agonist reduces hyperalgesia caused by a surgical incision in rats: a pertussis toxin-sensitive G protein-dependent process. *Anesthesiology*, Vol. 107, No. 5, (November, 2007), pp. (797-806)

Zhang, Y., Li, A., Lao, L., Xin, J., Ren, K., Berman, BM. & Zhang, RX. (2011). Rostral ventromedial medulla mu, but not kappa, opioid receptors are involved in electroacupuncture anti-hyperalgesia in an inflammatory pain rat model. *Brain Research*, Vol. 1395, (June, 2011), pp. (38-45)

Zylka, MJ. (2010). Needling adenosine receptors for pain relief. *Nature Neuroscience*, Vol. 13, No. 7, (July, 2010), pp. (783-784), ISSN: 1546-1726

Zylka, MJ. (2011). Pain-relieving prospects for adenosine receptors and ectonucleotidases. *Trends in Molecular Medicine*, Vol. 17, No. 4, (April, 2011), pp. (188-196)

10

Ethanol Interference on Adenosine System

Silvânia Vasconcelos et al.*
Federal University of Ceará, Department of Physiology and Pharmacology
Brazil

1. Introduction

It is well documented in literature a wide range of behavioral and physiological effects arising from ethanol intake (Spinetta et al., 2008; Soares et al., 2009; Brust, 2010). Because it is a substance that affects differently and simultaneously several neurotransmitter systems, covering different brain areas (Dahchour & De Witte, 2000; Vasconcelos et al., 2008; Vengeliene et al., 2008), it becomes complex to reveal the mechanism of action that governs its effects, being still a challenge for researchers. In addition, ethanol has a biphasic behavioral presenting an excitatory feature in the early stages and a depressant feature in its chronic use.

Among the wide range of pathways in central nervous system that are modified by ethanol, it is important to highlight those that explain ethanol diverse effects, like the ones releasing gamma-amynobutiric acid (GABA), glutamate, dopamine and norepinephrine (Kaneyuki et al., 1991; Vasconcelos et al., 2004). Moreover, another pathway that is rising on researches about ethanol effects is the adenosinergic system (Prediger et al., 2006; Thorsell et al., 2007).

Adenosine was described as a potent depressor of neuronal activity (Dunwiddie & Haas, 1985), and acts mainly via A1 receptor, which is a presynaptic inhibitor of the release of neurotransmitters such as dopamine, GABA, glutamate, acetylcholine and norepinephrine (Fredholm et al., 2001; Dunwiddie & Masino, 2001). Moreover, adenosine is involved in behavioral processes like motor function, anxiety, depression, reward and drug addiction, and human disorders such as Parkinson disease and schizophrenia (Moreau and Huber, 1999).

In addition, there is strong evidence of an involvement of the adenosinergic system on ethanol effects, including the extracellular increase of adenosine after acute exposure to ethanol (Krauss et al., 1993; Nagy et al., 1990), the accentuation or blockade of ethanol-induced motor incoordination provided by adenosine receptor agonists or antagonists, respectively (Dar, 2001; Soares et al., 2009), and the reduction of anxiogenic-like behavior in acute ethanol withdrawal (Prediger et al., 2006). Adenosine antagonists, like caffeine, are implicated in alcohol tolerance (Fillmore, 2003), and retrograde memory impairment caused by ethanol (Spinetta et al., 2008). Thus, adenosine receptors seem to modulate some of the

* Sarah Escudeiro[1], Ana Luíza Martin[1], Paula Soares[1], Antônio Vieira Filho[2], Larissa Silva[2],
Kátia Cilene Dias[1], Danielle Macêdo[1], Francisca Cléa Sousa[1], Marta Fonteles[1]
and Manoel Cláudio Patrocínio[2]
[1]*Federal University of Ceará, Department of Physiology and Pharmacology, Brazil*
[2]*College of Medicine Christus, Brazil*

pharmacological properties of ethanol, interacting with it by blocking or accentuating its properties.

2. Ethanol and adenosine relation in different neurotransmission systems

It's known in literature that ethanol alone interferes in different neurotransmitter systems, as GABAergic, glutamatergic, dopaminergic, serotonergic, noradrenergic, cholinergic and others, including adenosinic; however, its action on this last system has currently deserved more attention, due to its neuromodulator/neuroprotector action. Thus, in the present topic updates will be discussed on the relationship between ethanol and adenosine and its consequent interference in some systems above.

To better understand the association of ethanol and adenosine on different neurotransmitter systems, it is necessary to explore the likely hypotheses that explain how ethanol interferes with the adenosine system. Carmichael et al. (1991) suggested that a probable mechanism could occur via metabolism of ethanol by acetate, where this would be incorporated into acetyl-coenzyme A with subsequent formation of AMP, thereby directing the synthesis of adenosine.

Another possible mechanism of interaction between these two substances can be related to the fact that ethanol inhibits facilitated diffusion transporters, being the ENT1 (Equilibrative Nucleoside Transporter) an example, increasing the availability of extracellular adenosine (Diamond et al., 1991; Krauss et al., 1993). Finally, ethanol may facilitate the activation of receptors that have adenylate cyclase (AC) as intracellular signaling system (Rabin; Molinoff, 1981; Hoffman; Tabakoff, 1990), which is displayed by adenosine receptors. Therefore, there are different points of possible interference of the increased concentration of extracellular adenosine induced by ethanol on other neurotransmitter systems.

The GABAergic system in the striatum may be modulated by adenosine with regard to the effects of ethanol on motor coordination and sleep, involving cAMP (Meng; Dar, 1995; Meng et al., 1997). It was found that the use of adenosine agonists accentuate the reduction in the motor coordination induced by ethanol, whereas Ro15-4513, a weak partial inverse agonist of the benzodiazepine class of drugs, attenuated by blocking the effect of the first when used in combination (Meng; Dar, 1994, 1995), suggesting a participation via $GABA_A$ by an alteration in the conductance of chloride ions (Meng et al., 1997, Mohler et al., 1984). A mechanism suggested by Londos et al. (1980) and Van Calk et al. (1970) relates ethanol to alterations in the production of cAMP via AC through the A1 receptor, ie, increased availability of adenosine induced by ethanol leads to greater signs of adenosine on your receptor that has a higher affinity, which is related with inhibitory G protein, reducing cAMP production and concomitant modulation of the GABAergic system that increases chloride conductance.

This ratio adenosine/ethanol with the GABAergic system can still be related to opioid system, where ethanol induces the increased availability of β-endorphin which activates μtype receptors, altering the release of GABA in dopaminergic neurons in the ventral tegmental area, an area involved to reward behavior and abuse of ethanol (Mendez et al, 2003; Marinelli et al, 2004; Lam et al, 2008; Jarjour et al, 2009).

Indirectly, this relationship can also occur through ionotropic ATP receptors, that has the function of specific subtypes (P2X4R and P2X2R) inhibited by ethanol (Davies et al., 2002, 2005), altering the modulation of release of different substances such as GABA, glycine and glutamate (Mori et al., 2001; Papp et al., 2004).

Concerning the glutamatergic system, this one demonstrates relationship with the two subtypes of adenosine receptors A_1 and A_{2A}, once these receptors appear hetero-dimerized in glutamatergic nerve terminals in the striatum, modulating the concentration of glutamate in accordance with the availability of adenosine, where a lower concentration activates A_1R inhibiting glutamate release, and a higher concentration activates $A_{2A}R$, stimulating the release of glutamate and greater activation of the NMDA receptor. This regulates the release of dopamine in the nucleus accumbens stimulating higher consumption of ethanol (Ciruela et al., 2006; Quarta et al., 2004).

Another finding that reinforces the relationship ethanol/adenosine/glutamate is the synergic interaction that occurs between A_{2A} and mGluR5 receptors (which is related to the consumption of ethanol in the nucleus accumbens) in the striatum, that is, the co-activation of these receptors increases the phosphorylation of proteins regulated by dopamine and cAMP, increased ethanol consumption (Nishi et al., 2003). In addition, NMDA and A_1 receptors present a cross modulation on the negative effects of ethanol, like a reduction on motor coordination in the cerebellum, striatum and motor cortex (Mitchell; Neafsey; Collins, 2009). This relationship could be involved with the altered activity of Protein Kinase C (PKC) (Othman et al., 2002). This enzyme has a modulating function against the concentration of glycine, GABA internalization, externalization of NMDA expression of 5-HT3 (Chapell et al., 1998; Lan et al., 2001; Zhang et al., 1995; Sun et al., 2003).

Regarding the dopaminergic system, A_{2A} and D_2 receptors (as well as A_1 and D_1) exhibit dimerization between them, relating to the reward system in the striatum probably by modulation of AC activity by ethanol, leading to an increase in the concentration of cAMP and the activity of PKA, desensitizing D_2, and thus leading to an increased consumption of ethanol (Ferre et al., 2008; Mailliard & Diamond, 2004; Yao et al., 2002; 2003). A possible mechanism of the final response of the dimerized activation of these receptors is that ethanol desensitizes receptors linked to the stimulatory G protein (α subunit), modulating the coupling of D_2 with the AC pathway, which may be related to PKA (Yao et al., 2001; Batista et al., 2005). Inoue et al. (2007) found that co-activation of A_{2A} and D_2 mediates the transient interaction between nicotine and ethanol, showing an indirect relationship with the cholinergic system, where the use of antagonists of this co-activation can prevent, mitigate or even reverse the use of smoke and ethanol.

Indirectly, the adenosine system also maintains relation to the dopaminergic system via receptors P2XR which were identified in mesolimbic dopaminergic neurons, modulating their activity and, equivalently, the consumption of ethanol (Heine et al., 2007; Xiao et al., 2008).

Adenosine and serotonin systems are related in regard to ethanol via P2X receptors (P2XR). That is, 5-HT3 and P2XR are functionally coupled and both have their actions modulated by ethanol (inhibits P2X2 and P2X4 and stimulates 5-HT3), besides being involved with other neurotransmitter systems such as glycine, GABA, glutamate (mentioned above) and dopamine in the nucleus accumbens and ventral tegmental area (Davies et al., 2006).

Other neurotransmitters still present a few studies involving ethanol and the adenosine system, such as glycine, where ethanol inhibits their specific receptors probably via PKC (Tao & Ye, 2002), and taurine, which normalizes the activity of ATPases in tissues pretreated with ethanol (Pushpakiran et al., 2005), showing some indirect relationship with the system in focus.

3. Adenosine agonists and antagonists in the responses induced by ethanol

As widely described, ethanol affects several mechanisms of transmission on the central nervous system, bringing a wide range of behavioral and neurochemical responses. To reduce the risks and to prevent the damages arising from ethanol intake, many researches are engaged in finding other substances that could inhibit or reduce the responses of ethanol in the organism. An alternative for this proposition is to study the relationship of the mechanism of action of ethanol effects and substances that may interfere in these pathways. Adenosine system, as already mentioned, interacts with many effects induced by ethanol, affecting their responses as being influenced by them. This system has gained remarkable interest in research because of its neuromodulator/neuroprotective action (Halbach & Dermietzel, 2006; Wardas, 2002), and may bring about a new target for developing drugs that can interfere with the effects caused by ethanol.

Among the wide range of adenosine receptor agonists and antagonists used in experiments involving ethanol treatment, we will focus on the most common substances, like adenosine, N6-[2-(3,5-dimethoxyphenyl)-2-(2-methylphenyl)ethyl]adenosine g(DPMA), 2-chloro-N6-cyclopentyladenosine (CCPA), R(−)-N6-phenylisopropyladenosine (R-PIA) as agonists, and caffeine, theophylline, 1,3-dipropyl-8-cyclopentylxanthine (DPCPX), 3,7-Dimethyl-1-propargylxanthine (DMPX) as antagonists, these last being well described and characterized in a review performed by Muller & Jacobson (2011).

A moderate alcohol intake may not be harmful and has even beneficial effects in prevention of cardiovascular diseases, for example (Di Castelnuovo et al., 2010), but heavy alcohol consumption could be associated with some risks to the body, like reduced brain mass, neuronal loss, neuropathological changes, and impairment of cognitive functions, amnesia, dementia and even a significant increase in mortality. Furthermore, the consumption of significant quantities of ethanol during pregnancy is responsible for the Fetal Alcohol Syndrome (FAS), and prenatal alcohol exposure in humans, as well as in rodents, leads to an impaired cognitive and behavioral function, resulting from damage to the central nervous system (Chen et al., 2003; Riley et al., 2004; Hamilton et al., 2003). Thus, taking into account the substantial importance of this system, studies looking for the lessening of these various damages caused by ethanol intake are strictly necessary.

High amount of experimental studies, involving ethanol administration, use a chronic treatment as methodology protocol; but subchronic and acute treatments are also well used (Soares et al., 2009; Prediger et al., 2006). While acute treatment simulates hangover, chronic treatment usually refers to the withdrawal symptoms and body's adaptive responses to prolonged consumption of ethanol.

Although many studies have consistently demonstrated increases in anxiety-like behavior during the withdrawal period after chronic exposure to ethanol in rodents (Lal et al., 1991; Knapp et al., 1993; Gatch & Lal, 2001), there are limited experimental findings regarding this symptom after a single ethanol challenge dose. Prediger et al. (2006) designed an experimental study of acute ethanol withdrawal (hangover) in mice, in which a time-dependent development of anxiety-like behavior after an intraperitoneal administration of a single dose of ethanol (4 g/kg) in mice was assessed, and the potential of adenosine A_1 and A_{2A} receptor agonists in reducing this behavior was evaluated. They presented evidence that acute administration of 'nonanxiolytic' doses of adenosine (5–10 mg/kg, i.p.) or the selective adenosine A1 receptor agonist CCPA (0.05–0.125 mg/kg, i.p.), but not the adenosine A_{2A} receptor agonist DPMA (0.1–5.0 mg/kg, i.p.), which reduces the anxiety-like behavior during ethanol hangover in mice, as indicated by a significant increase in the exploration of the open arms of the elevated plus maze. In addition, the effect of CCPA (0.05 mg/kg, i.p.) was prevented by the pretreatment with the selective adenosine A_1 receptor antagonist DPCPX (3.0 mg/kg, i.p.), demonstrating that the activation of adenosine A_1 receptors, but not adenosine A_{2A} receptors, reduces the anxiogenic-like behaviour observed during acute ethanol withdrawal in mice.

In general, sensitivity to the adverse effects of ethanol is inversely correlated with alcohol consumption. In a study with mice lacking the A_{2A} receptor, Naassila et al. (2002) showed that these animals are less sensitive to the acute effects of ethanol as hypothermia and sedation, and consume more ethanol in a two-bottle choice paradigm compared with wild-type littermate control mice, demonstrating that the $A_{2A}R$ is involved in the sensitivity to the hypothermic and sedative effects of ethanol playing a role in alcohol-drinking behavior.

Furthermore, caffeine presents an ability to decrease sensitivity to the stumbling and tiredness associated with drinking large quantities of ethanol. Thus, adenosine receptors antagonists also appear to mediate some of the reinforcement effects of ethanol. This reinforcement is in part mediated via $A_{2A}R$ activation and probably associated with intracellular A_2 activation of cAMP/PKA signalling cascades in the nucleus accumbens (Thorsell, et al., 2007; Adams et al., 2008), but the exact mechanism of action remains unclear. Studies in humans examining methylxanthine and ethanol interactions have mostly focused on the influence that caffeine exerts on ethanol intoxication, and have yielded mixed results (Liguori and Robinson 2001; Drake et al. 2003); but a point that needs further attention is the fact that these studies converge upon the point that caffeine consumed in association with ethanol, rather than improving ethanol-induced impairments, would reduce the self-perception of ethanol intoxication (Morelli & Simola, 2011), since human data also show that caffeine enhances tolerance to ethanol (Fillmore, 2003).

In addition to reinforcing effects, adenosine also appears to be related to locomotive effects of ethanol at high dose (6 g/kg) in subchronic treatment during 5 days, as shown in the experimental study of Soares et al. (2009), in which the administration of Aminophylline, a non-selective adenosine receptor antagonist, at low doses (5 and 10 mg/kg) produced some degree of locomotion stimulation, and was able to reverse the depressive effects produced by ethanol on the number of falls and time spent in the bar, in the Rota rod test, suggesting a partial blockage of the action of ethanol. The selective A_1R agonist N^6-cyclohexyladenosine (CHA) has also been found to potentiate, and the antagonist DPCPX attenuates ethanol-induced motor incoordination in mice (Meng et al., 1997).

Chronic ethanol intake leads to several changes in the balance of neurotransmitter pathways and its receptors, being studied oftentimes focusing withdrawal symptoms. Accordingly

Concas et al. (1994), the adenosine receptor agonist CCPA produces inhibition of these symptoms, such as tremors and audiogenically induced seizures in rats treated repeatedly with ethanol (12–18 g/kg daily for 6 days), an effect prevented by DPCPX. Similar results about the specificity of the adenosine receptor in the responses of ethanol effects have been reported by Kaplan et al (1999) in mice receiving a 14-day liquid diet containing ethanol and treated with the adenosine A_1 receptor agonist R-PIA during the withdrawal period, indicating the adenosine A_1R modulate anxiety-like responses in mice, not only in acute, but also in chronic treatment with ethanol.

Thus, adenosine receptor activation seems to be strongly linked with sensitivity and reinforcement properties of ethanol either in A_1, or in $A_{2A}R$, with an opposite relation of activation, whereas the adenosine A_1R agonists reduce sensitivity, $A_{2A}R$ antagonists demonstrate to play this role. Despite A_{2A} knockout mice showed reduced conditioned place preference for ethanol. Houchi et al. (2008) showed that the increased propensity to drink ethanol in A_{2A} knockout mice was associated with an increase in sensitivity to the motor stimulant and anxiolytic effects of ethanol. Contrasting with these findings, the administration of A_{2A} antagonist DMPX reduced ethanol reward and consumption, in a study performed by Thorsell et al. (2007), in which a decreased lever-pressing for ethanol in an operant chamber was observed.

Caffeine and selective adenosine receptor antagonists may also reduce the duration of ethanol-induced loss of the righting reflex (El Yacoubi et al., 2003), reverse deficits in motor coordination induced by ethanol (Barwick & Dar, 1998; Connole et al., 2004) and reverse retrograde memory impairment caused by a high dose of ethanol (3 g/kg) (Spinetta et al., 2008). Indeed, the combination of caffeine and ethanol produces a beneficial effect after experimental traumatism brain injury (Dash et al., 2004), projecting its effect on stroke (Aronowski et al., 2003; Belayev et al., 2004) and indicating the importance of the interaction between caffeine and ethanol.

Beyond neurotransmission/neuromodulation, it is important to give attention to other factors that contribute to the relationship between adenosine system and ethanol effects, as indicated in a review performed by Ruby et al. (2011) about adenosine signalling in anxiety, which underlies the importance of the adenosine transporter ENT1. Many aspects of ethanol-related behaviors and anxiety appear to be involved in genetic factors as polymorphism and in the gene encoding ENT1 could be associated with alcoholism and depression in women (Gass et al., 2010). Further, acute ethanol inhibits ENT1, while chronic ethanol treatment leads to decreased ENT1 expression (Short et al., 2006; Sharma et al., 2010). Also, mice lacking this adenosine transporter displayed a decreased A_1 adenosine tone in the nucleus accumbens and elevated levels of ethanol consumption compared with wild-type mice (Choi et al., 2004). In contrast, it has been shown that ethanol operant self-administration is not altered by an A_1R antagonist while it is bimodally affected by an $A_{2A}R$ antagonist (Arolfo et al., 2004).

4. Conclusion and future prospects

As noted above, there are many different points of adenosine system interference on the effects of ethanol administration. This interaction is of fundamental importance because it could be a new target for developing drugs that may interfere, reducing the damage caused by ethanol.

5. Acknowledgment

This work was sponsored by the Conselho Nacional de Desenvolvimento Científico e Tecnológico - CNPq, Coordenação de Aperfeiçoamento de Pessoal de Nível Superior – CAPES, and Fundação Cearense de Apoio ao Desenvolvimento Científico e Tecnológico FUNCAP Grants.

6. References

Adams CL, Cowen MS, Short JL, & Lawrence AJ. (2008). Combined antagonism of glutamate mGlu5 and adenosine A2A receptors interact to regulate alcohol-seeking in rats. *International Journal Neuropsychopharmacol*, 11: 229-241.

Arolfo MP, Yao L, Gordon AS, Diamond I, & Janak PH. (2004). Ethanol operant self-administration in rats is regulated by adenosine A2 receptors. *Alcohol Clin Exp Res*, 28: 1308-1316.

Aronowski J, Strong R, Shirzadi A, & Grotta JC (2003). Ethanol plus caffeine (caffeinol) for treatment of ischemic stroke: preclinical experience. *Stroke*, 34: 1246-1251.

Barwick VS, & Dar MS. (1998). Adenosinergic modulation of ethanol induced motor incoordination in the rat motor cortex. *Prog. NeuroPsychopharmacol. Biol. Psychiatry*, 22: 587– 607.

Batista LC, Prediger RD, Morato GS, Takahashi RN, (2005). Blockade of adenosine and dopamine receptors inhibits the development of rapid tolerance to ethanol in mice. Psychopharmacology, 181: 714-721.

Belayev L, Khoutorova L, Zhang Y, Belayev A, Zhao W, Busto R, & Ginsberg MD. (2004). Caffeinol confers cortical but not subcortical neuroprotection after transient focal cerebral ischemia in rats. *Brain Res*, 1008: 278-283.

Brust JCM. (2010). Ethanol and Cognition: Indirect Effects, Neurotoxicity and Neuroprotection: A Review. *Int. J. Environ. Res. Public Health*, 7: 1540-1557.

Carmichael FJ, Israel Y, Crawford M, Minhas K, Saldivia V, Sandrin S, Campisi P, Orrego H. (1991). Central nervous system effects of acetate: contribution to the central effects of ethanol. *J Pharmacol Exp Ther*, 259: 403-408.

Chapell R, Bueno OF, Alvarez-Hernandez X, Robinson LC, Leidenheimer NJ. (1998). Activation of protein kinase C induces gamma-aminobutyric acid type A receptor internalization in Xenopus oocytes. *J Biol Chem*, 273: 32595-32601.

Chen WJ, Maier SE, Parnell SE, & West JR. (2003). Alcohol and the developing brain: neuroanatomical studies, *Alcohol Res. Health*, 27: 174–180.

Choi DS, Cascini MG, Mailliard W, Young H, Paredes P, McMahon T, Diamond I, Bonci A., & Messing R.O. (2004). The type 1 equilibrative nucleoside transporter regulates ethanol intoxication and preference. *Nat Neurosci*, 7: 855–861.

Ciruela F, Casado V, Rodrigues R, Lujan R, Burgueno J, Canals M, Borycz J, Rebola N, Goldberg SR, Mallol J, Cortes A, Canela EI, Lopez-Gimenez JF, Milligan G, Lluis C, Cunha RA, Ferre S, Franco R. (2006). Presynaptic control of striatal glutamatergic neurotransmission by adenosine A1-A2A receptor heteromers. *J Neurosci*, 26: 2080-2087.

Concas A, Cuccheddu T, Floris S, Mascia MP, & Biggio G. (1994). 2-Chloro-N6-cyclopentyladenosine (CCPA), an adenosine A1 receptor agonist, suppressed ethanol withdrawal syndrome in rats. *Alcohol Alcohol*, 29: 261–264.

Connole L, Harkin A, & Maginn M. (2004). Adenosine A1 receptor blockade mimics caffeine's attenuation of ethanol induced motor incoordination. *Basic Clin Pharmacol Toxicol*, 95: 299-304.

Dahchour A, & De Witte P. (2000). Ethanol and amino acids in the central nervous system: assessment of the pharmacological actions of acamprosate. *Prog. Neurobiol*, 60: 343-362.

Dar MS. (2001). Modulation of ethano-induced motor incoordination by mouse striatal A1 adenosinergic receptor. Brain Res. Bull, 55: 513-520.

Dash PK, Moore AN, Moody MR, Treadwell R, Felix JL, & Clifton GL. (2004). Post trauma administration of caffeine plus ethanol reduces contusion volume and improves working memory in rats. *J Neurotrauma*, 21: 1573-1583.

Davies DL, Asatryan L, KuO ST, Woodward JJ, King BF, Alkana RL, Xiao C, Ye JH, Sun H, Zhang L, Hu XQ, Hayrapetyan V, Lovinger DM, Machu TK. (2006). Effects of ethanol on adenosine 5'-triphosphate–gated purinergic and 5-hydroxytryptamine3 receptors. *Alcohol Clin Exp Res*, 30: 349-358.

Davies DL, Kochegarov AA, Kuo ST, Kulkarni AA, Woodward JJ, King BF, Alkana RL. (2005). Ethanol differentially affects ATP-gated P2X(3) and P2X(4) receptor subtypes expressed in Xenopus oocytes. *Neuropharmacology*, 49: 243-253.

Davies DL, Machu TK, Guo Y, Alkana RL. (2002). Ethanol sensitivity in ATPgated P2X receptors is subunit dependent. *Alcohol Clin Exp Res*, 26: 773-778.

Diamond I, Nagy L, Mochly-Rosen D, Gordon A. (1991). The role of adenosine and adenosine transport in ethanol-induced cellular tolerance and dependence. Possible biologic and genetic markers of alcoholism. *Ann NY Acad Sci*, 625: 473-487.

Di Castelnuovo A, Costanzo S, Donati MB, Iacoviello L, de Gaetano G. (2010). Prevention of cardiovascular risk by moderate alcohol consumption: epidemiologic evidence and plausible mechanisms. *Intern Emerg Med*, 5(4):291-7.

Drake CL, Roehrs T, Turner L, Scofield HM, Roth T. (2003). Caffeine reversal of ethanol effects on the multiple sleep latency test, memory, and psychomotor performance. *Neuropsychopharmacology*, 28: 371-378.

Dunwiddie TV, & Haas HL. (1985). Adenosine increases synaptic facilitation in the in vitro rat hippocampus: evidence for a presynaptic site of action. *J Physiol*, 369: 365-77.

Dunwiddie TV, & Masino SA. (2001). The role and regulation of adenosine in the central nervous system. *Annu. Rev. Neurosci.*, 24: 31–55.

El Yacoubi M, Ledent C, Parmentier M, Costentin J, & Vaugeois JM. (2003). Caffeine reduces hypnotic effects of alcohol through adenosine A2A receptor blockade. *Neuropharmacology*, 45: 977–985.

Ferre S, Ciruela F, Borycz J, Solinas M, Quarta D, Antoniou K, Quiroz C, Justinova Z, Lluis C, Franco R, Goldberg SR. (2008). Adenosine A1-A2A receptor heteromers: new targets for caffeine in the brain. *Front Biosci*, 13: 2391-2399.

Fillmore MT. (2003). Alcohol tolerance in humans is enhanced by prior caffeine antagonism of alcohol induced impairment. *Exp Clin Psychopharmacol*, 11: 9-17.

Fredholm BB, Ijzerman AP, Jacobson KA, Klotz K, Linden J. (2001). International Union of Pharmacology XXV – Nomenclature and classification of adenosine receptors. *Pharmacol Rev*, 53: 527-52.

Gass N, Ollila HM, Utge S, Partonen T, Kronholm E, Pirkola S, Suhonen J, Silander K, Porkka-Heiskanen T, & Paunio T. (2010). Contribution of adenosine related genes to the risk of depression with disturbed sleep. *J Affect Disord*, 126: 134-139.

Gatch MB, & Lal H. (2001). Animal models of the anxiogenic effects of ethanol withdrawal. *Drug Dev Res*, 54: 95–115.

Halbach OB, & Dermietzel R. (2006). Neuromodulators, In: *Neurotransmitters and neuromodulators*. 2ed, pp. (320-325), WILEY-VCH Verlag GmbH & Co. KGaA, ISBN 978-3-527-31307-5, Weinheim, Germany.

Hamilton DA, Kodituwakku P, Sutherland RJ, Savage DD. (2003). Children with Fetal Alcohol Syndrome are impaired at place learning but not cued-navigation in a virtual Morris water task, Behav. Brain Res. 143: 85– 94.

Heine C, Wegner A, Grosche J, Allgaier C, Illes P, & Franke H. (2007). P2 receptor expression in the dopaminergic system of the rat brain during development. *Neuroscience*, 149:165-181.

Hoffman PL, & Tabakoff B. (1990). Ethanol and guanine nucleotide binding proteins: a selective interaction. *FASEB J*, 4: 2612-2622.

Houchi H, Warnault V, Barbier E, Dubois C, Pierrefiche O, Ledent C, Daoust M, Naassila M (2008). Involvement of A2A receptors in anxiolytic, locomotor and motivational properties of ethanol in mice. *Genes Brain Behavior*, 7(8): 887-98.

Inoue Y, Yao L, Hopf FW, Fan P, Jiang Z, Bonci A, Diamond I. (2007). Nicotine and ethanol activate protein kinase A synergistically via G(i) betagamma subunits in nucleus accumbens/ventral tegmental cocultures: the role of dopamine D(1)/D(2) and adenosine A(2A) receptors. *J Pharmacol Exp Ther*, 322: 23-29.

Jarjour S, Bai L, & Gianoulakis C. (2009). Effect of acute ethanol administration on the release of opioid peptides from the midbrain including the ventral tegmental area. *Alcohol Clin Exp Res*, 33: 1033-1043.

Kaneyuki T, Morimasa T, Okada H, Shohmori T. (1991). The effect of acute and repeated ethanol administration on monoamines and their metabolites in brain regions of rats. *Acta Med Okayama*, 45: 201-8.

Kaplan GB, Bharmal NH, Leite-Morris KA, Adams WR. (1999). Role of adenosine A1 and A2A receptors in the alcohol withdrawal syndrome. *Alcohol*, 19: 157–162.

Knapp DJ, Saiers JA, & Pohorecky LA. (1993). Observations of novel behaviors as indices of ethanol withdrawal-induced anxiety. *Alcohol Alcohol (Suppl)*, 2: 489–493.

Krauss SW, Ghirnikar RB, Diamond I, & Gordon AS. (1993). Inhibition of adenosine uptake by ethanol is specific for one class of nucleoside transporters. *Mol Pharmacol*, 44: 1021-1026.

Lal H, Prather PL, Rezazadeh SM. (1991). Anxiogenic behavior in rats during acute and protracted ethanol withdrawal: reversal by buspirone. *Alcohol*, 8: 467–471.

Lam MP, Marinelli PW, Bai L, Gianoulakis, C. (2008). Effects of acute ethanol on opioid peptide release in the central amygdala: an in vivo microdialysis study. *Psychopharmacology*, 201: 261-271.

Lan JY, Skeberdis VA, Jover T, Grooms SY, Lin Y, Araneda RC, Zheng X, Bennett MV, Zukin RS. (2001). Protein kinase C modulates NMDA receptor trafficking and gating. *Nat Neurosci*, 4: 382-390.

Liguori A, & Robinson JH. (2001). Caffeine antagonism of alcohol induced driving impairment. *Drug Alcohol Depend*, 63:123 129.

Londos C, Cooper DMF, & Wolff J. (1980). Subclasses of external adenosine receptors. *Proc Natl Acad Sci USA*, 77: 2551-2554.

Mailliard WS, & Diamond I. (2004). Recent advances in the neurobiology of alcoholism: the role of adenosine. *Pharmacol Ther*, 101:39-46.

Marinelli PW, Quirion R, & Gianoulakis C. (2004). An in vivo profile of beta-endorphin release in the arcuate nucleus and nucleus accumbens following exposure to stress or alcohol. *Neuroscience*, 127: 777-784.

Mendez M, Leriche M, & Carlos Calva J. (2003). Acute ethanol administration transiently decreases [3H]-DAMGO binding to mu opioid receptors in the rat substantia nigra pars reticulate but not in the caudate-putamen. *Neurosci Res*, 47: 153-160.

Meng ZH, Anwer J, & Dar MS. (1997). The striatal adenosinergic modulation of ethanol-induced motor incoordination in rats: possible role of chloride flux. *Brain Research*, 776: 235-245.

Meng ZH, & Dar MS. (1994). Intrastriatal Ro15-4513 functionally antagonizes ethanol-induced motor incoordination and striatal adenosinergic modulation of ethanol-induced motor incoordination in rats. *J Pharmacol Exp Ther*, 271: 524-534.

Meng ZH, & Dar MS. (1995). Possible role of striatal adenosine in the modulation of acute ethanol-induced motor incoordination in rats. *Alcohol Clin Exp Res*, 19: 892-901.

Meng ZH, Pennington SN, & Dar MS. (1998). Rat striatal adenosinergic modulation of ethanol-induced motor impairment: possible role of striatal cyclic AMP. *Neuroscience*, 85: 919-930.

Mitchel RL, Neafsey EJ, & Collins MA. (2009). Essential involvement of the NMDA receptor in ethanol preconditioning–dependent neuroprotection from amyloid–beta in vitro. *J Neurochem*, 111: 580-588.

Mohler H, Sieghart W, Richards JG, & Hunkeler W. (1984). Photoaffinity labeling of benzodiazepine receptors with a partial inverse agonist. *Eur J Pharmacol*, 102: 191-192.

Morelli M, & Simola N. (2011). Methylxanthines and Drug Dependence: A Focus on Interactions with Substances of Abuse, In: *Methylxanthines, Handbook of Experimental Pharmacology*, Ed. Fredholm BB, pp. 483-508, Springer, ISBN 978 3 642 13442 5, London.

Moreau J-L, & Huber G. (1999). Central adenosine A$_{2A}$ receptors: an overview. Brain Res *Brain Res Rev*, 31: 65–82.

Mori M, Heuss C, Gähwiler BH, & Gerber U. (2001). Fast synaptic transmission mediated by P2X receptors in CA3 pyramidal cells of rat hippocampal slice cultures. *J Physiol*, 535: 115-123.

Muller CE, & Jacobson KA. (2011). Xanthines as Adenosine Receptor Antagonists. In: *Methylxanthines, Handbook of Experimental Pharmacology*, Ed. Fredholm BB, pp. 151-200, Springer, ISBN 978 3 642 13442 5, London.

Naassila M, Ledent C, Daoust M. (2002). Low Ethanol Sensitivity and Increased Ethanol Consumption in Mice Lacking Adenosine A2A Receptors. *The Journal of Neuroscience*, 22(23): 10487–10493.

Nagy LE, Diamond I, Casso DJ, Franklin C, Gordon AS. (1990). Ethanol increases extracellular adenosine by inhibiting adenosine uptake via the nucleoside transporter. *J Biol Chem*, 265: 1946-1951.

Nishi A, Liu F, Matsuyama S, Hamada M, Higashi H, Nairn AC, Greengard P. (2003). Metabotropic mGlu5 receptors regulate adenosine A2A receptor signaling. *Proc Natl Acad Sci USA*, 100: 1322-1327.

Othman T, Sinclair CJ, Haughey N, Geiger JD, Parkinson FE. (2002). Ethanol alters glutamate but not adenosine uptake in rat astrocytes: evidence for protein kinase C involvement. *Neurochem Res*, 27: 289-296.

Papp L, Vizi ES, Sperlagh B. (2004). Lack of ATP-evoked GABA and glutamate release in the hippocampus of P2X7 receptor-/- mice. *Neuroreport*, 15: 2387-2391.

Prediger RDS, Silva GE, Batista LC, Bittencourt AL, Takahashi RN. (2006). Activation of Adenosine A1 Receptors Reduces Anxiety-Like Behavior During Acute Ethanol Withdrawal (Hangover) in Mice. *Neuropsychopharmacology*, 31: 2210–2220.

Pushpakiran G, Mahalakshmi K, Viswanathan P, Anuradha CV. (2005). Taurine prevents ethanol-induced alterations in lipids and ATPases in rat tissues. *Pharmacol Rep*, 57: 578-587.

Quarta D, Borycz J, Solinas M, Patkar K, Hockemeyer J, Ciruela F, Lluis C, Franco R, Woods AS, Goldberg SR, Ferre S. (2004). Adenosine receptor-mediated modulation of dopamine release in the nucleus accumbens depends on glutamate neurotransmission and N-methyl-D-aspartate receptor stimulation. *J Neurochem*, 91: 873-880.

Rabin RA, & Molinoff PB. (1981). Activation of adenylate cyclase by ethanol in mouse striatal tissue. *J Pharmacol Exp Ther*, 216: 129-134.

Riley E.P., McGee C.L., Sowell E.R. (2004). Teratogenic effects of alcohol: a decade of brain imaging. *Am. J. Med. Genet.*, 127: 35– 41.9

Ruby CL, Adams CA, Mrazek DA, & Choi D. (2011). Adenosine Signaling in Anxiety, In: *Anxiety Disorders*, Ed. Kalinin VV, pp. 51-68, InTech, ISBN 978-953-307-592-1, Croatia.

Sharma R, Engemann S, Sahota P, & Thakkar MM. (2010). Role of adenosine and wakepromoting basal forebrain in insomnia and associated sleep disruptions caused by ethanol dependence. *Journal of Neurochemistry*, 115: 782-794.

Short JL, Drago J, & Lawrence AJ. (2006). Comparison of ethanol preference and neurochemical measures of mesolimbic dopamine and adenosine systems across different strains of mice. *Alcoholism: Clinical and Experimental Research*, 30: 606-620.

Soares PM, Patrocínio MC, Assreuy AM, Siqueira RC, Lima NM, Arruda MO, Escudeiro SS, de Carvalho KM, Sousa FC, Viana GS, Vasconcelos SM. (2009). Aminophylline (a theophylline-ethylenediamine complex) blocks ethanol behavioral effects in mice. *Behav Pharmacol*, 20: 297-302.

Spinetta MJ, Woodlee MT, Feinberg LM, Stroud C, Schallert K, Cormack LK, Schallert T. (2008). Alcohol-induced retrograde memory impairment in rats: prevention by caffeine. *Psychopharmacology*, 201: 361-371.

Sun H, Hu XQ, Moradel EM, Weight FF, Zhang L. (2003). Modulation of 5-HT3 receptor-mediated response and trafficking by activation of protein kinase C. *J Biol Chem*, 278: 34150-34157.

Tao L, & Ye JH. (2002). Protein kinase C modulation of ethanol inhibition of glycine-activated current in dissociated neurons of rat ventral tegmental area. *J Pharmacol Exp Ther*, 300:967-975.

Thorsell A, Johnson J, & Heilig M. (2007). Effect of the adenosine A2a receptor antagonist 3,7- dimethyl-propargylxanthine on anxiety-like and depression-like behavior and alcohol consumption in Wistar Rats. *Alcoholism: Clinical and Experimental Research*, 31: 1302-1307.

Van Calker D, Müller M, & Hamprecht B. (1978). Adenosine inhibits the accumulation of cyclic AMP in cultured brain cells. *Nature*, 276: 839-841.

Vasconcelos SM, Cavalcante RA, Aguiar LM, Sousa FC, Fonteles MM, Viana GS. (2004). Effects of chronic ethanol treatment on monoamine levels in rat hippocampus and striatum. *Braz J Med Biol Res*, 37: 1839-46.

Vasconcelos SM, Sales GT, Lima NM, Soares PM, Pereira EC, Fonteles MM, Sousa FC, Viana GS. (2008). Determination of amino acid levels in the rat striatum, after administration of ethanol alone and associated with ketamine, a glutamatergic antagonist. *Neurosci Lett*, 444: 48-51.

Vengeliene V, Bilbao A, Molander A, & Spanagel R. (2008). Neuropharmacology of alcohol addiction. *British Journal of Pharmacology*, 154: 299–315.

Wardas J. (2002). Neuroprotective role of adenosine in the CNS. *Pol. J. Pharmacol.*, 54: 313–326.

Xiao C, Zhou C, Li K, Davies DL, Ye JH. (2008). Purinergic type 2 receptors rat GABAergic synapses on ventral tegmental area dopamine neurons are targets for ethanol action. *J Pharmacol Exp Ther*, 327:196-205.

Yao L, Arolfo MP, Dohrman DP, Jiang Z, Fan P, Fuchs S, Janak PH, Gordon AS, Diamond I. (2002). Betagamma Dimers mediate synergy of dopamine D2 and adenosine A2 receptor-stimulated PKA signaling and regulate ethanol consumption. *Cell*, 109:733-743.

Yao L, Asai K, Jiang Z, Ishii A, Fan P, Gordon AS, Diamond I. (2001). Dopamine D_2 receptor inhibition of adenylyl cyclase is abolished by acute ethanol but restored after chronic ethanol exposure (tolerance). *J Pharmacol Exp Ther*, 298: 833-839.

Yao L, Fan P, Jiang Z, Mailliard WS, Gordon AS, Diamond I. (2003). Addicting drugs utilize a synergistic molecular mechanism in common requiring adenosine and Gi-beta gamma dimers. *Proc Natl Acad Sci USA*, 100: 14379-14384.

Zhang L, Oz M, & Weight FF. (1995). Potentiation of 5-HT3 receptor-mediated responses by protein kinase C activation. *Neuroreport*, 6: 1464-1468.

Permissions

The contributors of this book come from diverse backgrounds, making this book a truly international effort. This book will bring forth new frontiers with its revolutionizing research information and detailed analysis of the nascent developments around the world.

We would like to thank Luca Gallelli, for lending his expertise to make the book truly unique. He has played a crucial role in the development of this book. Without his invaluable contribution this book wouldn't have been possible. He has made vital efforts to compile up to date information on the varied aspects of this subject to make this book a valuable addition to the collection of many professionals and students.

This book was conceptualized with the vision of imparting up-to-date information and advanced data in this field. To ensure the same, a matchless editorial board was set up. Every individual on the board went through rigorous rounds of assessment to prove their worth. After which they invested a large part of their time researching and compiling the most relevant data for our readers. Conferences and sessions were held from time to time between the editorial board and the contributing authors to present the data in the most comprehensible form. The editorial team has worked tirelessly to provide valuable and valid information to help people across the globe.

Every chapter published in this book has been scrutinized by our experts. Their significance has been extensively debated. The topics covered herein carry significant findings which will fuel the growth of the discipline. They may even be implemented as practical applications or may be referred to as a beginning point for another development. Chapters in this book were first published by InTech; hereby published with permission under the Creative Commons Attribution License or equivalent.

The editorial board has been involved in producing this book since its inception. They have spent rigorous hours researching and exploring the diverse topics which have resulted in the successful publishing of this book. They have passed on their knowledge of decades through this book. To expedite this challenging task, the publisher supported the team at every step. A small team of assistant editors was also appointed to further simplify the editing procedure and attain best results for the readers.

Our editorial team has been hand-picked from every corner of the world. Their multi-ethnicity adds dynamic inputs to the discussions which result in innovative outcomes. These outcomes are then further discussed with the researchers and contributors who give their valuable feedback and opinion regarding the same. The feedback is then collaborated with the researches and they are edited in a comprehensive manner to aid the understanding of the subject.

Apart from the editorial board, the designing team has also invested a significant amount of their time in understanding the subject and creating the most relevant covers. They scrutinized every image to scout for the most suitable representation of the subject and create an appropriate cover for the book.

The publishing team has been involved in this book since its early stages. They were actively engaged in every process, be it collecting the data, connecting with the contributors or procuring relevant information. The team has been an ardent support to the editorial, designing and production team. Their endless efforts to recruit the best for this project, has resulted in the accomplishment of this book. They are a veteran in the field of academics and their pool of knowledge is as vast as their experience in printing. Their expertise and guidance has proved useful at every step. Their uncompromising quality standards have made this book an exceptional effort. Their encouragement from time to time has been an inspiration for everyone.

The publisher and the editorial board hope that this book will prove to be a valuable piece of knowledge for researchers, students, practitioners and scholars across the globe.

List of Contributors

Daniel Garcia and Lin Chau Ming
Universidade Estadual Paulista – Faculdade de Ciências Agronômicas, Brazil

James R. Reed
Department of Pharmacology, Louisiana State University Health Sciences Center, New Orleans, LA, USA

Yanier Nuñez Figueredo and Alicia Lagarto Parra
Center for Research and Development of Pharmaceuticals, CIDEM, Cerro, Ciudad Habana, Cuba

Juan E. Tacoronte Morales, Olinka Tiomno Tiomnova and Jorge Leyva Simeon
Center for Engineering and Chemical Researches, CIIQ, Cerro, Ciudad Habana, Cuba

Jorge Tobella Sabater
Pharmaceutical Laboratories MEDSOL, La Lisa, Ciudad Habana, Cuba

Luana de Jesus Reis Rosa, Gleidy Ana Araujo Silva, Jorge Amaral Filho, Magali Glauzer Silva and Yoko Oshima-Franco
University of Sorocaba/UNISO, Brazil

Patricia Santos Lops
Federal University of São Paulo/UNIFESP, Brazil

José Carlos Cogo
University of Vale do Paraiba/UNIVAP, Brazil

Adélia Cristina Oliveira Cintra
University of São Paulo/USP, Brazil

Maria Alice da Cruz-Höfling
University of Campinas/UNICAMP/I.B./D.H.E., Brazil

Eva Kovacs
Cancer Immunology Research, Switzerland

Metoda Lipnik-Štangelj
University of Ljubljana, Faculty of Medicine, Department of Pharmacology and Experimental Toxicology, Slovenia

Beril Anilanmert
Istanbul University, Institute of Forensic Sciences, Turkiye

Indu Dhar and Kaushik Desai
Department of Pharmacology, College of Medicine, University of Saskatchewan, Saskatoon, SK, Canada

Francisney Pinto Nascimento and Adair Roberto Soares Santos
Department of Pharmacology, Department of Physiological Sciences, Universidade Federal de Santa Catarina, Brazil

Francisney Pinto Nascimento, Sérgio José Macedo Jr. and Adair Roberto Soares Santos
Laboratory of Neurobiology of Pain and Inflammation, Department of Physiological Sciences, Universidade Federal de Santa Catarina, Brazil

Sarah Escudeiro, Ana Luíza Martin, Paula Soares, Kátia Cilene Dias, Danielle Macêdo, Francisca Cléa Sousa, Marta Fonteles and Silvânia Vasconcelos
Federal University of Ceará, Department of Physiology and Pharmacology, Brazil

Antônio Vieira Filho, Larissa Silva and Manoel Cláudio Patrocínio
College of Medicine Christus, Brazil

Printed in the USA
CPSIA information can be obtained
at www.ICGtesting.com
JSHW011813301024
72690JS00002B/68